24.95

D0710301

EAT, DRINK AND BE HEALTHY

EAT, DRINK AND BE HEALTHY

A Guide to Healthful Eating and Weight Control

Janet M. Chiavetta
in collaboration with
Carolyn Barrett, R.D., M.S., M.P.H.
Stephen V. Chiavetta, M.D.

Piedmont Publishers
1992

Graphics: Yolanda Martini
Cover design: April Higgins

Printed in the United States of America

Library of Congress Catalogue Card Number: 92-60883

ISBN 0-9633991-0-1

For information, contact Piedmont Publishers, 2512 Ridge Road, P.O. Box 32296, Raleigh, NC 27622. For ordering information, refer to the last page.

Cover photo: Joseph Bronzino
On the cover: Fettucine with Shrimp and Mussels (recipe, page 334)
Escargots (recipe, page 167)

Dedicated with love
to my sons, Stephen and John.
This book should enable them and others
to enjoy the pleasures of good foods,
while at the same time, protecting their health.

Contents

Chapter 9

Chapter 10

Part II: The Cookbook

Preface

*". . . and yet the true creator is necessity, which is
the mother of our invention."*

—Plato (circa 375 B.C.)

This maxim is as true today as it was over 2000 years ago. This cookbook and guide to healthful eating was created because of our family's *need* to change our diet. Because of my own struggle to learn what constitutes a healthy diet, I saw the need for a practical, comprehensive book on healthy eating. I also realized the need for a collection of tasty low-fat recipes that would appeal to typical American families.

Our family's need to change our diet became evident 5 years ago when my husband's cholesterol measured 330. We were shocked because we thought we were following a healthy diet. Furthermore, he was at his ideal body weight and jogged 4 miles a day. It was only after I did considerable research —on the amount of fats in foods, learned how misleading food labels could be, and found out that all the so-called "heart-healthy" fats can also contribute to heart disease —that I realized our diet was indeed not so healthy after all.

In the beginning, my main priority was to significantly reduce the fat in our diet, especially saturated and hydrogenated fats. The results were very promising. After less than three months on our new diet, my husband's cholesterol dropped over 100 points to 210. At that time, I decided I would write a book on what I had learned through my research and our own personal experience, hoping others would benefit from it.

More research led to more questions. Why did the American Heart Association recommend a diet of less than 30% of calories from fat? Why not 25% or 20%? What foods constitute a diet of 20% or 30% of calories from fat? Can one consume too little fat, and not get enough essential nutrients? If so, can this increase the risks for cancer or other diseases? What exactly constitutes a healthy, balanced low-fat diet? How important are exercise and other lifestyle factors?

After months of reading and research, and after studying nutrition at a nearby college, the answers to these questions and others began to unfold. While writing the book, I consulted on a regular basis with Carolyn Barrett, clinical assistant professor of nutrition at the University of North Carolina at Chapel Hill. My husband, a physician, was also invaluable to me as a consultant. The information presented in the book is medically and nutritionally sound and includes the most current scientific data on diet and lifestyle as a form of preventive medicine—not just for heart disease, but for cancer, stroke and intestinal disorders.

After learning what constituted a healthy low-fat diet, I was ready to begin compiling a recipe collection that met the approval of my family, which included two teenage sons. Since my teenagers were hooked on high-fat junk food like others their age, it was a real challenge. The recipes needed to meet the approval of the entire family, or be discarded or altered until they met the test. Friends and members of my extended family also tested recipes.

My goal was to produce a collection of recipes with enough variety to meet the needs of all anticipated occasions. Now, I am able to entertain formally or casually, plus prepare foods for my family, using only this cookbook. All the recipes have been tested at least twice and most of them many more times. I hope your families and friends will be as fond of these recipes as mine are.

Acknowledgements

I would like to express my gratitude to a number of people who were a tremendous help to me in preparing this book. Without their assistance, this book would not have been possible. To begin with, my sister Delaine Moe, a dietitian, was invaluable when I first began, providing me with both encouragement and first-hand information on her experiences with diet counseling.

I would also like to thank Harriet Hill, Fran Preston and Barbara Smith who were willing to read the text of the book and offer their comments and suggestions. Their input was most helpful in making the text more readable.

Testing over 240 recipes was made easier and more enjoyable with the help of my sister, Joanne Johnson, and friend, Mary Scarantino. Mary also provided me with some of her own family recipes, which have been included in the book and are among my favorites.

My husband, Steve Chiavetta, M.D. and Carolyn Barrett, R.D., M.S., M.P.H., provided their valuable assistance, which helped ensure that the information presented is both nutritionally and scientifically sound.

My son John assisted in typing and entering nutritional data into the computer. His computer experience was a real asset.

Finally, the production of the book could not have been accomplished without the able direction of Kaye Lasater and Susan McDonald. It was truly a joy working with them, because of their expertise and high standards of excellence.

Introduction

Many health-conscious Americans are changing the way they eat. They are especially concerned with reducing saturated fat and cholesterol in their diet to lower blood cholesterol levels. They also are paying closer attention to monitoring their blood pressure and are taking the time to exercise regularly. For many, these efforts are paying off. The death rate from heart disease has decreased by nearly 30% since 1978.

Still, based on current statistics, one third of Americans will suffer a heart attack, stroke, or blockage of an artery in a leg before the age of 65. Eventually, slightly over half of us will die as a result of heart disease.

One of the problems is that many Americans still are not aware of the *extent* of dietary changes necessary to make a significant difference in health risks—not only for heart disease, but also for cancer and other diseases. A recent national food survey shows that many Americans who are trying to eat "right" are making unhealthy food choices without realizing it. Many have substituted margarine for butter, cut down on red meats, or added more fish to their diet. But, are they doing enough? Are **you** doing enough to reduce your risks for heart disease and cancer? In many cases, the answer may be no. The diet changes mentioned above clearly are beneficial, but the diet still may be too high in cholesterol, fat, or salt, and too low in fiber.

This book will show you how the typical American diet plays a major role in many common diseases. It will help you achieve a healthier diet by giving you a better idea of how much fat, cholesterol, salt, sugar and fiber is optimum for you. You will learn obvious as well as hidden sources of these food components. Knowing this, you can monitor the amounts in your diet more closely. You will learn about different kinds of fat and how to read food labels. Sample daily menus will demonstrate tasty, healthy meal planning.

Once you know and understand the importance of certain foods to your body, and the bad effects of other foods, changing to a healthier diet becomes much easier. Finally you have the **motivation** to make gradual and permanent diet changes, knowing that it will reduce your risks for a wide array of the most common diseases.

Other lifestyle changes to promote good health will also be addressed, including weight control and exercise. All these changes together will significantly reduce your risks for heart disease, cancer, high blood pressure and intestinal diseases. Perhaps, even more important, these diet and lifestyle changes, by helping you maintain better health, should improve the *quality* of your life during your middle and later years.

Part I

A Guide to Healthful Eating and Weight Control

1

The Relationship Between Diet and Disease

Atherosclerosis, Heart Disease and Stroke

These three terms—atherosclerosis, heart disease and stroke—are closely related. Atherosclerosis occurs when plaque, made up primarily of cholesterol, is formed on artery walls. This restricts the opening of the arteries and causes a dangerous impediment to blood flow. One of the most common sites for this to occur is in the three pencil-thin coronary arteries which carry blood to the heart. When atherosclerosis affects these arteries, the term coronary heart disease (CHD) or coronary artery disease is used. If one of these arteries is severely blocked, a small clot can totally cut off the blood supply to the heart, resulting in a heart attack. If this happens in a clogged artery leading to the brain, a stroke results. A coronary artery spasm, often a result of severe stress, can also damage the heart by temporarily reducing or shutting off blood flow.

Sometimes when a coronary artery becomes severely blocked, smaller arteries upstream from the blockage open up and take over, actually bypassing the blockage. This is referred to as collateral circulation. Circulation to the heart is maintained, but with less than ideal blood flow. This phenomenon is what enables some people to function fairly normally with nearly total blockage of one or more coronary arteries. Figure 1.1 shows the cross-section of a coronary artery with no atherosclerosis, and progressive stages of the disease.

Atherosclerosis and its related diseases cause 51% of all the deaths in the United States each year—more than all other diseases and accidents combined! Each year 1.5 million Americans have heart attacks and over one-third of these die as a result of their first heart attack. Over 750,000 suffer strokes, which account for approximately 250,000 deaths annually. Many survivors do not fully recover—71% of stroke victims and 24% of heart attack victims find themselves with physical or mental limitations. Even more distressing is the fact that 16% of stroke victims and 11% of

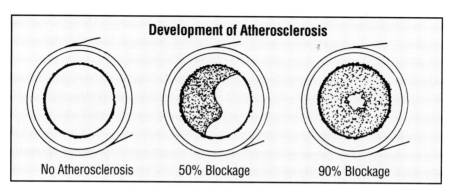

Figure 1.1 The cross-section of a coronary artery showing the progression of athero-sclerosis.

heart attack victims are left incapacitated.

Heart disease develops silently, over a period of many years. Often no symptoms appear until one of the coronary arteries is over 90% closed. In most cases, a physical exam will not disclose the disease until it is in its advanced stages. A resting EKG (electrocardiogram), for example, often records a "normal" pattern unless there is a blockage greater than 90%. A vigorous stress treadmill EKG test usually picks up coronary artery disease earlier, but not until a blockage obstructs about 65 to 90% of an artery.

Atherosclerotic Changes Begin in Early Life

Atherosclerotic changes begin to develop at a much earlier age than most people are aware. In 1,600 autopsies conducted by the Louisiana State University School of Medicine, it was found that fatty streaks (the earliest visible sign of atherosclerosis) were found in all children over 3 years old. Plaque deposits were present in some individuals in the second decade of life and were more frequent in the third decade, with males having greater evidence of disease than females. By the end of the fourth decade (age 39), plaque deposits of varying degrees were present in a **majority** of subjects, both male and female. It was found that our population cannot be divided into those individuals having or not having atherosclerosis, but rather, it must be divided according to the degree of severity of the disease.

Autopsy studies done on American soldiers who died in Korea and Vietnam also demonstrate the early onset of this disease. In 1953, Dr. William Enos published the results of his studies on 300 American soldiers killed in the Korean War. The autopsies showed that 77% of the men had evidence of coronary artery disease, ranging from minimal thickening to total closure of one or more of the three main coronary arteries. Three percent of these men had complete closure of one or more coronary vessels. Their average age was 22. In autopsies performed on soldiers killed in action in Vietnam, it was found that 5% had severe atherosclerosis.

Cholesterol Levels—Key Indicators of Coronary Heart Disease

Cholesterol levels have proven to be reliable indicators of the extent of atherosclerosis present in the body. Autopsy studies have shown a direct correlation between elevated cholesterol levels and the degree of atherosclerosis. Cholesterol levels are also excellent predictors of the likelihood of developing heart disease; the higher the levels, the greater the chance of suffering a heart attack or other heart related problems.

On the other hand, reducing cholesterol levels lowers the risk for heart disease. In 1984, after a 10-year study, an advisory panel of the National Institutes of Health came to this conclusion: "For every 1% reduction in blood cholesterol, there is a 2% reduction in the risk of coronary heart disease." Thus, if you lower your blood cholesterol level by 25% and maintain it (using diet, drugs or a combination of both), you will lower

Relationship Of Blood Cholesterol Levels To Increased IncidenceOf Coronary Heart Disease

Figure 1.2 Risk of coronary heart disease (includes heart attack or angina resulting from physical exertion or excitement) over a six year period, in men aged 30 to 49 years, based on total cholesterol levels.

your risk of heart attack and other complications of heart disease by 50%. Dr. Daniel Steinberg, chairman of the advisory panel, stated that if Americans would change their diets to reduce cholesterol levels by just 10%, then ultimately 100,000 fewer would die each year. Changes at any point in life are beneficial, but the earlier the changes are made, the better. Figure 1.2 shows the relationship of blood cholesterol levels to an increased risk of coronary heart disease, based on the reputable Framingham Heart Study.

Population studies, comparing the mean cholesterol levels and fat intake between nations, further verify the relationships between cholesterol levels, diet and the risk of CHD. Western countries, where the majority of people consume a high-fat diet (approximately 40% of calories from fat), have higher cholesterol levels and are at greater risk for heart disease. Oriental countries and Third World nations, where a low-fat diet is the norm (10 to 20% of calories from fat), have low cholesterol levels and lower incidence of heart disease. The mean cholesterol level for adults in Japan is 163 milligrams per deciliter (mg/dl), while in the U. S., it is 250. Our incidence of heart disease is 10 times greater than in Japan. Eastern Finland has the world's highest mortality rate from heart disease and its mean cholesterol level is 270. Its people consume a very high-fat diet (40+% of calories from fat) and much of the fat is highly saturated. Other population studies further document this relationship.

Significance of Diet vs. Genetics

In an attempt to see if genetics played a role in the wide discrepancies in cholesterol levels between nations, Dr. Ancel Keys of the University of Minnesota studied three groups of Japanese—each living in a different environment, with totally different diets. The first group lived in Japan and consumed a low-fat Asian diet consisting of about 10% of calories from fat. The second group lived in Hawaii and had a combination of the oriental diet and the American diet. The third group lived in Los Angeles and ate a typical American diet of about 40% of calories from fat. The blood cholesterol levels and incidence of heart attack rose with each group. The Japanese living in Los Angeles suffered 10 times as many heart attacks as those who lived in Japan! Their incidence of heart attack became the same as the average American.

According to the Journal of the American Medical Association, 80% of middle-aged men in America probably run a sizeable risk of dying prematurely from heart disease because the cholesterol level in their blood is too high. Research has indicated that *over 50% of all middle-aged adult males in the United States have a serious blockage of one or more of their coronary arteries.* A woman's development of heart disease is slower than a man's, due in part to her production of estrogen during the reproductive years. Estrogen is a sex hormone produced by the ovaries which seems to lower blood cholesterol and the risk of coronary artery disease. However, shortly after menopause when estrogen production decreases, women experience heart attacks at approximately the same rate as men.

Reversal of Disease

The most promising news is that by reducing blood cholesterol levels, we not only lower the risk of suffering from heart disease, but, in some cases, can actually **reverse** the disease process. Lowering cholesterol levels can reduce plaque deposits and increase blood flow to the heart in some individuals. This fact was announced in June 1987, by David Blankenhorn and colleagues at the University of Southern California, when they released the results of their two-year study. They reported that by lowering total blood cholesterol levels (an average of 26%) with diet and drugs over a two-year period, vessel disease was decreased in 16.2% of the men studied. The others receiving the drug/diet therapy showed significantly less progression of disease than the control group (no treatment).

In another study published in 1990, 82% of a small group of heart patients (28 patients) experienced reversal of disease (a reduction in plaque deposits) after following a strict vegetarian diet in combination with comprehensive life style changes. This reversal occurred after just one year's time and without the use of cholesterol lowering drugs.

The participants in this study, conducted by Dr. Dean Ornish of the University of California at San Francisco, followed a diet containing only 10% of calories from fat and 5 milligrams of cholesterol per day. In addition, they refrained from smoking and drinking caffeinated beverages; exercised moderately 30 minutes per day, six days a week; and participated in stress management training (including yoga and meditation) at least one hour a day. Salt was restricted only for those who had hypertension. Cholesterol levels were lowered significantly, in some cases by as much as half. Chest pains disappeared in nearly all those who had complained of them prior to the study.

In studies with Rhesus monkeys, severe coronary artery disease was produced through feeding these animals a high-fat, high-cholesterol diet. (Extensive disease was found in all the monkeys fed this diet. Ordinarily, these animals consume a low-fat diet and heart disease is rare.) On the other hand, after three years of feeding the monkeys a low-fat, cholesterol-free diet, the arterial blockages were reduced from 60% to only 20%.

From these studies, it becomes apparent that diet is a two-sided coin—It can either work for you or against you, depending on the choices made. The best research to date has shown that if cholesterol levels are kept below 150 (mg/dl) throughout a lifetime, heart attacks are virtually nonexistent. From 150 to 180, significant atherosclerosis and related diseases are extremely rare. From 180 to 200, the incidence of heart disease increases only slightly; and above 200, it increases more dramatically (See Figure 1.2). The National Institutes of Health recommends that all adults over 20 should strive to keep cholesterol levels below 200. Children's cholesterol levels should be less than 170.

Since most people are not willing to follow a diet as restrictive as in the Ornish study, prevention should be the primary goal. For most, this can be accomplished with a lifelong program of following a low-fat diet (20% or 30% of calories from fat) and adopting other aspects of a healthy lifestyle. Additional information on cholesterol appears in Chapters 2, 3 and 8.

High Blood Pressure

High blood pressure, or hypertension, as it is sometimes called, occurs when the heart is forced to pump harder to move the blood throughout the body. Its causes are not fully understood, but the main factors affecting the disease are age, stress, genetics and diet. The most important dietary factors are too much sodium (found in greatest concentration in table salt and other condiments and processed foods), obesity, too little potassium and calcium, and too much alcohol.

High blood pressure increases the risk for heart disease, heart attacks and strokes. When the blood is pumped with greater pressure through the blood vessels, it gradually weakens them or causes cracks to develop in the lining of the vessels. Cholesterol, circulating in the blood stream, is deposited in these cracks. Smooth muscle tissue develops at these sites, and together with the cholesterol, form atherosclerotic plaque. Thus, the atherosclerotic process is accelerated when hypertension is accompanied by high cholesterol. In addition, the damaged arteries are more susceptible to forming blood clots, increasing the risk of a heart attack or a stroke. The heart muscle itself weakens and enlarges as a result of hypertension, causing greater stress to the heart. Figure 1.3 shows how the risk factors for heart attack are cumulative. For each additional risk factor —smoking, high cholesterol and high blood pressure—the overall risk increases significantly.

Hypertension, like high cholesterol, can go unnoticed for years because there are no symptoms until the damage is excessive. Nearly 25% of the adult population over the age of 40 has high blood pressure. The incidence increases with age, affecting more than 50% of Americans over the age of 65.

Source: Framingham Heart Study, 16-Year Follow-up. Section 27, Government Printing Office, 1971.

Figure 1.3   The danger of heart attack increases with the number of risk factors present (using the example of a 45-year-old male). Numbers represent the incidence per 100,000 population.

Dietary Influences on Blood Pressure

Numerous studies have indicated a definite link between a high-salt diet and the incidence of high blood pressure. Cultures that consume high amounts of salt, such as in Northern Japan (20,000 milligrams of sodium or about 9 teaspoons of salt per day)*, have the highest incidence of elevated blood pressure, and societies such as the Alaskan Eskimos, who eat very little sodium (less than 2000 milligrams per day), have almost no hypertension. The same correlation was found by Dr. Lot Page of Harvard, who studied six primitive tribes in the Solomon Islands. Three of the tribes ate a high-salt diet and it was only in these three that high blood pressure existed. The other three tribes consumed a low-salt diet (less than 2000 milligrams of sodium per day) and had virtually no hypertension.

Researchers have found that high blood pressure among adults is rare when sodium consumption throughout a lifetime is less that 2000 milligrams per day. The average American consumes 3000 to 6000 milligrams daily, equivalent to one-and-a-half to three teaspoons of salt. The Recommended Dietary Allowance (RDA) for sodium is a minimum of 500 milligrams and a maximum of 2400 milligrams per day; well below the average American intake. The RDA includes sodium from all sources—table salt, processed foods, and the sodium that occurs naturally in foods. (The sodium present naturally in foods accounts for only 10% or less of total sodium intake.)

High blood pressure also has been produced in laboratory animals by feeding them a high-salt diet. Some strains of animals are more

* One teaspoon salt contains approximately 2300 milligrams sodium.

susceptible, suggesting genetic factors. This is also the case with humans, because about half are not salt-sensitive; that is, their blood pressure is not adversely affected by salt consumption.

Obesity can also contribute to high blood pressure. Obese adults (weight greater than 20% above desired weight) have double the incidence of high blood pressure as non-obese individuals. Overweight people with high blood pressure who lose 50% of their excess weight often experience a significant reduction in blood pressure.

Studies have also shown a steady increase in blood pressure as alcohol consumption increases. More than one or two drinks per day, or about an ounce of alcohol, causes blood pressure to rise in some individuals. Those who have high blood pressure, therefore, should be careful to limit their alcohol intake.

Cancer

Cancer accounts for 20% of all deaths in the United States each year. Dr. Peter Greenwald, director of the National Cancer Institute (NCI), estimates that diet is a significant factor in about one-third of all cancers. Other researchers have estimated the figure to be even higher—from 40 to 60%.

The main factors in the diet that lead to an increased incidence of cancer are excessive fat and too little fiber. Added substances such as preservatives and pesticides are also a concern, but food substances such as fat cause an estimated 35 times as much disease as added substances, according to a report by Tufts University Nutrition Department.

In both animal experiments and population studies it has been shown that the higher the intake of fat, the greater the likelihood of malignant tumors; especially of the colon, prostate and breast. Fiber intake primarily affects colon cancer rates; populations that eat a high fiber diet have a lower incidence of colon cancer.

One of the most convincing population studies linking cancer with fat intake involves a comparison of breast cancer rates between Japanese and American women. Both groups live in highly industrialized societies with similar amounts of environmental pollution, which eliminates pollution as a probable cause of the discrepancies. Nevertheless, Japanese women have less than one quarter the incidence of breast cancer as American women. Prior to World War II, their incidence was only one-tenth that of Americans. At that time, their fat consumption was only about 12% of total calories, but now it is about 24%, compared to our approximately 40%.

In addition, when Japanese migrate to the United States, the second generation's breast cancer death rate equals the rate of Americans. This suggests that the differences are not due to genetics. Other international studies show that although there may be large differences in the incidence of cancer between nations, after one or more generations, the migrant groups experience the same cancer rate as the host country. A change in dietary habits is considered the primary reason for this occurrence.

Even within a country, studies have shown that as fat intake increases, so does the incidence of cancer. Since World War II, there have been dramatic increases in cancer rates in Japan, Greece and Iceland, which coincides with an increase in fat consumption. Figure 1.4 shows the relationship between breast cancer rates and fat consumption of 40 different countries.

The International Fat–Breast Cancer Link

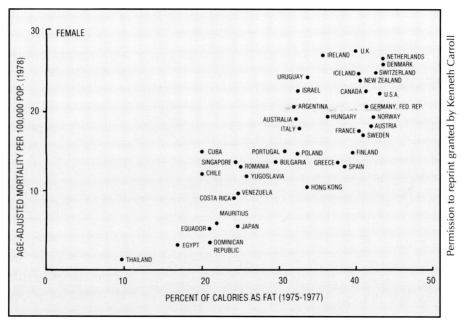

Figure 1.4   A high-fat diet, in countries such as the U.S., is associated with higher rates of death from breast cancer.

High-fat diets also produce more malignant tumors in laboratory animals than low-fat diets. In at least 25 different studies in different countries, it was shown that animals fed a low-fat diet (10 to 20% of calories), exhibited one-third to one-half fewer breast tumors than those fed a high-fat diet (40% of calories.) This is the case regardless of the type of fat used.

Colon Cancer: Excessive Fat & Insufficient Fiber

Colon cancer is linked to **both** excessive fat and insufficient fiber in the diet. Recent population studies suggest that the concentration of bile acids in the feces (body's waste products) is the most significant factor in predicting the incidence of colon cancer in population groups. The higher the fat intake, the higher the amount of bile acids in feces, and consequently, the greater the incidence of cancer. Bile acids are made in the liver, stored in the gall bladder, and are secreted into the intestines to help digest fat.

Dietary fiber, researchers say, helps protect against cancer by increasing the volume of feces and thereby diluting the concentration of bile acids in the stool. It is not known whether the bile acids irritate the colon wall, leaving it more vulnerable to cancer-causing agents, or if the bile acids are converted into carcinogens by fecal bacteria.

Whatever the case, epidemiologic studies have shown that fat is a stronger cancer promoter than fiber is a protector. For example, the Finnish diet is high in fat and fiber, and Finns have half the colon cancer rate of Americans. Japanese, on the other hand, consume a low-fat, low-fiber diet and their colon cancer rate is only one-fourth that of the U.S.

Dietary Factors to Lower Risk of Cancer

Just as choosing the wrong foods can increase the risk of developing certain types of cancer, choosing the right foods can decrease risk. Foods which have demonstrated a protective effect against cancer (in addition to fiber, previously mentioned) are the fruits and vegetables that contain vitamin C, and/or beta carotene; and the cruciferous vegetables, which include broccoli, cauliflower, cabbage, Brussels sprouts, and others. Beta carotene, found in deep green and yellow fruits and vegetables, especially carrots, pumpkin and sweet potatoes, is a "pre-vitamin," which is converted to vitamin A during digestion. (Preformed vitamin A occurs only in animal foods, mainly liver and dairy products.)

Research in this area is still in its early stages, but at this point the most conclusive evidence on a food component's role in reducing cancer risk involves beta carotene. Smokers who consume a lot of beta carotene-rich foods have half the rate of lung cancer as those who consume few of these foods. Numerous population studies also have demonstrated an overall decreased cancer risk for populations with greater consumption of foods high in beta carotene.

Beta carotene also is effective in inhibiting tumors in animals. Animals, exposed to a carcinogen and subsequently given beta carotene injections, did not develop mouth tumors as did the control group not treated with beta carotene. Dr. Gerald Sklar, of the Harvard School of Dental Medicine, stated that beta carotene and vitamin E are the first nontoxic agents that have been shown to both prevent and reverse cancer in experimental animals. (In preliminary studies, drug-level doses of vitamin E have been shown to enhance the immune system of older adults, which may in turn reduce their risk for cancer and heart disease.)

To date, foods with beta carotene, not supplements, have produced the positive results in the studies. Beta carotene supplements also may be beneficial, but until that is proven, be sure to eat foods with beta carotene, regardless of whether you are taking supplements. Beta carotene supplements appear to be harmless. Vitamin A supplements, on the other hand, can reach toxic levels, which can produce serious side effects. See Chapter 6 for more information on cruciferous vegetables and the fruits and vegetables that contain vitamin C and/or beta carotene and the recommended dietary intakes of each.

How Beta Carotene and Vitamin C Work

A normal cell can become cancerous if the DNA in the cell is damaged. The DNA can be damaged by free radicals or singlet oxygen, both of which are dangerous unstable molecules, produced in the body as a result of smoking, chemicals, viruses or certain types of radiation. Beta carotene and vitamin C attach to these potentially harmful molecules, rendering them harmless. For this reason, they are called antioxidants because they prevent harmful oxidation from occurring, just as a rust-preventive prohibits rusting, also a form of oxidation.

Intestinal Disorders

A low fiber diet contributes to a number of intestinal disorders in addition to colon cancer. These include diverticulosis, irritable bowel syndrome, constipation and hemorrhoids.

Fiber's role in disease prevention first became apparent early in this century. British physicians Denis Burkitt and Hugh Trowell found that rural Africans, consuming a diet of unprocessed, unrefined foods, were virtually free of the intestinal disorders that plagued Western cultures. Decades after the Africans moved to the cities and changed to a more refined diet, their incidence of these diseases rose significantly. Numerous studies on other population groups have confirmed the relationship between a high fiber diet and low incidence of intestinal disorders.

Intestinal diseases are common in the United States. Colon cancer is the second most prevalent type of cancer and the number one cause of cancer death in people who do not smoke. Constipation and diverticulosis were rare in Western cultures 60 years ago—before refined grains replaced whole grain products; when meat consumption was lower; and when beans, fruits and vegetables were consumed in greater quantities. Now diverticulosis affects one in three U.S. adults over the age of 60, and constipation is common among all ages but especially among older adults. Irritable bowel syndrome, which causes abdominal pain, accompanied by either diarrhea or constipation, affects nearly 15 to 20% of the adult population. Hemorrhoids affect approximately one-half of all adults over the age of 50.

Fiber's Role in Disease Prevention

Fiber is the indigestible portion of plant food. There are two kinds—insoluble and soluble, and both play an important role in the body's health. Insoluble fiber, found primarily in wheat bran, beans, and the peelings of fruits and vegetables, helps prevent constipation. It does this by adding bulk to the feces and attracting water into the digestive tract, which helps move it through the colon at a faster rate. Because fiber attracts water, it is very important to drink an adequate amount of liquid to allow fiber to work properly. (Eight cups of liquid per day is recommended.) The increased volume from fiber and water dilutes the bacteria and bile acids present in feces.

Diets low in insoluble fiber, on the other hand, produce firm fecal material within the large intestine, which is difficult to propel through the colon. This often results in constipation. It is thought that chronic constipation leads to diverticulosis. This occurs when excess pressure, exerted to move the fecal matter, builds up within the bowel and causes small pouches (diverticula) to form in the weakened walls of the colon. Diverticulitis occurs when these pouches become inflamed and cause intestinal pain. Hemorrhoids are also a common result of constipation.

Soluble fiber is a special type of fiber that is water soluble and found primarily in oat bran, beans and certain fruits and vegetables. It is beneficial to the body in two ways. First, it binds fatty compounds, including cholesterol, and carries them out of the body with the feces. This lowers blood cholesterol concentration and helps reduce the risk of heart disease. Soluble fiber also has a positive effect on the body's response to glucose. It delays the absorption of nutrients from the intestine, causing a gradual increase in blood sugar rather than a rapid one. This is especially important for people with diabetes.

Obesity

Obesity is a serious health problem in our country. Fifteen per cent of the American population, or 34 million people, are 20% or more over their "ideal" body weight. An additional 10 to 15% are overweight to a lesser degree. "Ideal" body weights are based on the 1983 Metropolitan Life Insurance Company table of desirable body weights. (See Table 1.1, page 15.)

According to a study by the Provident Mutual Life Insurance Company of male policyholders, it was found that mortality rates increased

1983 Metropolitan Height and Weight Tables for Men and Women
According to Frame, Ages 25–59

Weight In Pounds (in Indoor Clothing)*

Height (in Shoes)†		Small Frame	Medium Frame	Large Frame
Feet	Inches	**Men**		
5	2	128–134	131–141	138–150
5	3	130–136	133–143	140–153
5	4	132–138	135–145	142–156
5	5	134–140	137–148	144–160
5	6	136–142	139–151	146–164
5	7	138–145	142–154	149–168
5	8	140–148	145–157	152–172
5	9	142–151	148–160	155–176
5	10	144–154	151–163	158–180
5	11	146–157	154–166	161–184
6	0	149–160	157–170	164–188
6	1	152–164	160–174	168–192
6	2	155–168	164–178	172–197
6	3	158–172	167–182	176–202
6	4	162–176	171–187	181–207
		Women		
4	10	102–111	109–121	118–131
4	11	103-113	111–123	120–134
5	0	104–115	113–126	122–137
5	1	106–118	115–129	125–140
5	2	108–121	118–132	128–143
5	3	111–124	121–135	131–147
5	4	114–127	124–138	134–151
5	5	117–130	127–141	137–155
5	6	120–133	130–144	140–159
5	7	123–136	133–147	143–163
5	8	126–139	136–150	146–167
5	9	129–142	139–153	149–170
5	10	132–145	142–156	152–173
5	11	135–148	145–159	155–176
6	0	138–151	148–162	158–179

* Indoor clothing weighing 5 pounds for men and 3 pounds for women.
†Shoes with 1-inch heels

Source of basic data: *Build Study*, 1979 (Society of Actuaries and Association of Life Insurance Medical Directors of America, 1980).
Copyright 1983 Metropolitan Life Insurance Company.

Table 1.1

with weight. The more overweight, the more likely to die prematurely. "The weights associated with the greatest longevity, according to the National Institutes of Health, are *below the average* weights of the population, as long as such weights are not associated with illness."

"Obesity is as powerful a risk factor as any that we know, including smoking and high blood pressure," according to Dr. William Castelli, a highly respected medical researcher and director of the Framingham (Massachusetts) Heart Study. Obesity is an added risk factor for all the diseases discussed previously—cardiovascular disease, hypertension, and cancer. In addition, it contributes significantly to the development of adult onset diabetes mellitus.

Obesity is a major problem in cultures where a high percentage of calories come from fat. It is a rarity in countries where fat intake is 20% or less. The reason for this is fairly simple. Protein and carbohydrates provide 4 calories per gram. Fat yields 9 calories per gram. That means that you can eat **twice** as much in quantity of protein and carbohydrate than you can fat, and still ingest the same number of calories. On a 20% fat diet, 1000 calories provides the same amount of bulk as 1600 calories in a diet of 40% fat. This bulk, without excess calories, provides you with a feeling of fullness or satisfaction, making it easier to maintain an ideal body weight. If the typical American diet were composed of approximately 20% fat, far fewer people would be overweight. In Chapter 3, we will show you how to plan a diet of *either* 20 or 30% of calories from fat.

Summary

Diet truly does play a crucial role in overall health. By eating the right foods, we *can* greatly reduce the risk of dying prematurely from heart disease or cancer. We can also reduce the chances of being plagued by intestinal disorders. We have greater control over our health than many people are aware, as the numerous research studies have shown.

If we exercise this control by eating right, we practice "preventive medicine." The food we consume will be nourishing our body and helping to prevent disease, rather than clogging our arteries, adding excess fat, or promoting high blood pressure, cancer and intestinal diseases.

Necessary changes are not difficult to make, but first you need to know *what* you are eating. To do this, you must understand some basics; in particular, the different types of fat, and how to read and interpret food labels. These topics will be explained in the next chapter.

2

Understanding the Basics: Types of Fat and Reading Food Labels

The Different Types Of Fat

Cholesterol

Cholesterol is a special type of fat present only in foods of animal origin—red meats, fish, poultry and dairy products. Vegetables and vegetable products do not contain cholesterol. Cholesterol is not all bad—it is a vital component in the body's production of cell membranes, hormones, and bile acid, which is needed for fat digestion.

Despite its important role in the body, there is no *dietary* need for cholesterol; that is, we do not need to eat foods containing cholesterol. Whatever cholesterol the body needs is manufactured in the liver. The health problems associated with cholesterol occur when too much is present in the blood and the excess is deposited on the artery walls forming atherosclerotic plaque.

How Cholesterol Travels in Your Bloodstream

Cholesterol is transported through the bloodstream in special protein packages called lipoproteins. ("Lipo (fat) + protein = lipoprotein.) Since cholesterol is a type of fat, it is insoluble in water, and therefore must have a water soluble material to carry it through the bloodstream. Water-soluble protein molecules surround cholesterol and other fat particles, and carry them via the bloodstream to all parts of the body. The two lipoproteins that are the principle transporters of cholesterol are: *high-density lipoproteins*, also referred to as HDL or "good" cholesterol, and *low-density lipoproteins*, commonly referred to as LDL or "bad" cholesterol.

HDL cholesterol moves cholesterol out of the body, transporting it from the blood vessels and tissues to the liver. There much of it is converted to bile acids to aid in fat digestion, and later excreted in the stools. The higher the HDL levels in the blood, the lower the risk of developing heart disease.

LDL cholesterol, on the other hand, moves cholesterol in the opposite direction—from the liver to the various organs and tissues, including the artery walls. High levels of this cholesterol promote atherosclerosis. Although heredity plays some role in the level of LDL in the blood, the high-fat American diet is the principle reason that so many Americans (over 50% of the adult population) have high cholesterol levels.*

Saturated, Polyunsaturated and Monounsaturated Fats

All the fats and oils we consume contain a combination of saturated, polyunsaturated and monounsaturated fats. The fat may be visible, such as cooking oils and butter, or "hidden" in the foods we eat, such as in peanuts, meats and baked goods.

Although all the fats in our diet contain a combination of these three types, they are generally classified by the primary type of fat present. For example, the fat of sirloin steak is commonly referred to as saturated fat. This fat is indeed highly saturated (52%), but it also contains monounsaturated fat (44%) and polyunsaturated fat (4%). A "highly polyunsaturated" oil such as corn oil contains 61% polyunsaturated, 26% monounsaturated, and 13% saturated fat.

These three types of fats have different chemical structures which give them different characteristics. Saturated fats are harder at room temperature and far more stable chemically. The greater stability means that the fats will not spoil or turn rancid for a much longer period of time.

Polyunsaturated fats are less stable chemically which makes them vulnerable to attack by oxygen. When this happens, the oils become rancid, causing the foods made with them to spoil. The more unsaturated a fat, the more liquid it is at room temperature.

Monounsaturated fats differ in chemical structure from polyunsaturated fats, but their characteristics are similar. They are liquid at room temperature and have a shorter shelf life than saturated fats.

Highly saturated fats are the ones responsible for elevating blood cholesterol levels, which can lead to atherosclerosis, heart attack or stroke. The research to date shows that monounsaturated and polyunsaturated fats do not raise blood cholesterol levels.

Knowing that all fats and oils are a combination of the three types of fats is important, especially when trying to lower cholesterol levels. If you *substitute* highly polyunsaturated fat for highly saturated fat, e.g., substitute margarine for butter, your cholesterol levels should drop to some degree because you are consuming less saturated fat. But, the important

*Additional information on cholesterol, medical tests, and ways to improve blood cholesterol levels appears in Chapter 8.

point to remember is that all the highly monounsaturated and polyunsaturated fats and oils contain some saturated fats. Therefore, the most effective way to lower blood cholesterol levels is to reduce **total fat** intake.

Some recent studies have shown that the highly monounsaturated oils (olive, canola and peanut oils), are slightly better than polyunsaturated oils in reducing cholesterol levels. When used instead of saturated fats, both oils lowered LDL cholesterol about the same, but the monounsaturated oil did not lower the HDL or "good cholesterol," as the polyunsaturated oil did slightly. Therefore, in light of these preliminary findings, it would be prudent to use monounsaturated oils when suitable. Olive oil is excellent with stir-fry dishes and on salads; while canola oil, with a milder flavor, works well in baking.

The good news is that our bodies have no need for saturated fat. The only fat essential to our diet is polyunsaturated fat. The total amount of fat adults need is only three to five teaspoons (15 to 25 grams) per day from all sources, including the fat already present in foods. Eating a well balanced diet with a variety of foods guarantees that at least the minimum requirement is met. The majority of Americans consume between 16 and 26 teaspoons (80 to 130 grams) of fat per day.

Hydrogenated Fats

Hydrogenated fats are polyunsaturated fats that have been transformed to more highly saturated fats. Chemists found a simple way to do it: in a large processing vat, liquid oil is bombarded with hydrogen atoms, and the result is shortening—a man-made saturated fat!

Why do manufacturers do this? Remember the commercial advantage of saturated fat just mentioned—a much longer shelf life. The cookies and potato chips on grocery store shelves will stay fresh much longer—for weeks, months, and in some cases years. This greatly reduces the chances of dissatisfied customers returning spoiled merchandise.

Another advantage is that hydrogenated fats have a higher smoking point, which means foods don't scorch as easily at the high temperatures used for frying. This results in significant monetary savings to the food service industry, especially for fast food restaurants, which don't have to change the grease as often in their deep-fat fryers.

The hydrogenation process produces trans fatty acids, a unique type of fat that in preliminary studies has been shown to raise cholesterol levels. This means that hydrogenated fats such as margarine and shortening may raise cholesterol levels more than previously thought. However, margarine is still a better choice than butter because it has *fewer* cholesterol-raising fats. The bottom line is to go light on all fats, margarine included, and select the softer margarines (in a tub) because they are less hydrogenated and thus have fewer trans fatty acids.

Animal vs. Vegetable Fat

Many people think of vegetable fat as liquid and heart-healthy, and animal fat as the type responsible for clogging arteries. The distinction between these two is not that simple, however. Most vegetable fats are indeed liquid at room temperature and highly polyunsaturated or monounsaturated, but some are hard at room temperature and highly saturated. Highly saturated vegetable oils include palm oil, palm kernel oil, coconut oil, cocoa butter, and some hydrogenated vegetable oils. See Figure 2.1 for a classification of vegetable oils.

On the other hand, most animal fats are more highly saturated, which means they are more solid at room temperature. The degree of saturation varies, with poultry fat less saturated, and beef fat and butter fat much more so. Fish oil, an unusual animal fat, is in a class by itself. It is less saturated than poultry fat, (most varieties range from 15–25% saturated) and in addition, it contains a unique type of polyunsaturated fat, called omega-3 fatty acids. Fish oil actually has been shown to have a *protective* effect against heart disease, but only if it is used *in place of* highly saturated fats. (See next section on fish oils.)

Refer to Figure 2.2 for a breakdown of the percentage of saturated, polyunsaturated, and monounsaturated fats in various vegetable and animal fats/oils.

Types of Vegetable Oils		
Highly Polyunsaturated	**Highly Monounsaturated**	**Highly Saturated***
Corn Oil Safflower Oil Sunflower Oil Sesame Oil Soybean Oil Cottonseed Oil	Olive Oil Peanut Oil Canola Oil Cocoa butter	Coconut Oil Palm Oil Palm Kernel Oil
*Have greatest cholesterol-raising effect.		

Figure 2.1 Vegetable oils are classified by the type of fat most prominent in their chemical composition. Actually all fats and oils include a combination of polyunsaturated, monounsaturated and saturated fats.

Fish Oils

Fish oils contain a unique type of polyunsaturated fat known as omega-3 fatty acids. (It is sometimes sold in health-food stores under a specific name or abbreviation, such as EPA for eicosapentaenoic acid or DHA for docosahexaenoic acid.) These fish oils, *when consumed in large quantities in place of saturated fat,* have been shown to lower both LDL

Comparison of Dietary Fats

Dietary Fat	Fatty Acid Content Normalized to 100%		
Canola oil	6%	32%	62%
Safflower oil	10%	77%	13%
Sunflower oil	11%	69%	20%
Corn oil	13%	62%	25%
Olive oil	14%	9%	77%
Soybean oil	15%	61%	24%
Peanut oil	18%	33%	49%
Margarine	19%	32%	49%
Cottonseed oil	27%	54%	19%
Vegetable shortening*	28%	28%	44%
Chicken fat	31%	22%	47%
Lard	41%	12%	47%
Beef fat	52%	4%	44%
Palm oil	52%	10%	38%
Cocoa butter	61%	5%	34%
Butter (fat)	66%	4%	30%
Palm kernel oil	86%	2%	12%
Coconut oil	92%	2%	6%

Saturated Fat   Polyunsaturated Fat   Monounsaturated Fat

*Crisco shortening
Source: Agriculture Handbook No. 8-4. Washington, D.C., U.S. Department of Agriculture.

Figure 2.2 Breakdown of dietary fats into percentage of saturated, polyunsaturated and monounsaturated fats.

cholesterol levels and triglycerides. (Triglycerides are other fats circulating in the blood, which may also contribute to heart disease.) In addition, fish oils affect the blood in a similar way to aspirin—they "thin" the blood, making the blood platelets less sticky and thus less likely to form blood clots. They also appear to inhibit the formation of atherosclerotic plaque, which reduces the risks of heart attack and stroke.

These beneficial properties of fish oils first came to light through studies with the Greenland Eskimos. Scientists were puzzled by their low incidence of heart disease. Even though their diet was very high in animal fat from seal meat, fish, and whale blubber, their incidence of heart attack was about 100 times lower than in the United States.

When these same Eskimos moved to Denmark and ate the typical Western diet, their incidence of heart disease rose dramatically, to match that of the Danes and other Western Europeans. It was determined that it was the specific *type* of polyunsaturated fat in the fish oil that made the difference. The effectiveness of these fish oils as a protective influence against heart disease was further verified in studies with Japanese fishermen and with animals in the laboratory.

Does this mean that we should eat one pound of fish per day as the Eskimos do, or its equivalent of over two tablespoons of fish oil supplements per day? The answer is no, because of the associated health hazards and because more research still needs to be done to determine what, if any, are **safe and effective** doses of the supplements. Although the Eskimos have an extremely low incidence of heart disease, they have other health problems resulting from their high consumption of fish oils. They bruise easily, have frequent nosebleeds, and have prolonged bleeding times, which can lead to a variety of health problems.

Taking supplements of cod-liver oil or other fish oils in quantities of a tablespoon a day or more could lead to problems similar to those mentioned above. In addition, some fish oil supplements (cod-liver oil, especially) can cause vitamin A and D toxicity, because these vitamins are stored in the body and the amounts build up over time. Toxic levels of these vitamins cause serious side effects, and may even cause death.

Preliminary studies on fish oil supplements appear promising, but, so far, there is no definitive proof that they are effective. Several studies now underway are scheduled to be completed by the middle 1990's, and at that time the safety and effectiveness of these supplements will probably be determined. Most physicians are waiting for these studies to be completed before making recommendations.

It is heartily recommended now to *eat* more fish instead of foods with a high saturated fat content. Fish is an excellent low-fat protein source; and the type of fat present in fish may actually help reduce your risk of heart disease.

Because of the small amount of total fat in fish (the highest fat fish have about the same total fat as the leanest red meats), and the beneficial effects of fish oil, the recommended fish portion per day (4–6 ounces) is greater than that of meats (3–4 ounces). (See Figure 7.1, page 88, for the recommended daily servings and guidelines of the "Food Guide Pyramid.")

Table 2.1 lists the amount of omega-3 oils present in selected seafood. Other excellent sources of Omega-3 fatty acids are cooked beans, especially soybeans.

Simplesse—The Fat Substitute

Available to the public only since February 1990, Simplesse is a fat substitute made of egg whites and milk protein. These two ingredients are cooked and blended into a smooth thick fluid that resembles the creamy texture of fat.

The Food and Drug Administration (FDA) classified this new fat

Content of Omega-3 Fatty Acids of Selected Seafood
(in 5.25 ounces of fish, uncooked)

Food Item	Omega-3 Oil Content
Mackerel, Atlantic	3.8 g
Mackerel, king	3.3 g
Herring, Pacific	2.6 g
Herring, Atlantic	2.4 g
Trout, lake	2.4 g
Tuna, bluefin	2.4 g
Sturgeon, Atlantic	2.3 g
Anchovies	2.2 g
Sabelfish	2.1 g
Tuna, Albacore	2.1 g
Whitefish, lake	2.0 g
Bluefish	1.8 g
Salmon, sockeye	1.8 g
Mullet	1.7 g
Salmon, pink	1.5 g
Halibut, Greenland	1.4 g
Bass, striped	1.2 g
Oysters	0.6 to 1.2 g
Smelt, rainbow	1.1 g
Pompano	0.9 g
Mussels, blue	0.8 g
Trout, rainbow	0.8 g
Rockfish	0.8 g
Shrimp	0.3 to 0.8 g
Halibut, Pacific	0.6 g
Haddock	0.3 g
Lobster, Maine	0.3 g
Perch, Ocean	0.3 g
Red Snapper	0.3 g
Swordfish	0.3 g
Scallops	0.3 g

(Source: *Journal of The American Dietetic Association*, June, 1986.)

Table 2.1

substitute as (GRAS) "generally regarded as safe," when it was released for public use. It can only be used in products that do not require heating, such as sour cream, mayonnaise, yogurt and ice cream, since baking or frying destroys its creamy texture.

The fat and calorie savings with Simplesse, as with other low-fat and nonfat foods, can be substantial. For example, an 8-ounce serving of ice cream (11% fat) has about 14 grams of fat and 270 calories, while a similar serving of nonfat ice cream made with Simplesse has less than 1 gram of fat and only 144 calories. A tablespoon of regular mayonnaise has 6 grams of fat and 65 calories, compared to less that one gram of fat and only 9 calories in mayonnaise made with Simplesse.

Simplesse makes it possible to enjoy the creamy textures of ice cream and other foods without the high fat and high calories. Still, it is best to reserve these foods for occasional use, and to choose primarily nutritious foods that do not need a rich texture to taste good, like fruits, vegetables and whole grain products.

Interpreting Food Labels

The nutritional claims which appear on food packaging can often confuse even the most careful consumer. One of the reasons for this is that the manufacturers see the food label as the primary means of influencing consumers to buy their product. They are aware that many Americans have become more health conscious and consequently are trying to cut down on one or several of the following: calories, cholesterol, fat, salt, sugar and food additives. Often they attempt to make their products attractive to the consumer by appealing to these health concerns.

It is important to know exactly what the nutritional claims on food labels mean or do not mean. Here are three examples to show how misleading some can be. A food labeled "light" may be loaded with calories; one with "no cholesterol" can contain large amounts of cholesterol-raising saturated fat; and a "natural" food may contain many artificial ingredients.

Because of concern that consumers are being misled by these claims, Congress authorized the Food and Drug Administration (FDA) in 1990 to make widesweeping changes in regulations governing food labels. The objectives are to curb advertising hype and provide meaningful nutrition information so that health-conscious consumers can make informed food purchases.

In November 1991, the FDA announced a proposed set of strict guidelines governing food labels. Industry has been given two years to comment and make suggestions regarding the proposals. By May 1994, they must comply with the much stricter labeling laws.

The proposed changes will put restrictions on the marketing terminology used on food labels. It will also require that all foods (of meaningful nutritional value) include certain nutrition information, including calories per serving; amounts of carbohydrates, total fat, saturated fat, fiber, protein, sugar and sodium per serving; and information on vitamins and minerals. Currently, only about half of all packaged foods provide nutrition information. The U. S. Department of Agriculture (USDA) has jurisdiction over meat and poultry, and is working with the FDA to establish similar guidelines for meat and poultry products.

There are some government regulations, now in effect, regarding the terminology appearing on food labels. The following provides an explanation of the most commonly used terms and the regulations (effective until May 1994) that govern the use of these words. With the proposed new regulations, there will be fewer changes in the terms that are already strictly defined, such as "enriched" and "fortified." The greatest changes will be in the use of terms loosely defined; i.e. "fresh," "natural," and "lite" or "light."

Common Terminology Appearing On Food Labels

Cholesterol-free: Foods must have fewer than 2 milligrams, or no more than a trace, of cholesterol per serving. In addition to the cholesterol in foods, however, it is equally important to know the amount of saturated or hydrogenated fats, which elevate blood cholesterol levels to a greater extent than cholesterol from foods. Cholesterol is found only in animal products, not vegetable products. The proposed changes would require that the saturated fat content also be taken into account before a "no cholesterol" claim can be made.

Low cholesterol: These foods have fewer than 20 milligrams of cholesterol per serving. (Recommended daily levels range from 100 to 300 milligrams of cholesterol.

Cholesterol reduced: Products have been reformulated so that they have at least 75% less cholesterol than the original foods.

Enriched: Nutrients lost during processing are partially replaced by the manufacturers. For example, when wheat is turned into white flour, it loses at least 50 to 80% of many nutrients. Of these, iron, niacin, thiamin and riboflavin are replaced; but other nutrients lost in the milling process, such as fiber, zinc and copper are not restored.

Fortified: These foods contain added vitamins and minerals that were not originally in the food or were present in lower amounts. Commonly fortified foods include breakfast cereals, salt with iodine added, and milk with vitamins A and D added.

Natural: This term has different meanings for different foods. When applied to meat or poultry, it means the food is minimally processed and free of artificial ingredients. But for other foods, "natural" has no legal meaning. Many "natural" foods are highly processed, packed with fat and sugar, and loaded with preservatives. A "natural flavor," however, must come from a juice, oil, leaf, herb, or spice, but foods containing "all natural flavor" may still have artificial colors and preservatives. "Natural" should be interpreted with caution rather than reassurance. The FDA's proposed changes call for this term to be more strictly defined.

Organic: Most people are under the impression that organic foods are grown without the use of pesticides or chemical fertilizers. However, only 22 states have defined how foods must be grown in order to be labeled "organic." In the remaining 28 states, foods sold as "organic" may contain pesticide residues at the same levels as conventional foods. However, the 1990 Congress passed a Farm Bill which mandates that a single national standard be established for organically grown produce. Until the law is fully implemented (perhaps mid-1990's) only a *certified* organic label will guarantee its authenticity. This is a guarantee from the grower that strict organic guidelines have been followed and monitored by an independent agency.

Low-calorie: This indicates that a food has fewer that 40 calories per serving **and** less than 0.4 calorie per gram. A salad dressing with 35 calories per tablespoon may seem to be "low calorie" because of its small serving size, but it does not qualify since it contains more than 0.4 calorie per gram.

Reduced-calorie: These foods must have at least one-third fewer calories than the regular preparations. The nutritional comparison must be shown on the label.

Light or **lite:** This term does not necessarily mean low-fat or low-calorie. When this word appears, it is a signal to read the label carefully. If it refers to reduced calories, full nutrition information must be provided. But "light" can also refer to pale color, low sodium, light taste, reduced alcohol, or fluffy texture. When applied to processed meats, "light" means that products have at least 25% less fat than usual. This term will be more strictly defined under the new labeling laws.

95% Fat Free: This nutrition claim appears most often on processed meats such as ham slices. It means that by weight, only 5% of the meat is fat. However, since a gram of fat contains more than twice as many calories as protein or carbohydrate; and since some of the weight of the meat is water which has no calories; the fat content, in percentage of total calories, is usually about 30 to 40%. The number of grams of fat per serving size is a more accurate indicator of the fat content.

Nutrition Information

In contrast to the bold nutritional claims prominently displayed on the front of food packaging, the more important nutrition information usually appears in small print on the side or back of the package. This may include just the list of ingredients or more complete standard nutrition information.

All packaged or canned foods, with one exception, must include a list of ingredients. Only those which meet certain "standards of identity," such as mayonnaise, are not required to do so. In this case, the product must contain certain ingredients that are present in a specific amount as specified by the Food and Drug Administration (FDA). Under the proposed new laws, all foods would have to include a list of ingredients.

Standard Nutrition Information

The more complete standard nutrition information appears on about half of all labels, listing the calories per serving, and the quantities of fat, carbohydrate, protein and certain vitamins and minerals. This information must be included if a nutritional claim is made, such as "fortified with 13 essential vitamins and minerals." Often it is provided voluntarily by the manufacturer for the benefit of the consumer.

The proposed labeling rules mandate that *all* food products, (under the FDA's jurisdiction) that are meaningful sources of nutrition, contain standard nutrition information, similar to what is provided on the soup label, Figure 2.3. We will examine this label to better understand the information provided.

Serving Size

The serving size is listed first and is important to note when comparing brands, or when trying to limit calories or certain ingredients. Make sure that you compare similar quantities of food and that the serving size corresponds with what you are planning to eat. It could be much smaller than you would expect. For example, a popular brand of frozen burritos lists a serving size as one-third of a burrito. Most would consider a serving size to be a whole burrito. If you plan to eat a whole burrito, you must multiply the nutrition data by 3, including calories, grams of fat, etc.

Another example of an unusually small serving size appears on one of the top brands of "low sodium" soy sauce. There the serving size is 1/2 teaspoon. Does anyone use only a 1/2 teaspoon of soy sauce in an Oriental dish? The proposed new labeling laws would establish set serving sizes for similar types of foods.

Fat, Carbohydrate, and Protein Content

All the calories from the foods we eat come from either fat, carbohydrate or protein. (Alcohol also supplies calories, but is not considered a food.) The quantities of these three nutrients are given in number of grams, as shown on the soup label (Figure 2.3).

The amount of fat is sometimes better understood by expressing it as a percentage of total calories. This is because reference is often made to the *percentage* of fat in our diet. Converting grams of fat to the percentage of fat is fairly simple as illustrated by the sample calculation in Figure 2.4. The basic information you need to know is that there are 9 calories in a gram of fat. (Carbohydrate has 4 calories per gram; protein has 4 calories

```
NUTRITION INFORMATION PER SERVING
SERVING SIZE              4 OZ.—CONDENSED
(8 OZ. AS PREPARED - 226 g)
SERVINGS PER CONTAINER.......................2 3/4
CALORIES.............................................100
PROTEIN (GRAMS)........................................2
CARBOHYDRATE (GRAMS)........................... 8
FAT (GRAMS)................................................ 7
POLYUNSATURATED (GRAMS)..................... 5
SATURATED (GRAMS).................................... 2
CHOLESTEROL................less than 5 mg/serving
SODIUM................................... 820 mg/serving
PERCENTAGE OF U.S RECOMMENDED
DAILY ALLOWANCES (U.S. RDA)
     PROTEIN .............2     RIBOFLAVIN............. 4
     VITAMIN A ..........*     NIACIN.....................2
     VITAMIN C ..........*     CALCIUM................. 2
     THIAMINE........... *     IRON........................*

*CONTAINS LESS THAN 2% OF THE U.S. RDA OF THIS
NUTRIENT.
INGREDIENTS: WATER, MUSHROOMS, VEGETABLE OIL
(CORN, COTTONSEED OR PARTIALLY HYDROGENATED
SOYBEAN OIL), WHEAT FLOUR, CREAM, SALT, CORN-
STARCH, DRIED DAIRY BLEND, (WHEY, CALCIUM CASEIN-
ATE), MODIFIED FOOD STARCH, WHEY, MONOSODIUM
GLUTAMATE, SOY PROTEIN ISOLATE, NATURAL FLA-
VORING, YEAST EXTRACT AND DEHYDRATED GARLIC.
```

Figure 2.3 Standard Nutrition Information which appears on the label of a popular brand of Cream of Mushroom Soup.

per gram; and alcohol contains 7 calories per gram.)

The computation involves a two-step process. First, you determine the number of fat calories per serving by multiplying the grams of fat, as shown on the label, by 9 calories per gram. (7 grams x 9 cal/gm = 63 fat calories.) Next you get the percentage of fat by dividing the fat calories by the total calories, as shown on the label. (63 fat calories ÷ 100 total calories = .63, or 63%.) This tells us that 63% of the calories in this soup comes from fat.

Computing Percentage of Fat Calories

Step 1:	Grams of Fat	x	Calories per gram	=	Calories of fat
	7	x	9	=	63 fat calories
Step 2:	Fat calories	÷	Total calories	=	Percentage of fat
	63	÷	100	=	.63 or 63% Fat

Figure 2.4 The two-step mathematical process to derive the percentage of calories from fat.

This computation makes it more obvious that the soup, with 63% of its calories from fat, is indeed a high-fat item. Many cream-based soups are high in fat, but there are commercial soups available which are much lower in fat. Read the labels to find them.

Cholesterol and Sodium

The cholesterol and sodium content of the food product is listed next.

You only need to note the serving size to determine if the quantity you will eat corresponds to the serving size. Explanations of the recommended daily amounts of cholesterol (100 to 300 milligrams per day) and sodium (500 to 2400 milligrams per day) will be given in Chapters 3 and 4 respectively. Knowing the recommended amounts per day will enable you to determine if a particular food item would keep you within your desired limit or cause you to exceed it.

Percentage of U.S.RDA

U.S.RDA stands for U.S. Recommended Dietary Allowance, the estimated amount of various nutrients needed each day to maintain good health for all persons over age four, except pregnant or lactating (breast feeding) women. Separate charts of RDA's are given for these women and for children under four. The nutrient contents of foods are expressed as a percentage of the U.S.RDA. Most RDA's vary slightly according to age and gender. Taking these differences into account, a margin of error is built into these amounts, so that most people will not be deficient unless they consistently consume less than 70% of the U.S.RDA.

List of Ingredients

The list of ingredients is given in descending order according to weight, so that whatever is listed first is the most abundant ingredient. At best, this enables you to only estimate the quantities of each ingredient. However, if you also consider the amounts of carbohydrate, protein, and fat, you can get a more accurate idea. For example, using the soup label (Figure 2.3), you already know that 63% of the calories come from fat. Looking at the list of ingredients, you realize that the fat comes from vegetable oil and cream, since those are the only items that contain fat. Since the ingredients are listed in descending order by weight, you can also determine that the majority of fat comes from the vegetable oil since it is listed third and the cream is listed fifth.

Many products do not include a breakdown of fat, carbohydrate, and protein, which makes it more difficult to estimate the amounts of ingredients. Once the proposed nutrition labeling laws go into effect in 1994, however, all foods will include this information. Until then, it is helpful to know what foods are generally high in fat, sodium, sugar, fiber or whatever other ingredient you may be trying to limit or increase. In the next several chapters, charts will show the amounts of fat, cholesterol, sodium, and fiber in many of the most commonly eaten foods.

Determining Types of Fat from Food Labels

A breakdown of fats into polyunsaturated and saturated fats is not required by law (prior to May, 1994), and therefore is often absent from food labels. For this reason, it is important to *know* which fats are highly saturated and which ones are not. The highly saturated fats are: fats of animal origin (including lard), hydrogenated shortenings, butter, coconut oil, palm oil, palm kernel oil, and cocoa butter. See Figure 2.2 for a comparison of the percentage of saturated fat of the various dietary fats and oils. The new labeling proposals call for listing the amount of saturated fat, which should eliminate the guesswork.

Until the proposed legislation goes into effect, however, it is sometimes impossible to determine whether the fat is saturated or unsaturated since many labels don't specify which oil is used, listing just "vegetable oil" instead. Many others list an array of oils—for example, "contains one or more of the following: soybean, hydrogenated cottonseed, and/or palm kernel oil." This gives manufacturers a choice when prices fluctuate. When this is the case, assume the worst, since the saturated oils are usually cheaper and have a longer shelf life.

Since many processed foods contain saturated or hydrogenated fat, it becomes even more important to consider the amount of fat in the product, especially if your cholesterol level is elevated, or you have a family history of heart disease. Most people do not have the time to make all their foods from scratch, so the purchase of some processed foods is a necessity. Therefore, avoid, as much as possible, those processed foods highest in fat content, such as most snack crackers, fried foods and many desserts. Select instead low-fat processed foods, including most breads and cereals, low-fat yogurt and canned fruits (preferably the low-sugar varieties); and fresh or frozen fruits and vegetables.

Determining Quantity of Sugars from Food Labels

In reading a label for its sugar content, it is important to know that sugar can be listed by many different names. It is possible for sugar to be the first or second most prominent ingredient in a food item; but because it is broken down into different types of sugar, such as brown sugar, corn syrup, sugar and honey, these may appear as the third through eighth items. (Remember that the ingredients must be listed in descending order according to weight.) By listing the sugars separately, manufacturers confuse the consumer about the real sugar content of the product.

Table sugar is listed as sucrose on a label. Concentrated sugar also can be listed under the following names: glucose, maltose, dextrose, lactose, fructose, malt, corn solids, corn syrup, honey, molasses and brown sugar. Although not always reliable, a recommended guideline is to consider the food a high sugar product if any type of sugar is one of the first two ingredients.

3

Pursuing a Healthy Diet: Reducing Fat and Cholesterol

One of the most important steps toward a healthier diet is to eat less fat, especially saturated fat, and cholesterol. Consuming too much fat and cholesterol increases the risks for heart disease, cancer and obesity.

As mentioned previously, the amount of fat adults need is very small—only 3 to 5 teaspoons a day from all sources, or about 10% of total calories. Also, the only **essential** fat in the diet is polyunsaturated fat.

Recommendations on Fat Consumption

The National Committee on Diet, Nutrition and Cancer and the American Heart Association recommend a diet in which *no more than* 30% of calories comes from fat. Furthermore, *no more than* 10% of total calories should come from saturated fat. The American Heart Association recommends a greater reduction in saturated fat—to *less than* 7% of total calories—if blood cholesterol levels remain above 200 (mg/dl). Keep in mind that these recommended levels are not targets, but ceilings.

Today, many leading nutritionists in diet and health research recommend a 20% fat diet (20% of total calories from fat) for everyone, because of the greater benefits shown in many studies. The 20% fat diet has demonstrated greater success in combating obesity, in reducing cholesterol levels, and in decreasing the risks of some cancers. It is also a diet on which the whole family can thrive, receiving abundant amounts of all the essential nutrients. (Exception: Children below the age of two need additional fat because of the tremendous growth that takes place during the first two years. Follow the advice of your pediatrician or dietitian for this age group.)

In a study sponsored by the National Institutes of Health (NIH), a 20% fat diet was found to be an approachable goal for typical Americans accustomed to a much higher fat diet. The 233 families who took part in the NIH study were educated about the merits of a lower fat diet. Eighty per cent of them remained in the study for the full five years. During that time, they gradually reduced their fat intake to between 20% and 30% of total calories. They made the necessary changes and stuck with them. By the end of the study, most had decided to make the lower fat diet a permanent part of their lifestyle.

Some adults have gone even further with fat reductions, following the recommendations of the late Nathan Pritikin. He recommended a very stringent diet consisting of approximately 10% of calories from fat, and very low salt and sugar. Many of these adults have experienced drastic reductions in cholesterol levels, and when exercising care in eating a balanced diet, have managed to be well nourished at the same time. Although very effective in reducing cholesterol levels, the Pritikin diet is not recommended for children of any age because they need more fat to achieve their full growth potential.

Later in this chapter, simple guidelines are listed which show how to limit fat to approximately 20% of total calories. A chart showing total daily fat intakes (based on calorie consumption) for diets of both 20% and 30% of calories from fat also is provided.

Recommendations on Cholesterol Consumption

The American Heart Association recommends that adults and children consume no more than 300 milligrams of cholesterol per day. For those with high cholesterol levels (above 200), their recommendation is less than 200 milligrams per day. Some leading nutritionists recommend only 100 milligrams of cholesterol per day for everyone, as a preventive measure, regardless of blood cholesterol levels.

The main point to keep in mind is that the less cholesterol you eat in foods, the lower your blood cholesterol levels should be. If your blood cholesterol level is already very low, your need to lower your cholesterol intake is not as great as for those with levels near 200 or above.

A word of caution for those who feel their cholesterol levels are low enough that they needn't worry about cholesterol and saturated fats in foods—in a study conducted by the National Institutes of Health, it was found that no one is totally free of the risk of heart disease, no matter what their cholesterol level is. However, the lower the level, the lower the risk. (See Figure 1.2.)

Since most foods high in saturated fat are also high in cholesterol, if you eat less saturated fat, you will also consume less cholesterol. The guidelines listed near the end of this chapter for the 20% fat diet will keep cholesterol intake to approximately 100–150 milligrams per day, provided whole eggs are not used. (It should also keep saturated fat intake to less than 7% of total calories.)

Step 1—Identify Sources of Fat and Cholesterol

Before you can effectively reduce fat and cholesterol in your diet, it is necessary to know the sources—both the obvious and the "hidden". Figure 3.1 identifies the sources of fat in the typical American diet. The largest amount (44%) comes directly from fats and oils, with half (22%) from visible fats added at the table in the form of spreads and dressings; and the other half (22%) from baked goods and cooking oils used in food preparation. The next largest amount is from red meats (30%), followed by dairy (11%), poultry (5%), eggs (3%), grains, beans, fruits and vegetables (6%), and fish (1%).

From this chart, it is evident that fat consumption can be reduced most effectively by limiting the fats and oils used in baking, cooking, in spreads and salad dressings; and by cutting down on fats from red meats and dairy products.

Figure 3.2 shows the sources of cholesterol in the typical American diet. The largest percentage comes from egg yolks (45%) with approximately half from visible eggs (2-3 per week), and half from eggs used in food preparation. The next largest percentage is from red meat (28%), followed by dairy products (20%). Cholesterol in dairy products comes from the following: 9% from milk, 5% from cheese, 4% from butter and 2% from ice cream. Poultry contributes 4.5% of the dietary cholesterol, and fish contributes 2.5%.

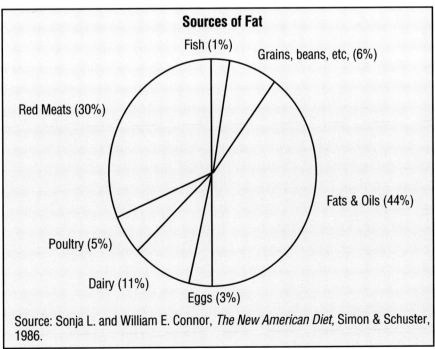

Source: Sonja L. and William E. Connor, *The New American Diet*, Simon & Schuster, 1986.

Figure 3.1 The sources of dietary fat in a typical American diet.

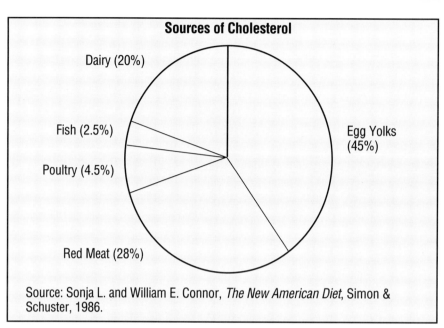

Sources of Cholesterol

Dairy (20%)

Fish (2.5%)

Poultry (4.5%)

Egg Yolks (45%)

Red Meat (28%)

Source: Sonja L. and William E. Connor, *The New American Diet*, Simon & Schuster, 1986.

Figure 3.2. The sources of cholesterol in a typical American diet.

Referring to Figure 3.2, it is easy to see that eliminating whole eggs would reduce cholesterol from foods by nearly one-half. The other major sources of cholesterol are red meats and dairy, which are also high fat sources, as shown previously. Therefore, if you cut down on red meats and high-fat dairy products, both fat and cholesterol will be reduced.

Cholesterol-Saturated Fat Index for Foods

Since **both** saturated fat and cholesterol are responsible for elevating blood cholesterol levels, the Cholesterol-Saturated Fat Index (CSI) for foods was devised, taking into account both these factors. The higher the number, the greater the cholesterol raising effect; and conversely, the lower the number, the less tendency to raise blood cholesterol levels. The CSI is particularly effective in making comparisons between foods from the same food group. See Table 3.1.

Comparisons of Meat, Fish and Poultry

In comparing the CSI of meat, fish and poultry, the better choices are obvious—fish, including shellfish, and poultry without skin, are preferable to red meats. That does not mean that red meats should necessarily be avoided, but definitely reduced. When eating red meats, be sure to choose the leaner cuts and trim the visible fat. Check with your butcher to find the leanest cuts. Also, on the days you eat red meat, make sure most of your other foods are lower in fat.

You may have heard in the past that shrimp and lobster are high in cholesterol and therefore should be avoided. It is true that they are relatively high in cholesterol, but the saturated fat content is so small that their CSI is similar to poultry without skin.

How does the presence of skin and manner of cooking affect the fat content of poultry? With the skin, the fat in poultry is roughly doubled. (To achieve the fat savings effect, the skin can be removed either before or after cooking.) If the poultry is dipped in batter with the skin on and deep fried, a common practice in many fast food restaurants, the fat content is approximately tripled, because of the extra fat absorbed by the batter. This means that a fried chicken breast from a fast food restaurant may contain as much, or more fat, than a large hamburger.

Processed Poultry Products

Many processed foods made with chicken or turkey are now available in supermarkets. These include chicken and turkey hot dogs, turkey bologna, and ground turkey. Are these any better than those made with beef and pork? One of the best ways to determine this is to compare the grams of fat on the food labels, if this information is given.

If this information is not provided, the following guidelines should be helpful. On the average, chicken and turkey dogs have 30% less fat than regular hot dogs. But this still does not put them in a low-fat category. They contain about 2 teaspoons of fat for a 2-ounce hot dog, as compared with 3 teaspoons of fat for their beef or pork counterparts. (1 teaspoon of fat equals approximately 5 grams of fat.) Turkey burgers have about one-fourth less fat than "lean" ground beef burgers. Again, however, the total fat is still quite high—2 1/2 teaspoons per 3-ounce patty. The fat content is high because the visible fat from the turkey is included when the meat is ground. If you grind your own turkey at home after removing the skin and visible fat, the same amount of ground turkey (3 ounces) has about one teaspoon of fat for the dark meat, and only 1/2 teaspoon (2.5 grams) for the light meat.

Comparisons of Fats and Oils

Comparing the CSI of fats and oils in Table 3.1 makes it apparent that there are vast differences in their effects on the heart and blood vessels. All of the highly polyunsaturated vegetables oils (CSI of 8) are far better than the highly saturated vegetable oils including coconut oil, palm oil, and cocoa butter (CSI of 47). So don't be fooled again by the claim "all vegetable oil"—find out what kind of vegetable oil! Even bacon grease is only half as harmful as the highly saturated vegetable oils.

These comparisons also show that, whenever possible, it is better to use soft margarines, which have a CSI of 10, than hard-stick margarines which have a CSI of 15. Mayonnaise has a CSI of 10, but there are tasty lower fat substitutes available, including those advertised as "light." Many of these have fewer calories and consequently less fat because they are more highly whipped, and therefore partly filled with air. Still, watch the quantity—a thin scraping is best.

Peanut butter should be used in moderation because 50% of its calories come from fat. It is fine to use in a sandwich as a protein source

The Cholesterol-Saturated Fat Index (CSI) and Calorie Content of Selected Foods

Fish, Poultry, Red Meat (3 1/2 ounces, cooked)	CSI	Cal.
White fish (snapper, perch, sole, cod, halibut, etc.), shellfish (clams, oysters, scallops)., water-pack tuna	4	91
Salmon	5	149
Shellfish (crab, lobster)	5	100
Poultry, no skin	6	171
Shrimp	7	105
Pork tenderloin; beef top round, lean	7	180
Beef, Pork and Lamb:		
10% fat (ground sirloin, flank steak)	9	214
15% fat (ground round)	10	258
20% fat (ground chuck, pot roasts)	13	286
30% fat (ground beef, pork, and lamb steaks, ribs, pork and lamb chips, roasts)	18	381

Cheeses (3 1/2 ounces)	CSI	Cal.
Low-fat cottage cheese, tofu (bean curd), pot cheese	1	98
Cottage cheese, Lite-line, Lite n' Lively, Weight Watchers, part-skim ricotta	6	139
Cheddar, Roquefort, Swiss, Brie, Jack, American, cream cheese, Velveeta, cheese spreads (jars) and most other cheeses	26	386

Eggs	CSI	Cal.
Whites (3)	0	51
Egg substitute (equivalent to 2 eggs)	<1†	91
Whole (2)	29	163

Fats (1/4 cup or 4 tablespoons)	CSI	Cal.
Peanut butter	5	353
Most vegetable oils	8	530
Mayonnaise	10	431
Soft vegetable margarines	10	432
Hard-stick margarines	15	432
Soft shortenings	16	530
Bacon grease	23	541

instead of meat or cheese, but if you eat large quantities as a snack, you will be consuming too much fat. The "partially hydrogenated" peanut butters available at the super market are not very hydrogenated (about 20%) and are therefore still very unsaturated. Some peanut butter lovers have found a way to reduce the fat in peanut butter, and still enjoy the peanut taste. They buy natural peanut butter, with the oil separated on the top, and pour this off, removing much of the fat. Some find this too dry, but others find it satisfies their peanut craving.

The Cholesterol-Saturated Fat Index (CSI) and Calorie Content of Selected Foods (cont.)

Fats (1/4 cup or 4 tablespoons) con't.	CSI	Cal.
Very hydrogenated shortenings	27	530
Butter	37	430
Coconut oil, palm oil, cocoa butter (chocolate)	47	530

Frozen Desserts (1 cup)	CSI	Cal.
Water ices, sorbets	0	245
Sherbet, low-fat frozen yogurt	2	290
Ice milk	6	214
Ice cream, 10% fat	13	272
Rich ice cream, 16% fat	18	349
Specialty ice cream, 22% fat	34	684

Milk Products (1 cupt)	CSI	Cal.
Skim Milk, (0.1 %), skim-milk yogurt	1†	88
1% milk, buttermilk	2	115
2% milk, plain low-fat yogurt	4	144
Whole milk, (3.5% fat), whole-milk yogurt	7	159
Liquid nondairy creamers: Mocha Mix, Poly Rich	4	326
Liquid nondairy creamers: store brands, Cereal Blend, Coffee Rich	22	344
Sour cream	37	468
Imitation sour cream (IMO)	43	499

*Cheeses made with skim milk and vegetable oils.
†< = less than.

Source: Adapted from Sonja L. and William E. Connor, *The New American Diet*, Simon & Schuster, 1986.

Table 3.1 *The Cholesterol–Saturated Fat Index (CSI) is a numerical value which shows the relative effect of particular foods in raising blood cholesterol levels. It takes into account both the cholesterol and saturated fat in foods. The higher the number, the greater the cholesterol-raising effect. (The CSI is calculated by using the following formula: 1.01 x Saturated Fat (gm) + 0.05 x Cholesterol (mg) = CSI)*

Comparison of Cheeses

Cheese has become an integral part of the American diet. We put it on hamburgers, in sandwiches and casseroles, and sprinkle it on pasta dishes. It is probably the most common appetizer served with crackers at a cocktail party or dinner party. The unfortunate thing about cheese, however, is that most of our favorites are loaded with saturated fat and cholesterol. Ounce for ounce, they have a cholesterol-saturated fat index well above the fattiest red meat—a CSI of 26 for cheese vs. 18 for the highest fat red meats (See Table 3.I.) Just one ounce of these high-fat cheeses contains between 7 and 10 grams of fat, or about 2 teaspoons of fat. *Approximately 90% of their calories come from fat.*

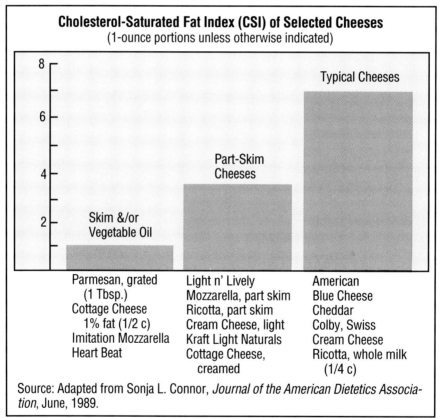

Cholesterol-Saturated Fat Index (CSI) of Selected Cheeses
(1-ounce portions unless otherwise indicated)

| Parmesan, grated (1 Tbsp.) Cottage Cheese 1% fat (1/2 c) Imitation Mozzarella Heart Beat | Light n' Lively Mozzarella, part skim Ricotta, part skim Cream Cheese, light Kraft Light Naturals Cottage Cheese, creamed | American Blue Cheese Cheddar Colby, Swiss Cream Cheese Ricotta, whole milk (1/4 c) |

Source: Adapted from Sonja L. Connor, *Journal of the American Dietetics Association*, June, 1989.

Figure 3.3 The Cholesterol-Saturated Fat Index (CSI) of selected cheeses.

There are several ways to reduce the fat intake from cheese. One way is to eat lower fat cheese. Refer to the list of lower fat cheeses in Figure 3.3. Some find these to be satisfactory substitutes, while others complain that they "miss the mark" for flavor. What works best for many is to find tasty *alternatives* to cheese and cracker appetizers. Some excellent choices are Hummous* or Tabouli* with plain toasted pita chips or low-fat crackers;

and Artichoke Relish* with pita chips or crackers. Seedless grapes and other fruits complement these appetizers nicely.

For casseroles or side dishes, grated Parmesan cheese is an excellent choice. It has a sharp, distinct flavor, so a little bit goes a long way. Using 1/4 cup in a casserole dish for a family of four amounts to just 1 tablespoon per person. One tablespoon has only 1.5 grams of fat—not much when compared to one ounce of the non-grated varieties (7 to 10 grams of fat). It is also very tasty sprinkled on pasta dishes.

Low-fat cottage cheese (1% milkfat) is another good choice, either eaten alone, or served with fruit or baked potatoes. It can also be mixed in a 1:1 ratio with a processed cheese spread to reduce the fat calories of the cheese spread by nearly one-half. The cheeses can be mixed by hand, or if a smooth mixture is preferred, in a food processor.

Comparison of Salad Dressings

A salad is not necessarily a low-fat food item. It can become a high-fat entree or side dish with the addition of salad dressings. This can be

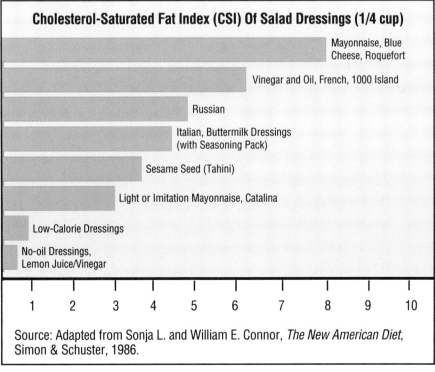

Cholesterol-Saturated Fat Index (CSI) Of Salad Dressings (1/4 cup)

Mayonnaise, Blue Cheese, Roquefort

Vinegar and Oil, French, 1000 Island

Russian

Italian, Buttermilk Dressings (with Seasoning Pack)

Sesame Seed (Tahini)

Light or Imitation Mayonnaise, Catalina

Low-Calorie Dressings

No-oil Dressings, Lemon Juice/Vinegar

1 2 3 4 5 6 7 8 9 10

Source: Adapted from Sonja L. and William E. Connor, *The New American Diet*, Simon & Schuster, 1986.

Figure 3.4 The Cholesterol-Saturated Fat Index (CSI) of selected salad dressings. The lower the CSI number the less cholesterol and saturated fat.

* Recipes appear in recipe section.

prevented either by using a smaller amount of dressing or by choosing a low-fat or nonfat variety.

The **quantity** of salad dressing can only be monitored if you add it yourself. Therefore, if you are eating out, be sure to ask for the dressing to be served on the side. Add just enough to lightly flavor the greens and vegetables. At a salad bar, be mindful that the small ladles usually hold about 2 tablespoons of dressing. This amounts to 150 or more calories if using the regular Blue Cheese, Italian or Thousand Island dressings.

In addition to being mindful of the quantity, it is just as important to be aware of the cholesterol-saturated fat content of dressings. The great differences in the CSI of the various salad dressings is due to the *amount* and *type* of fat in the dressings. The low-calorie commercial salad dressings generally have less than one-quarter of the fat and calories of the higher-fat varieties. The no-oil dressings have negligible fat content and often have fewer than 12 calories per 2-tablespoon serving. Read labels to make comparisons.

Low-fat salad dressings can also be made at home by using low-fat or nonfat mayonnaise, yogurt or sour cream bases. A comparison of the cholesterol-saturated fat index of some popular salad dressings is provided in Figure 3.4.

Step 2—How Much Fat Is Right for You:

Determining the Amount of Fat for Your Diet

To determine the specific amount of fat for your diet, you must first decide if your goal is to consume a diet of 20% or 30% of calories from fat. A diet of 20% of calories from fat is more optimum for most people, since there is a lower incidence of cancer, heart disease and obesity at this level. On the other hand, a diet of closer to 30% may be more practical for some. Less than 30% of calories from fat is still within the guidelines set by the American Cancer Society and the American Heart Association.

An important point to remember is that most preferences for certain types of food are acquired, and therefore it takes time to get used to different foods. Many people, after becoming accustomed to a lower fat diet, actually grow to prefer the lighter fare. They feel better and have lost the craving for many high fat foods.

Once you have decided on your goal, you need to determine your average daily calorie consumption. From this, you can figure how many grams or teaspoons of fat you should consume per day.

Estimate Daily Calorie Intake

Estimating how many calories you eat in a day can be done in one of two ways. First, you can refer to Table 3.2, which gives the average calorie consumption based on age and sex. You can adjust the number of calories higher or lower, depending on your size, your level of exercise, and your eating habits. Looking at the Table, if you are an average-size 30-year-old woman, you fall into the second category and probably consume about 2000 calories per day.

Average Daily Calorie Intake

	No. of Calories
Women (19 to 22 years)	2100
Women (23 to 50 years)	2000
Women (51 to 75 years)	1800
Men (19 to 22 years)	2900
Men (23 to 50 years)	2700
Men (51 to 75 years)	2400
Children (7 to 10 years)	2400
Girls (11 to 18 years)	2150
Boys (11 to 18 years)	2750

Table 3.2   U.S. RDA table showing average recommended calorie intakes for men, women,and children based on age. The usual calorie variation for maintaining weight at any age is ± 400 calories.

For a more accurate measure of your total calorie intake, keep an exact record of everything you eat and drink for three consecutive days (representative of your usual eating habits). Give this information to a dietitian, who can figure your average daily calorie consumption for you.

If you have access to a calorie chart, you can figure it yourself. You simply add up all the calories from the food and drinks you have recorded for the three day period, and divide this total by 3 to get the average number of calories you eat per day. Keep in mind that if you want to lose weight, you should set a goal of fewer calories than what you are now consuming.

Calculate Grams/Teaspoons of Fat per Day

After you know the approximate number of calories you eat in a day, you can determine how many grams or teaspoons of fat you should have to achieve a dietary goal of 20% or 30% of calories from fat. As an example, we will use a 2000-calorie diet, with 20% of the calories from fat. We will determine how many grams of fat we can have each day for this particular diet.

First, as shown in Figure 3.5, you calculate 20% of the total calories (2000) to get the total number of fat calories, which is 400. (.20 x 2000 = 400.) This first step tells you that if you consume 2000 calories a day, with 20% of the calories from fat, 400 of your total calories can come from fat.

Second, since there are 9 calories per gram of fat, you must divide the total fat calories (400) by 9 to get the grams of fat, which is 44 grams. (400 ÷ 9 = 44.) This means that approximately 44 *grams* of fat can be consumed each day on a 2000-calorie diet with 20% of the calories from fat.

For a diet of 30% fat, substitute .30 for .20 (2000 x .30 = 600 fat calories). Do the remaining calculations the same. (600 fat calories ÷ 9 cal./gm. = 66.6 grams of fat per day.)

Sample Calculation of Daily Fat Intake
(for 2000 calories/day with 20% of calories from fat)

Total Calories	x	Percentage of Fat	=	Total Fat Calories
2000	x	.20	=	400 Fat Calories
Fat Calories	÷	9(cal./gram)	=	Total Grams of Fat
400	÷	9	=	44 Grams of Fat

Figure 3.5 The calculations to determine the daily allowance of fat calories and grams of fat for a 2000 calorie diet with 20% of calories from fat.

The fat content of foods is also expressed in teaspoons of fat. Since one teaspoon of fat is equal to approximately five grams of fat, you simply divide the grams of fat by 5 to derive teaspoons of fat. For example, 44 grams of fat ÷ 5 equals 8.8 teaspoons of fat.

Converting Grams of Fat to Teaspoons of Fat

Grams of Fat	÷	5(grams fat/teas.)	=	Total Teas. of Fat
44	÷	5	=	8.8 Teas. of Fat

For those who shy away from mathematical calculations, Table 3.3 does the work for you. It gives the number of grams of fat per day you can consume depending on your total calorie intake (from 1200 to 3400 calories), and whether you prefer a 20% or a 30% fat diet.

To use the chart, first determine the approximate number of calories you consume per day. Next, look in either of the two columns to the right to find the grams of fat for a 20% or a 30% fat diet. Using 2000 calories as an example, you see that you can consume 44 grams of fat per day in a 20% fat diet, and 67 grams of fat in a 30% fat diet.

Step 3—Counting Grams/Teaspoons of Fat In Foods

As you may have guessed, knowing the approximate amount of fat (in teaspoons or grams) to include in your diet is useless, unless you also know the amount of fat in the foods you eat. For example, if you have decided to set a target of 36 grams of fat for your diet, you need to know what foods constitute that amount of fat.

Recommended Fat Consumption Based On Daily Caloric Intake		
Total Calories	Grams of Fat/Day Fat=20% of Calories Grams	Grams of Fat/Day Fat=30% of Calories Grams
1200	27	40
1400	31	47
1600	36	53
1800	40	60
2000	44	67
2200	49	73
2400	53	80
2600	58	87
2800	62	93
3000	67	100
3200	71	107
3400	76	113

Table 3.3 Grams of fat per day in diets of 20% and 30% of calories from fat, based on daily caloric intakes of 1200 to 3400 calories.

This is not as difficult as it seems. The grams of fat per serving are listed on many food labels, and are included with recipes in some cookbooks. By reading labels and also becoming familiar with the grams of fat in many basic foods, you can closely estimate the quantity of fat in the foods you eat and in the recipes you prepare. In a short period of time, you will become accustomed to what you can eat and what you should avoid in order to stay within your limit. Counting grams of fat will no longer be necessary.

The fat content of many of our most commonly eaten foods is listed in Table 3.4. As you can see from this, almost all fruits and vegetables without added sauces and most breads have little or no fat.

Comparing the grams of fat in various types and cuts of meats, trimmed and untrimmed, shows the wide differences in their fat content. The white meat of turkey and chicken are by far the lowest and the highest are the untrimmed red meats, especially ribs.

Dairy products also have great variations in fat content. Skim milk has all the calcium and protein of the higher fat milk, but without most of the fat. It's fairly easy to get used to, if you do it gradually—from whole milk, to 2% milk, to 1% milk and then to skim. If you can't get accustomed to skim, 1% or 2% is preferable to whole milk. Ice milk, frozen yogurt, sherbet and nonfat ice cream are good substitutes for regular ice cream. Different brands vary in fat content and flavor. Shop around until you find the one(s) that best suit your family's preferences. If you crave the creamy taste of ice cream but prefer less fat, try the ice creams made with the fat substitute "Simpless," which taste creamy, but contain almost no fat.

Fat Content of Selected Foods

Fruits and Vegetables	Fat(g)	Cal.
Fruits and Vegetables, canned, frozen, or fresh, with no added sauces (except avocado)	0.1	50-100
Breads		
Wheat, Raisin, Rye, White, Pumpernickel, etc. (1 slice)	1.0	50-80
Poultry (per 3 oz. cooked, 4 oz. uncooked)		
Turkey, light, without skin	2.7	135
Turkey, dark, without skin	6.2	160
Chicken, light, without skin	3.3	127
Chicken, dark, without skin	7.1	150
Duck, without skin	9.6	172
Ground Turkey, commercial	10.5	183
Chicken Hot Dog (2 oz.)	8.8	116
Beef (per 3 oz. cooked, 4 oz. uncooked)		
Top Round, trimmed,* braised	4.9	176
Eye of Round, trimmed, choice, roasted	5.7	156
Round Tip, trimmed, roasted	5.4	153
Top Sirloin, trimmed, broiled	6.6	170
Tenderloin (filet mignon), broiled	8.6	180
Beef Chuck Pot Roast, trimmed, braised	8.8	199
Rib Eye, trimmed, choice, broiled	9.9	191
Rib Eye, untrimmed, choice, broiled	17.7	250
T-Bone Steak, trimmed, choice, broiled	8.8	182
T-Bone Steak, untrimmed, choice, broiled	20.9	276
Ground Beef, lean, broiled	16.2	234
Beef Ribs, untrimmed, braised	35.7	400
Beef Bologna (1 oz.)	6.6	72
Hot Dog, Beef (2 oz.)	16.3	180
Veal (per 3 oz. cooked, 4 oz. uncooked)		
Veal Cutlet, trimmed, braised	4.3	172
Veal Loin Chop, trimmed, roasted	5.9	149
Veal Sirloin, untrimmed, braised	11.2	214
Veal Sirloin Chop, trimmed, braised	5.5	173
Veal Rib Roast, trimmed, choice	6.3	151
Lamb (per 3 oz. cooked, 4 oz. uncooked)		
Leg of Lamb, trimmed	6.6	162
Leg of Lamb, untrimmed	14.0	219
Lamb Loin Chop, trimmed, choice, broiled	8.2	183
Pork (3 oz. cooked, 4 oz. uncooked)		
Pork Tenderloin, trimmed	4.1	141
Center Loin Chop, trimmed, broiled	8.9	196
Center Loin Chop, untrimmed, pan-fried	25.9	318
Ham, boneless, regular (11% fat)	7.7	151
Ham, boneless, lean (5% fat)	4.7	123
Bacon, 3 slices	9.4	109
Pork Sausage (2 oz.)	16.2	184

*Trimmed indicates that all visible fat has been removed.
All meats are prepared with no extra fat.

Fat Content of Selected Foods

Seafood (3 oz. cooked w/no extra fat)	Fat(g)	Cal.
Flounder and Sole	1.3	99
Orange Roughy	6.0	107
Perch, Ocean	1.8	103
Salmon, Pink	5.1	118
Salmon, Sockeye or Red	9.3	183
Swordfish	4.4	132
Clams	1.7	126
Scallops	0.8	88
Shrimp	0.9	84
Dairy Products		
Cheese (1 oz.)*	8-10.0	105
Parmesan Cheese (1 tbsp.)	1.5	23
Cottage Cheese, regular (1/2 cup)	5.1	117
Cottage Cheese, 1% fat (1/2 cup)	1.2	82
Mozzarella, park skim (1 oz.)	4.5	72
Heavy Cream (2 tbsp.)	11.2	104
Sour Cream (2 tbsp.)	5.0	52
Milk, whole (1 cup)	8.2	150
Milk, 2% fat	4.7	121
Milk, 1% fat	2.4	104
Milk, skim	0.4	86
Buttermilk (1 cup)	2.2	99
Eggnog (1 cup)	19.0	342
Ice Cream, 10% fat (1 cup)	14.3	269
Ice Cream, rich, 16% fat (1 cup)	23.7	349
Ice Milk, hard (1 cup)	5.6	184
Sherbet (1 cup)	3.8	270
Fats, Oils		
Butter, Cooking Oils (1 tsp.)	4-5	40
Whipped Margarine (1 tsp.)	2.5-3	23-27
Mayonnaise (1 tbsp.)	10	100
Light Mayonnaise (1 tbsp.)	5	50
Salad Dressings, regular (2 tbsp.)	12-18	140-170
Salad Dressings, low-cal. (2 tbsp.)	2-5	30-50
Desserts		
Brownies (2" square)	6-8	150-170
Cookies, homemade (4 cookies)	10	180
Fruit Pies, homemade (1/8 pie)	12-14	280-300
Pecan Pie, homemade (1/8 pie)	23	431
Cake (from mix): Chocolate, White, Yellow (1/12 cake)	10-12	250-300
Muffins, homemade or from mix	3-4	100-120

*Includes Provolone, Swiss, Cheddar, American, Roquefort, Brie, etc.

Source: U.S. Dept. of Agriculture Handbooks No. 8-5, 8-10, 8-13, 8-15, 8-17, and Bowes and Church's *Food Values of Portions Commonly Used*, 15th Edition, revised by Jean A.T. Pennington, Harper & Row, New York, 1989.

Table 3.4 Fat and calorie content of selected foods.

Other healthy desserts are fruits or low-fat baked goods, such as those that appear in the dessert section of this book. Favorite high-fat pies and cakes are best avoided or reserved for special occasions.

Fat Content in Fast Foods

Since fast foods play such an important part in the typical American diet, it is important to be aware of the amount of fat in these foods. It is a rare family indeed that doesn't make an occasional stop at McDonald's, Hardee's, Burger King, Taco Bell, etc. Table 3.5 lists the fat content of a sampling of foods available at several fast food restaurants.

Fat Content in Selected Foods from Fast Food Restaurants

McDonalds	Fat(g)	Calories
Regular Hamburger	9	255
Big Mac	26	500
Filet of Fish	18	370
Quarter Pounder with Cheese	28	510
Grilled Chicken Breast Sand.	4	252
Chunky Chicken Salad	4	150
French Fries (medium)	17	320
Apple Pie	15	260
Strawberry Low-fat Shake	1	320
Kentucky Fried Chicken		
Original Recipe (breast)	15	283
Extra Crispy (drum & thigh)	44	610
Cole Slaw (one serving)	7	119
Mashed Potatoes with gravy	2	71
Burger King		
Whopper	36	614
Whopper, Double	53	844
Hamburger	11	272
BK Broiler Chicken Sand.	8	267
Saus. Egg, Cheese Crossanwich	40	534
Taco Bell		
Bean Burrito with red sauce	14	447
Beef Burrito with red sauce	21	493
Taco, hard shell, beef	11	183
Soft Taco, Chicken	10	213
Taco Salad, without shell	31	484
Domino's Pizza (16", 2 slices)		
Cheese Pizza	10	376
Pepperoni Pizza	17	460
Deluxe Pizza	20	498

Source: Michael F. Jacobson and Sarah Fritschner, *The Completely Revised and Updated Fast Food Guide*, 2nd Edition, Workman Publishing, New York, 1991.

Table 3.5 Fat and calorie content of selected foods from fast food restaurants.

Many of the foods from fast food restaurants are high in fat. However, this does not mean that these restaurants should be avoided entirely. There are wide variations in the fat content of foods that each restaurant serves. One simply has to learn which ones are the lowest in fat and order these when eating out. (Several fast food restaurants have nutrition information available upon request for all the foods they serve.) Some of the best meat choices are the regular hamburgers, grilled chicken breast sandwiches, and chicken taco. Chunky Chicken Salad (from McDonald's), is low in fat, whereas the Taco Salad (from Taco Bell) is high, so do not assume salads are always low-fat. The strawberry shake from McDonald's is made with ice milk so the grams of fat are not as high as one might expect—a good choice for an occasional treat for a child (or an adult who is not calorie conscious) because of the calcium content. A soft drink, however, would have no fat and fewer calories, so may be preferable if watching fat and calories very closely. (See Appendix A for more complete nutrition information on a wide variety of foods served at fast food restaurants.)

High Fat Dinners Are Not Limited to Fast Foods

High-fat meals are not limited to fast food restaurants. Let's analyze a menu from a typical steakhouse meal to demonstrate this point. (See Figure 3.6.) The menu includes the following:

T-Bone Steak, 10 ounces, trimmed
Baked Potato with Butter and Sour Cream
Tossed Green Salad with Italian Dressing
Hot Roll with Butter
Coffee with Cream
Cheesecake

The grams of fat are listed to show the amount of fat in each food item. As you can see, this one meal contains over 1700 calories, and 61% of the calories come from fat. Furthermore, the majority of the fat comes from foods high in saturated fat.

The menu can be altered to bring the fat content down to a much healthier 27% of calories. (See Figure 3.7.) It is important to keep in mind that this meal is a typical evening meal, including more meat and thus probably more fat than the other two meals of the day. Therefore, the *percentage* of fat calories for the *day* could be less, provided low-fat food selections were made at breakfast and lunch. Four ounces of meat per day is more than adequate to supply protein needs.

A low-fat salad dressing was used to keep the fat calories down. The margarine allotted for the bread (1/2 teaspoon) and baked potato

(1 teaspoon) is limited, but should be adequate. Nonfat sour cream was added to the potato to provide additional flavor without increasing the fat.

Fat Content of Typical Steak Dinner			
Food	Serving Size	Fat (g)	Calories
T-bone steak	10 oz	50	769
Baked potato	1 large	0	145
Butter	2 tsp	8	72
Sour cream	2 tbsp	5	52
Tossed green salad	2 cups	0	20
Italian dressing	3 tbsp	27	252
Dinner roll	1	2	80
Butter	1 tsp	4	36
Coffee	1 cup	0	0
Cream	1 tbsp	5	44
Cheesecake	1 piece	16	257
Totals		117 g.	1727 cal.

Figure 3.6 The fat and calorie content of a typical steak dinner. Most of the total calories (61%) come from fat.

Fat Content of Adjusted Steak Dinner			
Food	Serving Size	Fat (g)	Calories
Beef tenderloin	4 oz	11	233
Baked potato	1 large	0	145
Margarine	1 tsp	4	36
Nonfat sour cream	2 tbsp	0	20
Carrots, steamed	1/2 cup	0	35
Zucchini, steamed	1/2 cup	0	14
Tossed green salad	2 cups	0	20
Low-fat dressing	2 tbsp	2	40
Whole wheat bread	1 slice	1	70
Margarine	1/2 tsp	2	18
Coffee	1 cup	0	0
Sugar	1 tsp	0	15
Totals		20 g.	646 cal.

Figure 3.7 Fat and calorie content of lower-fat steak dinner. The percentage of calories from fat was reduced from 61% to 28%.

Tips for Reducing the Fat In Your Diet

Now that you know the sources of fat and cholesterol, and how much fat you should consume in a diet with 20% or 30% of calories from fat, you are ready to begin cutting down. The best and easiest way to begin is simple substitution. Figure 3.8 lists suggested lower fat/lower cholesterol substitutions.

Suggested Substitutions

Instead of . . .	Serving Size	Fat(g)	Use . . .	Serving Size	Fat(g)
Sour cream	1 cup	48	Plain yogurt (low-fat)	1 cup	4
Butter*	1 tbsp.	12	Margarine	1 tbsp.	12
1 Whole Egg	1 egg	6	2 Egg Whites or 1 Egg Substitute	2 whites	1
2 Whole Eggs	2 eggs	12	3 Egg Whites or 2 Egg Substitutes	3 whites	1
Milk, Whole	1 cup	8	Milk, 2%	1 cup	5
Milk, 1%	1 cup	1	Milk, Skim	1 cup	0
Evaporated Milk (canned)	1 cup	17	Evaporated Skim Milk (canned)	1 cup	1
Whipped Cream (over fruit, desserts)	1/4 cup	5	Vanilla Yogurt (low-fat)	1/4 cup	1
Ice Cream	1/2 cup	7	Ice Milk, 1% fat	1/2 cup	2
Yogurt, plain (whole milk)	1 cup	7	Yogurt, plain (skim milk)	1 cup	1
Cream (in coffee)	1 tbsp.	2	Skim Milk, Powdered Milk,	1 tbsp.	0
Cinnamon Danish	1.3 oz. (1)	9	Raisin & Honey Bagel	1 bagel	1
Croissant	1 oz. (1)	6	Whole Wheat Bread	2 slices	2
Cr. of Mushroom Soup (Campbell's)	10 oz. prepared	11	Minestrone Soup (Campbell's)	10 oz. prepared	2
Bologna	1 oz.	7	Ham slice, 5% fat	1 oz.	1
Italian Dressing	2 tbsp.	16	Italian Dressing, (reduced calorie)	2 tbsp.	0
Mayonnaise	1 tbsp.	11	Light Mayonnaise (Kraft)	1 tbsp.	5
Tuna, in oil, drained	3 oz.	10	Tuna, in water, drained	3 oz.	1
Butter or Margarine (on potatoes or vegetables)	1 tsp.	4	*Butter Buds* or *Molly McButter* (powdered)	1/2 tsp.	0

*The grams of fat are the same for butter and margarine, but margarine is far less saturated (19%) than butter (66%). Tub margarine is less saturated than stick margarine.

Figure 3.8 Suggested substitutions to reduce fat and cholesterol in your diet. The grams of fat in each food item are given to show you the fat savings that result from the substitutions.

Sample Daily Menu—Fat Limited to 20% of Total Calories

It's not difficult to follow a diet in which only 20% of the calories come from fat. To demonstrate this, let's examine a sample day's menu of about 1600 calories. Refer to Figure 3.9. The total fat must be limited to 36 grams to stay at 20% of the calories. The fat content of foods is shown in grams.

Breakfast	Fat(grams)	Calories
6 oz. orange juice	0	75
1/2 cup Shredded Wheat n' Bran	1	90
1/2 cup skim milk	0	5
1 1/2 Tbsp. raisins	0	40
Whole wheat toast (2 slices)	2	120
1 teaspoon margarine (1/2 t./slice)	5	35
Total Breakfast	**8 grams**	**405 calories**
Snack		
1 apple	0	80
Lunch		
Minestrone Soup (1 cup)	2	226
Ham Sandwich		
Lettuce leaf	0	0
Tomato slice	0	8
Ham (1 slice)	1	25
Mustard	0	5
2 slices whole wheat bread	2	120
Skim Milk (8 oz.)	0	90
Total Lunch	**5 grams**	**474 calories**
Snack		
Rye Crispbread (2 crackers 2 1/2" X 4 1/2")	0	50
Dinner		
Beef Tenderloin (4 oz.)	12	220
Baked potato (1 large)	0	140
Margarine, whipped (1 teas.)	4	35
Carrots, steamed (1/2 cup)	0	25
Green beans, steamed (1/2 cup)	0	25
Mixed green salad (1 cup)	0	0
French dressing, reduced cal. (2 Tbsp.)	2	40
Coffee (1 cup) w/ skim milk (2 tbsp.)	0	11
Fresh strawberries (1 cup) mixed w/	1	55
1/4 cup low-fat strawberry yogurt	1	58
Total Dinner	**20 grams**	**609 calories**
DAILY TOTALS	**33 grams**	**1618 calories**

Figure 3.9 A daily meal plan in which fat is limited to 20% of total calories.

The total fat consumed for the day was 33 grams. That's within the desired goal of 36 grams of fat, or 20% of the total calories. An example showing 30% of calories in fat will not be shown since it is very easy to increase the fat intake. For 1600 calories, fat consumption must be less than 53 grams per day to stay within 30% of total calories.

This sample daily menu, where fat intake is kept to just 20% of total calories, demonstrates several things:

1) Greater quantities of food can be eaten when fat is kept to a minimum. This sample menu includes three fairly large meals and two snacks, but contains just 1600 total calories. The quantity of food would be significantly greater for 2000 to 3000 calories, which is what most men consume daily.

2) It is important to choose lower fat food items in order to keep the fat allowance within the limits—for example, choosing skim milk (0 grams fat), instead of whole milk (8 grams fat/cup); and choosing a broth-based soup, such as minestrone (2 grams fat/cup) instead of a cream-based soup, such as cream of mushroom soup (11 grams fat/cup). Whole milk (1 7/8 cup) would have added 14 grams of fat and the cream of mushroom soup would have added 9 grams of fat. Just these two changes would have increased the fat content by 23 grams, or almost 5 teaspoons of additional fat. Even 2% milk (1 7/8 cups) would have added 8.5 grams of fat.

3) It is essential to *avoid very high fat foods*. For example, McDonalds "Big Mac" contains 32.4 grams of fat, a doughnut contains 10 grams of fat, and a medium order of French fries contains 17 grams of fat. These three items alone would bring you well over the fat limit on a 1600-calorie diet. The main point is to avoid the highest fat items entirely and choose the lower fat foods, whether you are eating at home or in a restaurant. Also, if you choose a moderately high-fat item at one meal, be especially careful the rest of the day to choose low-fat or nonfat foods.

Guidelines for Limiting Fat to 20% of Total Calories
Breakfast and Lunch

Limit breakfast and lunch to about 2 teaspoons (10 grams) of fat per meal, unless total calories are *much* higher than 1600 calories. In that case, eat low-fat foods, but increase the quantity. For example, eat two lower fat sandwiches or 2 cups of broth-based soup, rather than one thick hamburger or one cup of a cream-based soup. There is a great variety of breakfasts and lunches that remain within these limits. Some examples are shown in Figures 3.10 and 3.11.

Sample Low-Fat Breakfasts

Breakfast I	Grams of Fat
Pancakes (3)	6
1 teaspoon whipped margarine	3
Syrup (2 T.)	0
Orange juice (6 oz.)	0
Skim Milk (8 oz.)	0
Total	9 grams fat

Breakfast II	
Egg Substitutes (2 Eggbeaters)	0
Fried in 1 teas. whipped margarine	3
Toast (2 pieces)	2
With 1 teas. whipped margarine	3
Cantaloupe (1/4 cantaloupe)	0
Coffee (1 cup)	0
Total	8 grams fat

Breakfast III	
2 Whole bagels	2
With 2 teas. light cream cheese	2
Cantaloupe (1/2 cantaloupe)	0
Coffee (1 cup)	0
Total	4 grams fat

Figure 3.10 Three sample breakfasts where fat is limited to 10 grams or less per meal.

Sample Low-Fat Lunches

Lunch I	
McDonald's Regular Hamburger	9
Apple	0
Tossed Green Salad	0
With No-oil dressing	0
Skim milk or coffee	0
Total	9 grams fat

Lunch II	
Minestrone Soup (1 cup)	2
Turkey or Ham Sandwich	
1 slice lean ham or turkey	1
Whole wheat bread (2 slices)	2
Mustard (1 teas.)	0
Orange (1)	0
Skim milk or coffee	0
Total	5 grams fat

Figure 3.11 Two sample lunches where fat is limited to 10 grams or less per meal.

Guidelines—Dinner

1) Determine your remaining fat allowance after subtracting the fat consumed during breakfast and lunch. Plan the dinner meal accordingly. If you are cooking for a family, try to limit the fat for the dinner meal to no more than 30% of total calories. This would be approximately 20 grams of fat for a 600-calorie meal. See sample daily menu, Figure 3.9.

2) Use a low-calorie salad dressing with salads, and *Butter Buds* or another nonfat butter substitute on potatoes (instead of margarine), if this is necessary to keep fat allowance within the limit. It may not be necessary if the other foods served at the meal are low in fat.

3) Steam or microwave vegetables and serve without adding butter or high-fat sauces. Instead, sprinkle with herbs, dry *Butter Buds*, or *Molly McButter*. The butter substitutes provide the natural butter flavor without the added calories. When sprinkled over hot, steaming vegetables, including potatoes, these products appear to melt as butter.

4) Eat breads dry or with a thin scraping of soft spread tub margarine. (It is less saturated than stick margarine.) Measure the amount you use (1/4 teaspoon to 1 teaspoon) to accurately calculate it into your total daily fat intake.

5) Avoid high-fat casseroles. Keep in mind when preparing casseroles for a family of 4, that for every 2 tablespoons of fat (including cooking oils, butter and margarine) you add, you are adding 1 1/2 teaspoons of fat per person. If serving only two, you would be adding 3 teaspoons (15 grams) of fat per person.

6) Fat used in cooking is not limited to just cooking oils, butter and margarine. It is also present in concentrated amounts in cheese, sour cream, mayonnaise, Half & Half, cream, whole milk, cream-based soups and most salad dressings. Limit use of these foods or substitute with low-fat varieties. Read labels to be aware of the fat you are adding when using these foods.

7) Use low-fat sauces or nonfat gravy with meats or fish. See sauce recipes in book. For instructions on how to make a nonfat gravy, see recipe for Turkey Gravy, p. 262.

8) Whenever possible, serve fruits for dessert. They contain almost no fat, are low in calories (compared to cakes and pies), and are loaded with nutrients and fiber.

9) Begin to think of meat as a condiment at meals instead of the main food to fill up on. Limit meat portions to about 4 ounces, and fish portions to 6 ounces per day. Four ounces of meat is roughly equivalent to the size of a deck of cards. For chicken, a single chicken breast is about 4 ounces, and a leg and thigh together equal about 4 ounces. A list of lower fat meat choices is provided in Table 3.6.

Choose These Meats to Reduce Fat and Cholesterol

The meats listed below are good choices (some better than others) when you are limiting fat and cholesterol in your diet. Under each category of beef, pork and poultry, the cuts are listed in ascending order according to fat content, i.e. the lowest fat cuts are listed first. All the figures shown are for 3-ounce cooked servings (4 ounces uncooked), with all visible fat removed. None of the meats was prepared with added fat. (During cooking, meats lose approximately 25% of their weight, mostly in water and fat.)

Name of Cut	Cal.	Fat	Sat. Fat	Chol.
Beef (Choice grade)*				
Top Round Steak, braised	176	4.9	1.7	76
Round Tip, roasted	153	5.4	1.9	69
Eye of Round, roasted	156	5.7	2.0	59
Top Sirloin, broiled	170	6.6	2.6	76
Bottom Round, roasted	164	6.6	2.2	66
Chuck Arm Pot Roast, braised	187	7.4	2.7	86
Tenderloin, broiled	180	8.6	3.2	71
Flank Steak, broiled	176	8.6	3.7	57
Pork				
Tenderloin, roasted	141	4.1	1.4	79
Ham, canned, (4% fat)	116	4.1	1.4	35
Ham, canned, (5% fat)	123	4.7	1.5	45
Center Loin Chop, broiled	196	8.9	3.1	83
Poultry (roasted)				
Turkey, light meat, no skin	135	2.7	0.9	59
Chicken breast, no skin	127	3.3	0.9	62
Chicken, 2 drumsticks, no skn	152	5.0	1.3	82
Turkey, dark meat, no skin	160	6.2	2.1	73

*The three grades of beef (based on fat content) are prime, choice and select. Prime is the highest in fat, followed by choice and then select.

Source: U.S. Dept. of Agriculture Handbooks No. 8-5, 8-10, and 8-13.
Adapted From: *Mayo Clinic Nutrition Letter*, November 1988.

Table 3.6 Calories, total fat, saturated fat and cholesterol content of selected lower fat meats.

Summary of Tips for Reducing Dietary Fat

• Incorporate more beans into your diet in place of meat as a protein source. For example, when making chili, use less meat and more beans, or totally eliminate the meat and use just beans. (See recipe, Vegetarian Chili, page 305.) Beans are an excellent low-fat protein source, and provide generous amounts of fiber and iron.

• Instead of red meats, use more poultry and fish in the main meal. Limit portions of meat to about 4 ounces per day, and fish portions to about 6 ounces per day.

- Use turkey breast in recipes calling for beef or veal. Raw turkey breast can be sliced thin and used in recipes calling for veal cutlets. It can also be ground and made into meatballs, burgers, etc., preferably after the skin and visible fat have been removed. You can grind it yourself in a food processor, or take it to your butcher to be ground.
- Buy canned fish packed in water rather than oil. If not available, drain oil well.
- Use only lean meats and trim all visible fat before cooking. Roast meat on a rack so that fat can drip off and be discarded.
- Remove skin from poultry before eating. (You can leave it on while baking or roasting to retain moisture. This will not increase fat content because fat does not migrate inward.) If seasonings or sauces, such as barbecue sauce, are used during baking or roasting, remove the skin before cooking, so that the sauce or seasoning flavor is not lost when the skin is removed.
- When browning meat, especially ground meat, spoon off excess fat before adding other ingredients. Blot cooked patties with a paper towel.
- Before making gravy, refrigerate meat drippings so that chilled and hardened fat can be removed from the top and discarded. If time does not permit refrigeration, pour drippings into a tall glass and remove liquid fat from the top with a spoon. Discard the fat. Make nonfat gravy from the remaining juices, following directions for Turkey Gravy, page 262.
- When making tuna or chicken salad, replace the mayonnaise with nonfat mayonnaise, "light" mayonnaise and/or nonfat yogurt. Begin with half "light" mayonnaise and half nonfat mayonnaise and cut the fat further, i.e. increase the proportion of nonfat mayonnaise, if taste permits. Do the same when making potato salads or other mayonnaise-based dishes. Many have found that tuna salad tastes great using no mayonnaise—just nonfat yogurt, pickle relish, and chopped onions with the tuna.
- When selecting frozen dinners or entrees at the supermarket, look for ones with fewer than 10 grams of fat per dinner. These are likely to derive less than 30% of their calories from fat. Supplement these dinners with bread and fresh fruit or fruit salad.
- When opening canned soups, skim fat from the top if it is visible. If making your own soup or stew, do the same.
- Reduce oil (butter, margarine or shortening) in recipes by 25% to 50%. Start with 25% less and reduce it further if taste and texture permit.
- Make hot fruit sauces with no oil. Thicken by adding cornstarch to cool fruit juice mixture. It will thicken when sauce comes to a boil. Fruit sauces are delicious with desserts or served over meat or fish.

- If possible, use non-stick pans for baking. This usually eliminates the need to grease the pan. However, if you still experience some sticking, use a vegetable cooking spray. A small amount prevents sticking more effectively than other oils or shortening.
- When sautéing vegetables, use a non-stick pan, with a small amount of water or vegetable spray. If sticking occurs, add water and steam until water is gone. Watch carefully because water evaporates quickly and burning can occur. The water prevents the vegetables from sticking or burning. When browning meats in non-stick pans, it is usually not necessary to add grease or water.
- Use vegetarian baked beans with no added fat, rather than regular baked beans (with pork). There are several different brands available at most grocery stores.
- Instead of topping baked potato with sour cream, use nonfat sour cream, low-fat yogurt or cottage cheese.
- Use reduced-calorie or fat free salad dressings instead of regular salad dressings. Many of the reduced-calorie and fat free dressings have less than two grams of fat per 2-tablespoon serving, while the regular dressings have from 12 to 18 grams of fat per 2-tablespoon serving.
- In fruit salads, such as Waldorf salad (recipe, page 216), or over fresh fruit, use low-fat vanilla or fruit flavored yogurt rather than mayonnaise or whipping cream.
- Check grams of fat on cereal boxes. Some of those thought to be "healthy," such as granola cereals, are high in both sugar and fat compared to other cereals.
- Make crustless fruit pies for dessert. Most of the fat in fruit pies is in the crust. If served a pie with crust, you can reduce fat calories by not eating the crust.
- Use unsweetened cocoa powder instead of baking chocolate in recipes, since it is *much* lower in fat, especially saturated fat. Baking chocolate is loaded with cocoa butter, one of the highly saturated fats.
- Reduce the fat in cheese spreads by mixing the spread 1:1 with low-fat cottage cheese (1% fat) in a food processor. It will reduce the grams of fat by nearly one-half.

4

Sodium And Other Factors Affecting Blood Pressure

No one is born with a craving for salt. Babies respond no differently to salted or unsalted foods, although they do show a definite preference for sweetened foods. Our love of salt is an *acquired* taste. By eating foods with added salt, we grow to expect the salty taste in foods. That is why when we try to restrict salt, food tastes bland and unappetizing—at least at first.

Does Everyone Need to Restrict Salt?

There is not universal agreement on whether everyone should restrict salt because research has shown that only about half the population is salt sensitive, i.e. their blood pressure is affected by the amount of salt in their diet. Nevertheless, restricting salt is still recommended by many physicians and most government advisory committees for *both* the prevention and treatment of high blood pressure. As explained in Chapter I, population studies show that if sodium intake (one of the components of salt) is low enough (less than 2000 milligrams per day), hypertension (high blood pressure) rarely develops. On the other hand, in countries with very high consumption of sodium, such as Japan, about 60% of the population develops the disease. It makes sense to limit sodium to reduce the risk of hypertension, especially if this condition runs in your family.

Keep in mind, though, that sodium intake must be kept at a very low level (below 2000 milligrams per day) to inhibit the development of hypertension. Restricting it to a lesser degree will not necessarily reduce the risk of developing hypertension, but for those who are salt sensitive, it should minimize the rise in blood pressure.

If you have high blood pressure, salt restriction is especially important. Sometimes, reducing salt can eliminate the need for medication, particularly for those whose blood pressure is only slightly elevated. Cutting sodium by 50% results in an average drop of 5 millimeters of mercury (mm Hg) for systolic pressure (top number) and 4 mm Hg for diastolic pressure (bottom number). For example, a blood pressure of 140/90 would drop, on the average, to 135/86. If diet changes are not sufficient and drugs are still needed, limiting sodium can reduce the amount of medication needed. Also, certain medications work more effectively with fewer negative side effects when sodium is restricted.

If you do not have high blood pressure and choose not to limit sodium in your diet, be sure to have your blood pressure checked annually. This way, if hypertension develops, you can be treated with diet or drugs before major harm is done to your heart and blood vessels. (See Chapter 8 for additional information on medical tests for high blood pressure, normal blood pressure ranges, etc.)

Other Factors that Play a Role

Other factors that help lower blood pressure are losing weight (if overweight), regular aerobic exercise, and avoiding excessive use of alcohol (no more than two drinks per day). Increasing potassium and calcium in the diet also appears to have a positive effect on blood pressure in some individuals.

Potassium's Role

A diet rich in potassium has shown some promise in helping to reduce hypertension. A number of studies has shown that doubling potassium intake from foods, while sodium is kept constant, resulted in an average decrease in diastolic blood pressure (bottom number) of 3 to 5 mm Hg. (This is about the same as the average drop in blood pressure that results from restricting sodium by 50%.) In other words, if your blood pressure is 140/90, which is the upper limit of normal, you may be able to bring it down to 140/85 by eating enough foods high in potassium.

The amount of potassium that brought about this reduction was 4000 to 5000 milligrams per day, or about twice the average American intake of 2500 milligrams per day. See Table 4.1 for a list of potassium-rich foods. Try to incorporate more of these foods into your diet, especially the low-fat, high-fiber fruits, vegetables and beans. If done in combination with weight loss and restricting sodium, the drop in blood pressure could be even greater.

Adding supplements of potassium do not appear to be beneficial, and could result in an overdose, so this is *not* recommended. A study, reported in *The New England Journal of Medicine*, has shown that adding a potassium supplement (potassium chloride) to a low-salt diet had no effect on the blood pressures of those in the study group. Although these studies are not conclusive, adding potassium-rich foods is highly recommended as part of an overall healthy diet.

Choose Potassium-Rich Foods

	Potassium (mg)		Potassium (mg)
Beans (cooked, 1 cup)		**Meat, Fish, Poultry (3 oz)**	
Grt. Northern Beans	919	Beef, average, lean	317
Navy Beans	755	Pork, average, lean	300
Baked Beans	907	Haddock	296
Red Kidney Beans	658	Snapper	355
Lentils	731	Scallops (6 scallops)	428
Split Peas	710	Salmon, Sockeye	332
Fruits & Fruit Juices		Rainbow Trout	539
Apricots, fresh (3)	313	**Vegetables, (cooked)**	
Apricot Nectar (1 c)	214	Lima Beans (1/2 c)	476
Avocado, 1/2	651	Broccoli (1 stalk)	286
Banana (1 banana)	451	Carrot (1 carrot)	233
Dates, pitted (10)	541	Cauliflower (1/2 c)	200
Fruit Cocktail (1 c)	230	Collards (1/2 c)	214
Grapefruit Juice (6 oz)	300	Potato (1 potato)	844
Grape Juice (6 oz)	250	Pumpkin, canned (1/2 c)	251
Cantaloupe (1/2)	682	Spinach, raw (1 c)	312
Honeydew (1/4)	935	Spinach, frozen (1/2 c)	283
Orange	250	Sweet Potato (1)	397
Pear (1 pear)	208	Tomato (1)	254
Pineapple Juice (6 oz)	255	Tomato Juice (6 oz)	376
Prunes (5 large)	313	Mixed Vegetables (1/2 c)	248
Dairy Products		Brussels Sprouts (1/2 c)	247
Buttermilk (1 c)	371	Squash, Acorn (1/2 c)	446
Skim Milk (1 c)	406	Rutabaga (1/2 c)	244
Yogurt (1 c)	531	Zucchini (1/2 c)	228

Source: Bowes and Church's *Food Values of Portions Commonly Used*, 15th Edition, revised by Jean A.T. Pennington, Harper & Row, New York, 1989.

Table 4.1 The potassium content of selected foods. All the foods listed here are excellent sources of potassium.

Processed Foods Lose Potassium, Gain Sodium

There's a simple, painless way to increase potassium and decrease sodium in your diet—eat fewer processed foods and more natural foods. An unfortunate change occurs with many foods when they are processed—they gain sodium and lose potassium, and in some cases, not just a little, but a lot. See Table 4.2.

Nature did not intend for us to eat a lot of sodium, since all unprocessed foods—fruits, vegetables, grains and meats, are naturally low in sodium. So why do processed foods contain so much? The main reason is that processing often removes the natural flavors of foods, and salt is added to enhance what would otherwise be a bland product. Salt is also

How Processed Foods Gain Sodium and Lose Potassium

Food	Amount	Potassium (mg)	Sodium (mg)	Ratio
Milk	1 cup	370	122	3:1
Chocolate pudding (cooked from mix)	1 cup	354	343	1:1
Chocolate pudding (instant)	1 cup	335	820	1:2
Beef roast (cooked)	3 oz.	279	42	7:1
Corned beef (canned)	3 oz.	51	803	1:16
Chipped beef	3 oz.	170	3660	1:22
Corn (cooked)	1 cup	304	71	4:1
Creamed corn (canned)	1 cup	248	671	1:3
Sugar-coated corn flakes	1 cup	27	262	1:10

Reprinted by permission from *Nutrition: Concepts and Controversies, Third Edition* by Eva May Nunnelley Hamilton, et al; Copyright © 1985 by West Publishing Company. All Rights reserved.

Table 4.2 *When foods are processed, they often lose potassium and gain sodium as indicated by the values in this chart.*

added as a preservative for some foods, such as bacon, ham and sausage.

Calcium's Role

Adding calcium to the diet has been shown to lower blood pressure in some individuals, especially those whose calcium intakes are below recommended levels. In a number of studies, adding 800 to 1500 milligrams of calcium per day (1 glass of milk contains about 300 milligrams of calcium) lowered diastolic blood pressure by about 5 mm Hg in one-third or fewer of the participants.

In a Harvard study of 60,000 nurses, it was found that those who consumed very little calcium and magnesium had a 23% greater chance of developing hypertension than those who consumed the recommended amount. Adding calcium supplements for those who are already consuming sufficient amounts of the mineral has not been shown to lower blood pressure. The main concern should be to get *adequate* amounts of calcium in your diet, so you do not *increase* your risk for hypertension and to protect yourself from osteoporosis. This can be accomplished by eating a balanced diet, as explained in Chapter 7.

Advantages and Disadvantages of Medication

Medication is an important tool in treating high blood pressure. Some individuals with hypertension do not respond adequately to weight loss, sodium restriction and other dietary measures. Medication is their only choice. In the last 25 years, the use of blood pressure medication has helped reduce the number of premature deaths due to heart disease and stroke.

However, there are certain drawbacks to taking medication, and therefore, it should be used only if diet modification does not work. Some of the more common negative side effects include the following: Diuretics used in treating high blood pressure can raise cholesterol values 5-10% or roughly 20 points in some individuals. Diuretics can also cause blood sugar levels to become elevated and potassium to fall in 1/3 of those taking them. Other medications (beta blockers) can cause HDL, the "good" cholesterol, to decline. Newer drugs, known as ACE (angiotensis converting enzyme) inhibitors and calcium entry blockers, have slightly fewer side effects, but diet and weight reduction are still the best options if they work for you.

How Much Sodium is Ideal?

The Recommended Dietary Allowance (RDA) for sodium is a maximum of 2400 milligrams per day, or roughly 1 teaspoon of salt. (1 teaspoon salt contains about 2300 milligrams sodium.) Actually, our bodies only need 500 milligrams per day. Keeping sodium levels within the recommended guidelines calls for major changes for most Americans who consume an average of 3000 to 6000 milligrams per day.

Where Sodium Comes From

Where does all this sodium come from? Only about 10% occurs naturally in foods. Another 30 to 40% comes from the salt shaker, including salt used at the table and in cooking. Finally, the largest percentage (40–60%) comes from processed foods, with about 20% of this coming from breads, cereals and other grain products.

For a more specific idea of the sodium content in foods, refer to Table 4.3. Becoming aware of the amount of sodium in the foods you eat enables you to choose your foods more wisely.

Obviously, you could stay well within the suggested guidelines by only eating simple, unprocessed foods, with no added salt. In fact, you could keep your sodium intake to about 500 milligrams per day, but that is extremely difficult to do and it's not necessary. There is still a place for

Sodium Content Of Selected Foods

Naturally Low-sodium Foods	Amount of Sodium (in milligrams)
Fresh fruits & vegetables	
Frozen fruits & vegetables (plain)	
Hot cereal, pasta, rice	Generally less than
Dry beans, peas, lentils, nuts	50 mg. per serving
Canned or dried fruits, jellies	
Spices and herbs (no salt added)	
Eggs	

Foods with Low/Moderate Sodium

Milk (1 cup)	125
Yogurt (1 cup)	150
Cottage cheese (1/2 cup)	450
Cold breakfast cereals (average)	0-250
Meat, fish, poultry (3.5 oz.), unprocessed	50-80
Shellfish (3 oz. cooked) (without added salt)	50-250
Bread (1 slice)	150-200
Margarine (1 teaspoon, soft)	35

Condiments

Salt (sodium chloride)	2300/teaspoon
Seasoned salt mixtures	1200/teaspoon
Light salt*	1100/teaspoon
Monosodium glutamate (MSG)	600/teaspoon
Light seasoned salt	300/teaspoon
Baking soda	800/teaspoon
Baking powder	400/teaspoon
Soy sauce	825/tablespoon
Mild or lite soy sauce	600/tablespoon
Steak sauce, chili sauce	250/tablespoon
Mustard, worcestershire, tartar sauce	200/tablespoon
Catsup, BBQ sauce, seafood cocktail sauce	150/tablespoon
Mayonnaise, sweet pickle relish	100/tablespoon
Bouillon, broth, powdered soup base	900/cup

Processed Foods/Fast Foods

Frozen chicken TV dinner	1150
Pot pie	800
Fried chicken dinner (fast food)	2250
Small hamburger (fast food)	500
Large hamburger (fast food)	1500
Chicken sandwich (fast food)	700-1200
Large pickle	1450
Canned beans (3/4 cup)	550
Lunchmeat (1 oz.)	300
Cheese (1 oz.)	250-500
Quick breads	400
Cake (1 piece), cookies (4), brownies (1)	100-200

*Light salt contains a mixture of half sodium chloride and half potassium chloride.

Table 4.3

your favorite condiments and sauces if used in moderation. Keep in mind that the sodium content listed for condiments is in quantities of a teaspoon or a tablespoon. Catsup, for example, is not particularly high in sodium if just one tablespoon is used, but some catsup lovers use far more than that. Worcestershire sauce, BBQ sauce and seafood cocktail sauce are also moderate in sodium content (as well as low in fat). Mustard is only slightly higher, but since it has such a strong flavor, sometimes just a teaspoon is sufficient.

Lite Salt

Light salt contains a mixture of half sodium chloride and half potassium chloride. By using it in recipes instead of table salt, you will cut sodium intake in half, provided the same quantity is used. When used in cooking, many report that they cannot tell the difference from regular table salt.

Monosodium Glutamate (MSG)

What about monosodium glutamate and seasoned salt mixtures which contain MSG? Some people (1–2%) are allergic to MSG and suffer adverse effects, called Chinese Restaurant Syndrome, when eating foods with this additive. Thus, they should try to avoid it. For the vast majority of people, however, it is "generally regarded as safe," according to the FDA.

MSG is a natural compound, the sodium form of glutamate, an amino acid present in virtually all proteins. Glutamate is also naturally present in high levels in many vegetables, including mushrooms, tomatoes and peas.

MSG and seasoned salt mixtures can be added to foods to enhance their flavors without adding as much sodium as table salt. MSG has 600 milligrams of sodium per teaspoon, while table salt has 2300 milligrams. Generally speaking, just 1/2 teaspoon of MSG per four servings is an optimal amount for flavor. (It enhances flavor, but doesn't taste salty.) That would be only 75 milligrams of sodium per serving—not bad. A seasoned salt mixture (1200 milligrams of sodium per teaspoon) also can be effective in reducing sodium if used instead of table salt, since it has only about half the sodium. Light seasoned salt, with just 300 milligrams per teaspoon, is an even better choice.

Fast Foods and Processed Foods

The majority of fast foods and many processed foods are loaded with sodium. These should be eaten only occasionally if trying to keep sodium within the recommended guidelines. Read labels of processed foods, including canned foods, for sodium content. Some have low or moderate amounts of sodium. Be aware that there are sometimes great variations in sodium from one brand of food to another, even for the same food item. (See Appendix A for sodium content in selected Fast Food items.)

Meal Planning Guidelines to Limit Sodium to Less Than 2400 Milligrams Per Day

Breakfast: Limit sodium to less than 400 milligrams. This amount still enables you to choose a variety of breakfast foods. For example:
- Cereal and milk (Choose cereals with less than 200 milligrams of sodium per serving)
- 1 egg or egg substitute and toast (2 pieces) with one teaspoon margarine and/or jelly
- 2 pancakes with a pat of margarine (optional) and syrup

Fruit juices and/or fruits can be added to any of these breakfast choices without adding additional sodium.

Lunch: Limit sodium to less than 700 milligrams. If eating lunch out, this can be difficult, but not impossible. However, you may want to bring fruit from home to supplement the available food. Some food combinations that stay within this guideline include:
- Cold sandwich made with lunchmeat or turkey breast on two slices of bread or a bun, with lettuce, tomato and a thin scraping of mayonnaise or mustard; cup of yogurt, and soft drink
- Fast food hamburger (small), apple and glass of milk
- Salad with unlimited amount of fresh fruit or vegetables and 2 tablespoons salad dressing (less than 300 milligrams of sodium per 2-tablespoon serving); slice of bread or roll, and glass of milk.

Additional fruits and vegetables (no salt added) can be added to any of these lunches without adding sodium. (Salt is usually added to the cooked vegetables served in restaurants and cafeterias. You can request that they make no-salt or low-salt varieties available.)

Dinner: Limit sodium to less than 1000 milligrams. First consider the foods you always include at dinner and find out their sodium content. For example, it might be an 8-ounce glass of milk (125 milligrams) and one slice of bread (150–200 milligrams), totaling about 300 milligrams of sodium. That means you have 700 milligrams left for the remainder of the meal. Use the majority of that on a meat or casserole dish. Make allowance for dessert or salad dressing if having either one. Supplement with as many fruits and vegetables (no salt added) as desired.

The recipes in this book have moderate levels of sodium, and should help you meet the suggested guidelines. You may choose to further reduce the amount of sodium in some recipes. If so, reduce it gradually, unless you are already used to a low-sodium diet. We chose not to make all the recipes low-salt, because, as mentioned before, unless you gradually reduce salt, some foods will be bland and unappealing. The sodium content of all the recipes is provided for your information.

Tips for Reducing Sodium

It is important to remember that the fondness for salt is an acquired taste. Over the years, we have gradually grown to like salty, and sometimes very salty, foods. This did not happen overnight, and it is easier on almost everyone if the change to less salt is done gradually. It usually takes from 1–2 months for taste buds to adjust to a lower level of sodium. So give it a chance for at least that long.

- Reduce the salt (sodium) used in cooking by one-half. There are two relatively easy ways to restrict salt in cooking. The first is to use Lite salt instead of regular salt, which automatically reduces the sodium by one-half (provided the same quantity is used), without sacrificing much of the sodium taste. The second is to reduce regular salt in a two-step process. First, reduce it by 25%, which is hardly noticeable, and continue in this fashion for about a month. Then reduce it by another 25%. After three to four weeks, most people don't miss the extra salt. If they return to the amount of salt they had been using, it usually tastes too salty.
- Reduce or eliminate the salt used in non-yeast baking. With many baked goods, you can eliminate the salt and not miss it at all. When making yeast-raised breads or rolls, some salt is needed to react with the yeast. Still, the amount of salt can usually be reduced by one-third to one-half without making a noticeable difference.
- Decrease dependence on the salt shaker at the table. Start by eliminating salting vegetables, and then reduce the amount used on meat dishes. Use herbs, spices or low/moderate salt condiments in place of salt. Some especially good low-salt choices with lots of flavor are garlic powder, onion powder, lemon pepper, lemon juice, vinegar, chili sauce and Tabasco sauce. In addition, a tablespoon of catsup, BBQ sauce or seafood cocktail sauce adds only 150 milligrams of sodium, enabling you to stay within the guidelines if other foods are not high sodium.
- Eat more natural foods and fewer processed foods. This is one of the most important steps in a low or moderate sodium diet. In almost all cases, you get more flavor and less sodium with fresh natural foods.
- Use low-sodium soy sauce instead of regular soy sauce. This has only

about half the sodium of regular soy sauce.

- When choosing canned or frozen vegetables, choose those with no salt added.
- Choose cereals with less than 200 milligrams of sodium per serving.
- Choose salad dressings with less than 300 milligrams of sodium per 2-tablespoon serving.
- Reduce the salt in canned beans and tuna fish by rinsing for one minute. In an experiment at Duke University Medical Center, it was found that rinsing beans resulted in 40% less sodium, and rinsing tuna brought an 82% decline (from 418 to 74 milligrams of sodium).
- When a recipe calls for liquid from canned foods, use water or homemade stock instead.
- When cooking pasta or hot cereals, do not add salt to the water.
- "Cut" the sodium in prepared spaghetti sauces by adding an equal amount of "no salt added" tomatoes or tomato sauce to the spaghetti sauce mixture. To make 4 cups of sauce, use two cups of prepared spaghetti sauce and one can (16 oz.) "no salt added" tomatoes, chopped. This will result in about 50% less sodium.
- "Cut" the sodium in canned soups by adding two or three times as much water as it calls for. Add sliced carrots and diced potatoes for extra flavor and thickening. Campbell's "Bean and Bacon" soup works well with these additions. Add vegetables or extra pasta to other soups, such as chicken or turkey noodle soup. Most commercial soups contain 800 to 1000 milligrams of sodium for a 1-cup serving. Following this suggestion will bring the sodium level to about 400 to 500 milligrams per cup.
- Avoid obviously salty foods such as pickles, potato chips, sauerkraut and salted nuts.
- If you eat out frequently, find out if there are low or moderate sodium choices available on the menu. Fast foods are usually very high in sodium, as are most restaurant and cafeteria foods. Sometimes restaurants have menu items that are lower in sodium, and it's up to you to inquire if these choices are available. If you eat out only occasionally, don't worry about the salt content. Pay more attention to the amount of fat.
- When choosing processed foods at the grocery store, look for the sodium content on the label if given. Choose those food items that enable you to stay within the sodium guidelines for each meal.

In summary, if you have high blood pressure, you should definitely limit your sodium intake to within the recommended level. If you fail to do so, you will be putting your cardiovascular health in jeopardy.

If you do not have high blood pressure, you may or may not decide to limit sodium. It is prudent to do so to reduce the risk of developing hypertension later on. But, if you feel you are at low risk, or if you must eat out in restaurants frequently, it may be more practical for you to concentrate on all the other components of a healthy diet. In this case, be sure to get your blood pressure checked yearly, so if you develop hypertension, you can take the appropriate steps to protect your health.

Even if you do not reduce sodium as low as the RDA suggests, restricting it to some degree is still helpful. First of all, if you are salt sensitive, your blood pressure will not rise as high; and second, if you have to restrict it further because you develop high blood pressure, it will be easier since your taste buds will not be accustomed to as high a level of sodium.

5

Sugar—Is It Bad For You?

Sugar is the number one food additive today, and its widespread use is a recent phenomenon. We now eat more sugar in a week than our ancestors from the early 1800's ate in a year. Over the last 150 years, the methods of sugar production have improved dramatically, increasing the supply and bringing down the prices. Instead of being a rare commodity enjoyed primarily by the rich, it is affordable in seemingly unlimited quantities to almost everyone.

In the mid 1800's, sugar consumption was just 20 pounds per person per year; by 1913, it was 76 pounds per year; and now, *on the average, we eat about 125 pounds of caloried sweeteners a year.* This represents approximately 20% of our total calories. Even with the increased use of artificial sweeteners in the last 20 years, the use of calorie-containing sweeteners has continued to rise.

Sources of Sugar

Most of the concentrated sugar we eat (70%) has already been added to the processed foods we buy at the store. This is not only in the obviously sweet foods, but also in condiments, salad dressings, peanut butter, and many other foods. We add about 24% ourselves in baking or at the table; and about 6% is from institutional sources (restaurants, hospitals, etc.).

Unlike our acquired taste for salt, we have an inborn love of sugar. Anyone who has witnessed a baby's enthusiasm when eating fruit for the first time knows this is true. Although we are born with a natural sugar craving, the amount of sugar we desire is conditioned. The more sugar you eat, the more you crave in order to satisfy your "sweet tooth". The opposite is also true. The less you eat, over a long period of time, (at least two or three months), the less you will want. You can reduce the amount of sugar in foods you prepare, and then actually prefer that amount once you condition yourself to it.

Sugar—Natural vs. Concentrated

Are the natural sugars in fruits healthier than concentrated sugar used as an additive? All the different sugars, from those occurring naturally in fruits, to the concentrated sugar in candy bars, are broken down during digestion to glucose, the basic energy unit of carbohydrates. Even the starch in potatoes, rice and corn is broken down to this same glucose, which serves as the fuel for all the cells in the body. Strictly speaking, the body doesn't treat the natural sugar in fruits any differently than concentrated sugar.

Fruits and vegetables are healthier alternatives for another reason. Their diluted sugars come naturally packaged with vitamins, minerals and fiber, all essential to a healthy body. Also, they have less caloric density, which means that there are fewer calories in relation to the bulk of the food. Because of this, you are less likely to consume too many calories when eating fruit. For example, one apple has just 80 calories; whereas, a piece of apple pie has about 282 calories. You would have to eat three and one-half apples before you would consume as many calories as in that one piece of pie. Most people would feel satisfied after one, or at most, two apples.

Concentrated sugar in candy bars, etc. is also more likely to bring on an insulin response than the diluted sugars in fruits. Initially you feel a burst of energy because the sugar from the candy bar goes quickly into the blood stream in the form of glucose. This triggers the pancreas to produce insulin to drive the sugar (glucose) from the bloodstream into the cells. In some individuals, this results in an excess of insulin and a deficiency of glucose in the blood, which produces a tired and weak feeling. This occurs shortly after the initial burst of energy. It doesn't cause permanent harm but can keep you from feeling your best.

Recipes for baked goods, which call for concentrated fruit juices instead of granulated sugar, are not necessarily more nutritious. Most of the vitamin C from the juice is destroyed during baking. Vitamin A is not destroyed (by baking) but most concentrated juices contain little, if any, of this vitamin. Therefore, follow your taste buds in deciding what sweetener to use. Judge the nutritional value of baked goods by the other ingredients in the recipe, not by the type of sweetener.

Is Too Much Sugar Harmful?

Is it harmful to your health to derive 20% of your calories from sugar? A panel of scientists at the Food and Drug Administration (FDA) concluded after extensive study that sugar alone doesn't contribute to any health problems other than dental cavities. That's promising news to everyone who has a strong sweet tooth.

Keep in mind, though, that what accompanies the sugar, in many cases, is harmful. Most candy bars and many desserts are loaded with fat, which can increase our risks for heart disease, cancer and obesity.

There are three factors to consider in determining whether sugar as an additive is detrimental to your health. The first is to look at what accompanies the sugar. If sugar is used to enhance the flavors of nutritious foods, such as low-fat sweetened fruit sauces over lean meat, or a low-fat, low-cholesterol rice pudding, it can indeed be part of a healthy diet. The recipes in this book have combined good nutrition with the use of sugar— they are low in fat and contain other nutritious foods in combination with the sugar.

The second factor to consider is whether you can afford the empty calories in sugar. You may well afford the one teaspoon of sugar (16 calories) in your tea or coffee, but not the 5 teaspoons of sugar (and all the fat) in a chocolate bar. Approximately one in four Americans is overweight, and eating less sugar is a wise way to cut back calories without sacrificing needed nutrients. If you limit fat intake and exercise regularly, a moderate amount of sugar should not result in excessive weight gain.

The third consideration is whether the sugar is displacing more nutritious foods. For someone on a low-calorie diet, this can be an especially serious problem. Theoretically, it is estimated that with careful food selection, one needs close to 1500 calories a day to obtain all the needed nutrients with natural foods, i.e. without vitamin supplements.

Many teenage girls eat only 1200 calories a day to maintain their desired body weight. If they are "wasting" 20% or more of these calories on concentrated sugar, they will probably be nutrient deficient in some areas. Anyone on a low-calorie regimen should be extremely careful to eat only the most highly nutritious foods.

On the other hand, teenage boys and girls active in competitive sports may burn 3000 to 4000 calories a day. They can well afford some "empty" calories from sugar, if their nutrient needs have already been met.

Also, there are certain health conditions that warrant closer monitoring of sugar. Persons with diabetes, hypoglycemia and high levels of triglycerides in their blood need to watch their sugar intake more carefully.

Types of Sugar

Concentrated sugar is listed many different ways on food labels. When trying to limit sugar, it is important to recognize which ingredients represent sugar. Although the names change, the nutritional value of sugars used in processed foods is negligible, except for molasses. Refer to the "Miniglossary of Sugar Terms," page 71, for a description of the different types of sugar.

Miniglossary of Sugar Terms

Brown sugar: At 51 calories per tablespoon, brown sugar has no significant nutritive value. It is usually made by adding a small amount of molasses to white sugar.

Confectioner's sugar: This is finely powdered sucrose (table sugar), 99.9 percent pure.

Corn syrup: Corn syrup is made by breaking down corn starch with acids, resulting in a clear, sweet liquid. It is nutritionally equal to white sugar.

Corn sweeteners: These include corn syrup and sugars derived from corn.

Dextrose: A component of table sugar, dextrose is the technical name for glucose. Hundreds of dextrose (glucose) molecules make up starch molecules, or complex carbohydrates, found in vegetables, beans and grains.

Fructose: Fructose is one of several fruit sugars. It is made chemically by splitting sucrose into its components, fructose and dextrose. It does not raise blood sugar levels as much as dextrose and sucrose, and is therefore less of a problem for diabetics.

Glucose: One of the simple sugars, glucose is one of the components of sucrose, or table sugar. All carbohydrates are broken down to glucose during digestion.

High-fructose corn syrup: This sugar generally contains 42 to 90% fructose, and the remainder dextrose. Because it is inexpensive to make, high-fructose corn syrup, abbreviated HFCS on food and drink labels, is now used in nearly all soft drinks in place of sucrose.

Honey: Honey has erroneously been credited with being a healthier alternative to sugar. Actually, it is nutritionally equivalent to table sugar, although somewhat sweeter and more expensive. It causes blood sugar levels to rise more than sucrose (table sugar).

Lactose: This is the sugar found naturally in milk and other dairy products. It is less sweet than sucrose.

Maple sugar: This sugar is derived from the concentrated sap of the sugar maple tree. Although once a common sweetener, it is now rarely added to foods, and typically has been replaced by sucrose and artificial maple flavoring.

Molasses: A by-product of table sugar made from sugar cane, molasses is the only form of sugar that contains substantial amounts of nutrients. One tablespoon of blackstrap molasses supplies 12% of the U.S.RDA for calcium, and 18% of a woman's RDA for iron (32% of a male's RDA). Light molasses is a diluted form and has about one-third as much of the same nutrients.

Natural sweeteners: All of the sugars listed here are natural sugars.

Raw sugar: Raw sugar is a less refined version of white table sugar.

Sucrose: This is white table sugar, made from sugar cane or sugar beets. It is composed of one fructose molecule and one dextrose (glucose) molecule.

Artificial Sweeteners

The use of artificial sweeteners has skyrocketed since the 1950's when they first became popular in diet drinks. Since that time, there has been a lot of controversy concerning the safety of sugar substitutes, but most experts now agree that they are safe for most people. They are not recommended for children under the age of two, however, since its safety for that age group is still questionable.

The two principal artificial sweeteners are saccharin and aspertame. Aspertame is called "Nutra-sweet" in diet drinks, chewing gum, presweetened cereals, etc.; and is sold as "Equal" in a powdered form to be used in place of sugar. It is composed of two amino acids that occur naturally in foods, phenylalanine and aspartic acid. The safe daily limit, set by the FDA, is equivalent to about 16 cans of diet drinks (72 packets of Equal) for a 160-pound adult, or 4 cans of diet drinks for a 40-pound child. Most people consume 10% or less of this amount per day. Tests with animals have shown no ill effects when consumption levels are 100 times the acceptable level for humans.

Aspertame can pose a health risk for individuals who have a rare genetic condition called phenylketonuria (PKU). This disease, which is usually diagnosed at birth, involves a sensitivity to the amino acid phenylalanine, one of the components of aspartame. Those with PKU must restrict the amount of phenylalanine they consume. Aspertame may also cause headaches in some individuals.

There is more widespread concern over the use of saccharin than aspertame. It has been banned in Canada, except as a table-top sweetener sold only in pharmacies. The ban was imposed because of a study (March 1977) linking it with an increased incidence of bladder cancer in animals. In the U.S., beginning in February 1988, the FDA has required that foods containing saccharin carry a warning label stating that "use of this product may be hazardous to your health." To date, saccharin has not been shown to cause cancer in humans.

Many processed foods contain a combination of both sweeteners. Aspertame is much more expensive than saccharin and it breaks down and loses its sweetness more readily. Therefore, saccharin is added to reduce overall costs and to increase the product's shelf life. Be sure to carefully read the small print on the label if you want to avoid or limit foods sweetened with saccharin.

There are some benefits to using artificial sweeteners. They do not promote tooth decay and they have fewer calories for those who would like to lose weight. Using artificial sweeteners to help lose weight does not work for most people though, since the number of overweight Americans has increased since sugar substitutes were first introduced. Many of them consistently use artificial sweeteners in diet drinks, etc., and use that as a rationalization for eating other high-calorie foods. They may eat several times as many calories in the high-calorie food as they are saving by drinking a diet soda.

Suggestions for Reducing Sugar Consumption

Here are some suggestions for reducing the sugar in your diet or your family's diet:

- Reduce the sugar in recipes by one-fourth. When you are accustomed to that taste, try reducing it by another quarter. (Using less sugar in baked goods changes the texture slightly, causing the product to be more dense, less light and airy.)
- Keep fewer candies and desserts in the house and more fresh fruit. When you crave sweets, fruits are more likely to satisfy you when concentrated sweets are not available.
- Use sugar-free or low-sugar jams and jellies.
- Use unsweetened cereals and sweeten them by adding fresh or dried fruits.
- Try to limit high-sugar soft drinks. As an alternative, add spark to unsweetened fruit juices by adding seltzer or club soda.
- Make your own "frozen pops" by freezing fruit juices in plastic pop molds or in small paper cups. Insert stick into cup when juice is partially frozen.
- Choose frozen or canned fruits with little or no sugar added.

6

Adding Complex Carbohydrates– Fruits, Vegetables and Whole Grains

Up to this point we have discussed food components that should be limited in a healthy diet, i.e. fat, cholesterol, salt and sugar. With complex carbohydrates, the opposite is advised. More of these should be *added* to the diet, particularly, more fruits, vegetables and whole grain products. Calories lost by reducing fat should be replaced, all or in part, by complex carbohydrates. If your goal is to lose weight, then only some of the calories should be replaced, so that total calories are reduced.

Why Complex Carbohydrates are Important

As a whole, complex carbohydrates are low in fat and contain an abundance of natural vitamins, minerals and fiber. Therefore, eating a diet rich in these foods brings many health benefits. It reduces your risks for cancer, heart disease (in part, by replacing the fat), and intestinal disorders. Furthermore, it makes it easier to maintain ideal body weight, since complex carbohydrates (without added fat) are high in bulk, but relatively low in calories. Some complex carbohydrates, particularly beans and grains, are also excellent sources of protein, with only negligible fat. This is in contrast to protein from animal sources, which contains varying amounts of saturated fat.

The components in fruits and vegetables that appear to have a protective effect against cancer are beta-carotene (which is converted to vitamin A during digestion), vitamin C, and a nonvitamin compound called *indoles* found in cruciferous vegetables. (See Figure 6.1 for a list of cruciferous vegetables.) Some researchers suspect that other components of fruits and vegetables, still unidentified, may work in combination with these to produce the benefits. One study showed that the greater the "dose" of produce of any type, the greater the protective effect against cancer. The protective effect may be further enhanced if eating more produce means eating fewer fatty foods. (Several studies conducted in the early 1990's have shown that beta-carotene may also have a protective effect against heart disease and stroke.)

The fiber from complex carbohydrates is one of the factors that helps reduce the risk of colon cancer and other intestinal disorders, including diverticulosis, irritable bowel syndrome, constipation and hemorrhoids.

Complex Carbohydrates Are Not Fattening

Many people are under the mistaken notion that carbohydrates, especially starches, are fattening. Actually, the opposite is true—they are relatively low in calories. Perhaps they have acquired this reputation because of what is added to them. For example, a large plain baked potato contains only 145 calories. But, if you add two teaspoons of butter or margarine and two tablespoons of sour cream to it, you bring the total calories to 265. Sprinkle on a few bacon bits and one-half ounce shredded cheese and the total reaches 368—a hefty increase from the original 145 calories!

Bread is also relatively low in calories. Most varieties range from 65 to 70 calories per slice. One study demonstrated that a young man's diet could include as many as 12 slices of bread in a day (in addition to other foods to provide a balanced diet) and still allow him to lose more than a pound a week. The 12 slices of bread (780 calories) have about as many calories as just one Wendy's Double hamburger with cheese (800 calories).

For many, just eating more fruits and vegetables in place of higher fat foods enabled them to lose weight without feeling hungry or deprived.

How Many Fruits & Vegetables Should We Eat?

According to National Food Consumption Surveys, most of us fall far short of the number of fruits and vegetables we are advised to eat each day. On any given day, almost a third of Americans report eating no vegetables and almost two-thirds do not have a salad. Only about half report having at least one piece of fruit per day.

The U. S. Department of Agriculture recommends that we eat three to five servings of vegetables per day and two to four servings of fruit. A serving is either a half-cup portion or a medium-size fruit or vegetable. Ideally, at least one of the fruits or vegetables should be high in vitamin C, another should be high in vitamin A, and one a cruciferous vegetable. A six-ounce glass of fruit juice is acceptable as a fruit portion, but the nutrients and fiber in a fresh fruit are superior to those in juice.

Variety Is the Key

Nutritionally, all fruits and vegetables are not created equal. Some are better than others; some are high in one nutrient, but low in another; some

Fruit (serving)	Fiber (grams)	Vit. C (%USRDA)	Vit. A (%USRDA)	Calories
Apple (1)	3.0	13	1	81
Apple, w/o skin	2.4	8	1	72
Apple Juice (6 oz.)	0.6	3*	-	87
Apricots (3 med.)	1.4	18	55	51
Banana (1 med.)	1.8	17	2	105
Blackberries, raw (1/2 c)	4.7	25	2	37
Blueberries (1/2 c)	1.7	16	1	41
Cantaloupe (1/4)	1.1	113	103	57
Cherries (10)	1.1	8	3	49
Dates, dried (5 dates)	3.6	-	-	114
Grapefruit, pink (1/2)	0.7	78	6	37
Grapefruit, white (1/2)	0.7	65	-	39
Grapefruit Juice (6 oz)	0.4	90	-	70
Honeydew (1/10)	0.9	77	2	66
Mango (1)	3.7	95	161	135
Nectarine (1)	2.5	12	20	67
Orange (1)	3.1	133	5	65
Orange Juice (6 oz)	0.4	155	7	83
Papaya (1/2)	2.7	157	61	59
Peach (1)	1.4	10	9	37
Pear (1)	4.3	11	-	98
Pineapple (1/2 c)	1.4	20	-	39
Plum (1)	2.5	10	4	36
Prunes, dried (5 prunes)	3.0	3	17	101
Raisins (1/2 c)	4.0	4	-	225
Raspberries (1/2 c)	4.0	26	2	31
Strawberries (1 c)	3.9	141	-	45
Tangerine (1)	2.0	43	15	37
Watermelon (1 c)	0.6	25	11	50

*Fortified apple juice provides 75% of the USRDA for Vitamin C per serving.

(-) less than 1% of the USRDA
(NA) not available.

Sources: Bowes and Church's *Food Values of Portions Commonly Used*, 15th Edition, revised by Jean A. T. Pennington, Harper & Row, New York, 1989; and Human Nutrition Information Service, USDA, Provisional Table on the Dietary Fiber Content of Selected Foods, HNIS/PT-106, 1988.

Table 6.1   Fiber, vitamin C, vitamin A and calorie content of selected fruits and fruit juices.

have more fiber; etc. For this reason, it is important to vary the fruits and vegetables in your diet to get a balance of all the important nutrients. See Table 6.1 for a comparison of the fiber, vitamin C, vitamin A and calories in fruits and fruit juices.

The Value of Vegetables

Vegetable (serving)	Fiber (grams)	Vit. C (%USRDA)	Vit. A (%USRDA)	Calories
Asparagus, raw (1/2 c)	1.4	30	15	22
Beets (1/2 c)	1.4	9	-	26
Broccoli (1/2 c)	2.0	62	22	23
Brussels sprouts (1/2 c)	3.4	60	11	33
Cabbage, green (1/2 c shrd)	0.8	28	-	8
Carrots (1 raw)	2.3	12	405	31
Cauliflower (1/2 c)	1.4	57	-	15
Celery, raw (1 stalk)	0.6	5	1	6
Corn, canned (1/2 c)	2.5	10	4	66
Cucumber (1/2 c sliced)	0.5	3	-	7
Eggplant (1/2 c)	1.2	-	-	13
Green beans (1/2 c)	1.0	10	8	22
Lettuce, Romaine (1/2 c shrd)	0.5	12	14	4
Lettuce, iceberg (1 leaf)	0.3	-	1	3
Mixed vegetables (1/2 c frzn)	2.1	5	78	54
Mushrooms, boiled (1/2 c)	1.7	5	-	21
Onions, raw (1/2 c chopped)	1.3	12	-	27
Parsley, raw (1/2 c chopped)	1.3	45	32	10
Peas (1/2 c)	2.2	13	10	63
Peppers, sweet (1/2 c chpd)	0.8	106	5	12
Potato, no skin (baked)	2.3	37	NA	88
Pumpkin, canned (1/2 c)	3.4	8	538	41
Spinach, raw (1/2 c)	0.7	13	38	6
Spinach, cooked (1/2 c)	2.0	15	148	21
Squash, all varieties (1/2 c)	2.2	17	72	13
Sweet potato, mashed (1/2 c)	3.0	47	559	172
Tomato (1 raw)	1.6	37	28	24
Turnip, chopped (1/2 c)	1.2	15	-	14
Turnip greens, boiled (1/2 c)	2.2	33	80	15
Watercress, raw (1/2 c chpd)	0.4	12	16	2

(-) Less than 1% of the USRDA
(NA) Not available

Sources: Bowes and Church's *Food Values of Portions Commonly Used*, 15th Edition, revised by Jean A. T. Pennington, Harper & Row, New York, 1989; and Human Nutrition Information Service, USDA, Provisional Table on the Dietary Fiber Content of Selected Foods, HNIS/PT-106, 1988.

Table 6.2   Fiber, vitamin C, vitamin A and calorie content of selected vegetables.

Vegetables, like fruits, also vary in the nutrients present. Some are much better sources of vitamin A (beta-carotene) and others are high in vitamin C, or fiber. Vary your choices for optimal nutrition. Table 6.2 compares the fiber, vitamin C, vitamin A and calorie content of selected vegetables.

Cruciferous Vegetables

According to the American Cancer Society, cruciferous vegetables activate enzymes in the liver, which are thought to break down cancer-promoting chemicals. Research indicates that these vegetables reduce the risk of certain types of cancer, including esophageal, stomach, colon, rectal, lung and bladder cancer. Their effectiveness in combatting cancer is further enhanced by the fact that they are good sources of vitamins A and/or C. See Figure 6.1 for a list of cruciferous vegetables.

Cruciferous Vegetables

Bok choy	Kohlrabi
* Broccoli	Leaf mustard (Chinese spinach)
* Brussels sprouts	Radish greens
* Cabbage: napa, red, white	Rutabagas
* Cauliflower	Sea Kale
Chinese kale	Mustard
Collards	Spinach
Garden cress	Upland cress
Horseradish	Watercress
Kale, Southern curled	White mustard

*Animal research has shown that these starred vegetables offer special protection against some forms of cancer. The remaining vegetables, though not yet tested, are members of the cruciferous vegetable family and are expected to offer similar protection.

Figure 6.1 Cruciferous Vegetables.

How Safe Is Our Produce?

Occasionally, news stories question the safety of our fruits and vegetables, stating that there may be dangerous levels of pesticides and/or herbicides in supermarket produce. How valid are these concerns? According to the National Research Council (NRC), the health risks posed by eating the fruits and vegetables available in supermarkets are very small. It is far more hazardous to your health to avoid fruits and vegetables (for whatever reason), than it is to eat them, the NRC contends. It is recommended, however, that all fresh produce be washed thoroughly before eating to remove any surface pollutants.

Maximizing the Nutritional Value of Fruits and Vegetables

Many of the vitamins and minerals in fruits and vegetables are susceptible to being lost during the storage or cooking process. However, with proper methods, the majority of these nutrients can be preserved. The following information and suggestions should help you receive the maximum amount of nutrients from fruits and vegetables.

l) In most cases, fresh and frozen produce provide more nutrients than canned fruits and vegetables. Frozen foods may contain more nutrients than fresh fruits and vegetables that have been stored in the produce department for more than a day.

2) Fresh produce contains most nutrients when ripe—not underripe or overripe (soft, wrinkled). To keep fruits and vegetables from becoming overripe and losing nutrients, store in the refrigerator.

3) Cook vegetables over, not in, water. This minimizes the loss of water-soluble vitamins, which include vitamin C and the B vitamins. If cooked in water that is poured down the drain, as much as 50% of these vitamins may be lost, no matter if the food is cooked in 1/4 cup or 4 cups of water.

4) Avoid long cooking times. Cook only long enough to make vegetables "crisp-tender."

5) Cook potatoes with the skins on to preserve nutrients, especially if boiled in water. Nutrients lost in the water include vitamin C, the B vitamins, potassium, iron and zinc.

6) Try to use the liquid from steamed or boiled vegetables, rather than discarding it, because many water soluble vitamins and minerals are dissolved in the water. The liquid can be used in soups, in cooking rice, or to moisten casseroles.

7) If you store cut fruits or vegetables, or fruit juices, cover with an airtight wrapper or container and store in the refrigerator. If this procedure is followed for reconstituted orange juice, for example, it will retain 80% of its vitamin C after eight days of storage.

8) Avoid purchasing potatoes that are spongy, wrinkled, or sprouting eyes. If there is a green tinged area, cut it away.

9) Choose broccoli that has dark green, tight florets, with firm, not rubbery stalks. Yellow or enlarged florets are signs of overmaturity.

10) If a banana begins to turn brown, and you are not ready to eat it, refrigerate it. It will slow down the ripening process. Refrigeration causes the peeling to turn an unattractive black color, but that doesn't affect the banana, which will remain fresh inside for several days.

Fiber

Complex carbohydrates provide the primary source of fiber in the diet. If you are not getting enough fiber, the reason is very simple—you are not eating enough fruits, vegetables and/or whole grain products.

There are two types of dietary fiber—soluble and insoluble. Both play an important role in overall health. Soluble fiber is needed to remove fatty compounds (including cholesterol) from the body, and to help regulate blood glucose levels. Insoluble fiber is needed to ensure proper elimination of the body's waste products and a healthy digestive system. Soluble fiber is found primarily in oats, oat bran, beans, fruits and vegetables. The main sources of insoluble fiber are whole grain products, especially wheat bran, beans, and the peelings of fruits and vegetables.

How Much Fiber?

The National Cancer Institute and an expert panel convened by the Food and Drug Administration recommend 20 to 30 grams, and no more than 35 grams of dietary fiber per day. The Mayo Clinic Nutrition Department recommends the same minimal level, but with an upper limit of 50 grams of fiber. This is considerably more than the 10 to 15 grams per day consumed by the average American. The recommendation is considered adequate to reduce the risks for intestinal diseases including colon cancer, diverticulosis and irritable bowel syndrome. It should also be adequate to avoid constipation.

An upper limit of 35 to 50 grams per day is suggested because even fiber can have the potential for harm if consumed in excess. Too much fiber can cause mineral losses or dehydration (if you don't drink enough fluids). Mineral losses can occur if foods pass through the body too quickly before some minerals have the chance to be absorbed.

It is best to take in fiber from a variety of sources—whole grains, nuts (in moderation because of high fat content), fruits and vegetables—and to eat it throughout the day, rather than large doses of wheat bran once or twice a day. Not only do you need the nutrients from a wide variety of foods, but cancer studies suggest that the greatest benefits are realized when fiber-rich foods are eaten throughout the day. A pure bran cereal at breakfast is fine as long as you also get additional fiber from other sources. See Table 6.3 to compare the fiber content of selected foods.

Let's examine two sample daily meal plans for breakfast, lunch and dinner that equal 25 to 30 grams of fiber per day. This will give you a good idea of the combinations of foods that meet the recommended guidelines for fiber. See Table 6.4.

As the sample menus indicate, your fiber needs can be met in many different ways. The following suggestions should help you meet those

Dietary Fiber in Selected Foods			
	Fiber (gm)		**Fiber (gm)**
Breads and Rice			
Brown Rice (1 c)	3.0	Pear (1)	4.3
White Rice (1 c)	1.2	Strawberries (1 c)	3.9
Whole Wheat Bread (1 slice)	1.6	**Legumes**	
White Bread (1 slice)	0.6	Baked Beans (1 c)	6.6
Cereals (1 oz.)		Chickpeas (1 c)	5.7
All-Bran (1/3 c)	8.5	Blackeye Peas (1/2 c)	7.9
Fruit & Fiber (1/2 c)	4.3	Lentils (1 c)	7.9
Raisin Bran (1/2 c)	3.7	Navy Beans	6.6
Shredded Wheat (1 biscuit)	2.2	Chestnuts, roasted (3 nuts)	2.8
Wheat Chex (2/3 c)	3.7	**Vegetables**	
Fruits		Broccoli, cooked (1/2 c)	2.0
Apple (1)	3.0	Carrot, 1 raw	2.3
Banana (1)	1.8	Lima Beans, cooked (1/2 c)	6.1
Blueberries (1/2 c)	1.7	Mixed Veg. (1/2 c)	2.1
Dates, dried (5 dates)	3.6	Peas (1/2 c)	2.2
Mango (1)	3.7	Potato w/skin (1 med)	3.0
Orange (1)	3.1	Spinach, cooked (1/2 c)	2.0
Plum (1)	2.5	Sweet Potato, (1/2 c)	3.0

Sources: *Bowes and Church's Food Values of Portions Commonly Used*, 15th Edition, revised by Jean A.T. Pennington, Harper & Row, New York, 1989; and USDA Provisional Table on the Dietary Fiber Content of Selected Foods, HNIS/PT-106, 1988.

Table 6.3 Approximate dietary fiber content of selected foods.

needs. Eat a total of *at least* five fruits and vegetables per day. You can choose a variety of breads, but include some whole grain types. Include beans, and occasionally, nuts (in small quantities) for excellent high-fiber sources. Read the fiber content on cereal boxes to include some high-fiber choices (from 5 to 14 grams of fiber per serving). Sometimes, mixing a high fiber cereal with a lower fiber cereal enables you to get the fiber you need with the taste you prefer.

Benefits of Whole Grains vs. Refined Grains

In addition to fiber, whole grain products also have other benefits. They contain more protein and minerals than their refined counterparts, and have at least twice as much vitamin B6, vitamin E, magnesium and zinc. The additional nutrients are found in the bran and germ, the parts removed during refining. Figure 6.2 shows the components of a kernel of wheat.

Most breads and cereals are enriched, which means some of the

Daily Menus Demonstrating Recommended Fiber Intake

Day I Menu		Day II Menu	
Breakfast I	**Dietary Fiber (g)**	**Breakfast II**	**Dietary Fiber (g)**
Whole wheat toast (2 slices)	3.2	All-bran cereal (1/3 cup)	8.5
Margarine (1 teaspoon)	-	Milk (1/2 cup)	-
Orange juice (6 oz.)	0.4	Bagel, plain white	1.2
Banana	1.8	Light Cream cheese	-
		(2 teaspoons)	
Lunch I		Orange	3.1
Ham sandwich			
Hard roll	1.4	**Lunch II**	
Ham (1 oz.)	-	Salad	
Mayonnaise (1 teaspoon)	-	Lettuce (1 cup)	1.0
Lettuce	-	Tomato	I.6
Baked beans (3/4 cup)	5.0	Garbanzo beans (1/4 cup)	1.4
Apple	3.0	Salad Dressing	-
Milk shake	-	(2 tablespoons)	
		Whole wheat bread (2 slices)	3.2
Dinner I		Margarine (1 teaspoon)	-
Chicken breast (4 oz.)	-	Apple	3.0
Whole wheat bread (1 slice)	1.6	Iced tea	-
Potato (with skin)	3.0		
Broccoli (3/4 cup)	3.0	**Dinner II**	
Tossed Salad w/vegetables	1.5	Beef-Vegetable Stir Fry	
Strawberries (1/2 cup)	2.0	Beef (3 oz.)	-
Skim milk (8 oz.)	-	Cauliflower (1/4 cup)	0.7
Total Fiber for Day I	**25.9 (g)**	Broccoli (1/4 cup)	1.0
		Green pepper (1/4 cup)	0.4
		Brown rice (1 cup)	3.0
		French bread (1 slice)	0.6
		Frozen yogurt (1 cup)	-
		Skim milk (8 oz.)	-
		Total Fiber for Day II	**28.7 (g)**

Table 6.4 Two daily menus to show different combinations of food that meet the recommended guidelines for fiber.

nutrients lost in the refining process are restored, including iron, thiamin, riboflavin and niacin. Other minerals lost, but not replaced, are magnesium, manganese, chromium, zinc, folate, vitamin B6, and copper. Researchers are discovering that a substantial number of Americans may not consume enough of these nutrients, since they eat so few whole grain foods.

Don't Be Fooled by "Wheat Bread" Labels

Manufacturers seem to have caught on that Americans want to eat more whole grain bread but prefer the soft, fluffy texture of white bread. So they label some breads "wheat bread" and add caramel color to make

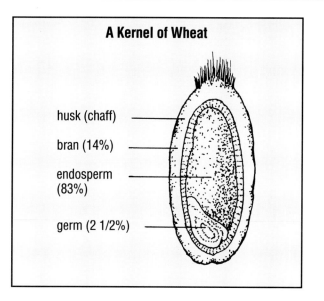

A Kernel of Wheat

husk (chaff)

bran (14%)

endosperm (83%)

germ (2 1/2%)

Figure 6.2 A kernel of wheat. The husk or chaff is inedible to humans and is usually fed to livestock. The remaining wheat kernel has three main parts: the endosperm, the germ and the bran. The endosperm is the soft, inside part of the kernel, which contains starch and protein, and is the only part of the kernel used to make refined white flour. The germ has high nutritive value since it contains the concentrated food, including vitamins and minerals, to support new life after the wheat seed is planted. The bran forms a protective coating around the kernel, and is also rich in nutrients and fiber. (Corn, oat and rice grains have similar structures.)

it look like whole wheat bread. In fact, the bread may be made primarily with refined flour, with only a small proportion of whole wheat flour added. Therefore, the texture is soft like white bread. It is fine to eat this bread occasionally, but be aware that the fiber and trace minerals of true whole wheat bread are not present.

If you want to buy whole grain wheat bread, look at the list of ingredients and buy those that list "whole wheat flour" as the first ingredient. If "wheat flour" is listed first, this usually means *refined* wheat flour, or "white flour."

Other Grain Products

Bread is just one source of whole grain foods. There are many other nutritious grain products that can bring interesting tastes and textures to your table. Try to incorporate more of these into your diet. These include barley, which is excellent in soups, salads or casseroles; oats and oat bran, which come in a variety of forms; brown rice and wild rice; and the many different types of wheat grain products, the most common being cracked wheat, bulgur and wheat germ. The following list describes a wide variety of grain products.

Types of Rice

Brown Rice is the whole rice grain. Only the outer husk has been removed from the kernel. It contains more fiber, protein, phosphorus and potassium than white rice. It has a nutty flavor and chewy texture.

Regular-milled White Rice or Polished Rice has had its husk, bran, aleurone (a thin layer under the bran) and germ removed during processing. It loses about 20% of its protein, more than half its minerals, and most of its vitamins in this process. Often it is enriched, replacing some of the lost nutrients.

Parboiled or Converted White Rice has undergone a special steam-pressure process that pushes some of the nutrients from the outer bran into the starchy center of the grain. This rice has less fiber and protein than brown rice but more nutrients than other forms of white rice.

Precooked or Instant Rice has been cooked, rinsed and dried by a special process. It is the least nourishing and the most highly processed. It is also the most expensive white rice.

Wild Rice is not true rice, but is the unmilled grain of an aquatic grass. It is relatively expensive, because its supply is limited. Wild rice is very nutritious because it is never refined.

Wheat Grains

Bulgur or cracked whole wheat, has been precooked, dried and cracked into small pieces. It comes in three sizes: small, medium and large. It has a nutty taste and is delicious by itself or mixed with salads, soup or rice. It contains all the nutrients of whole grain wheat.

Couscous is finely cracked wheat grain that has been steamed and dried. It is usually light in color and refined, so it does not contain the fiber and nutrients of a whole grain product. It can be substituted for rice in most dishes.

Wheat berries are whole wheat kernels. They are similar in appearance to rice but the grains are larger. They take a long time to cook (3 hours), but once cooked, they make a crunchy cereal with a naturally sweet taste. Wheat berries can also be used in breads and muffins.

Wheat Germ is the embryo or germ of the wheat kernel. It contains essentially all the fat of the kernel and is a good source of B vitamins, vitamin E and iron. Available as tan flakes in vacuum-packed jars, it should be refrigerated after opening to prevent oxidation.

Corn Products

Hominy is the endosperm of the corn kernel, without the bran and germ. It is milled into very fine pieces to make hominy grits. Because it does not include the bran or germ, it is comparable in nutrients to refined wheat.

Cornmeal is a granular product of corn which may be made either with or without the germ and most of the bran. Refined cornmeal and hominy grits may be enriched, improving the nutritional quality.

Other Grains

Barley can be purchased in two forms. Processed or "pearled" barley, which has had the hull and bran removed, but not the germ, is the more common variety available in grocery stores. Higher in protein than other grains, it is used primarily in soups. Unpearled barley, found mainly in health food stores, is a richer source of dietary fiber.

Buckwheat is actually not a grain but is used as one. Its seed contains a glutenous substance that can be made into flour so it is commonly considered in the grain family. Fine buckwheat flour is similar to refined white flour, but has somewhat less protein. It is used primarily in making griddle cakes and is valued for its distinctive flavor.

Rye is used chiefly as a flour-making grain. Darker in color than wheat flour, it is used to make pumpernickel bread. It is also combined with wheat flour to make rye bread. It is similar in quality and nutrients to wheat flour.

Oats are used chiefly in making oatmeal, including both rolled oats and ground or cut oats (oat bran). In processing, the outer hull is removed, but most of the germ and bran remain. Therefore, it retains the nutrients of a whole grain product, providing a good source of thiamin and other B vitamins and iron. Oat bran is one of the best sources of soluble fiber.

A Word About Beans

Some have called beans or legumes "the perfect food," because they contain an abundance of so many important nutrients—starch, high-quality protein, fiber, vitamins and minerals. They have been an important carbohydrate/protein staple for many civilizations throughout history. An adult's complete daily protein requirement can be met with just two cups of legumes served with a grain product, and two cups of milk or its equivalent.

From a nutrition standpoint, there are definite advantages to changing our protein sources, i.e., incorporating more beans, while eating less meat. This way, the diet is lower in fat and cholesterol and higher in fiber. Beans are an excellent source of both soluble and insoluble fiber.

When adding beans to your diet, start slowly to help alleviate problems with intestinal gas. Start by sprinkling them on salads, using them in soups, or otherwise eating small servings so your system can get accustomed to them. Split peas and lentils are easier for the body to adjust to than other types of beans. In research studies, it has been found that when eating beans on a daily basis, most people stop having excessive gas after two or three weeks.

Tips for Adding More Whole Grains and Beans

- In recipes calling for all-purpose flour, substitute 1/3 of the flour with whole wheat flour. The taste and texture of baked goods change very little with this amount of substitution. (Exceptions are very light angel food cakes, sponge cakes and some white cakes.)
- In some stir-fry dishes or casseroles, reduce or eliminate the meat and replace it with cooked beans. Black beans, kidney beans or garbanzo beans usually combine well with meat dishes.
- Use more whole wheat varieties of processed foods, such as English muffins, waffles or pasta. With pasta, try mixing whole wheat pasta with regular pasta at first, so the change in texture is not too great.
- Sprinkle bran flakes, wheat germ and/or bran on top of casseroles for crisp toppings. These also can be used as a filler with low-fat ground meats.
- Substitute brown rice for white rice or add wild rice to white rice dishes.
- When shopping for snack foods, look for whole grain products. There are some excellent low-fat, high-fiber varieties available, including Norwegian crispbreads and some of the 100% rye crackers and whole wheat crackers. Be sure to check the fat content on the labels.

Tips for Adding More Fruits and Vegetables

- When hungry for a snack, choose a fruit, either fresh or dried.
- Make fruit a regular dessert item.
- Add a variety of raw vegetables or fruit to salad greens.
- Have peeled, ready-to-eat, raw vegetables available in the refrigerator for snacks.
- Add fruits to cereal, ice milk, low-fat frozen yogurt, etc.
- Add raisins or shredded vegetables (carrots, zucchini or sweet potatoes) to muffins and spice cakes.

7

Putting It All Together—Meal Planning and Exercise

Changing to a healthier diet means altering eating habits that have been formed over many years. It is not difficult to do, but does require motivation and effort, especially in the beginning. The motivation should come from knowing the many long-term health benefits to be gained.

You have already learned many of the components of a healthy diet, which were discussed in the previous four chapters. Now you will learn how to combine all this information and work it into well-balanced meals.

In the past, planning well-balanced meals meant choosing a specified number of servings from the Basic Four Food Groups. The primary consideration was getting enough vitamins, minerals and protein in the diet. Little, if any, consideration was given to the amounts of fat, cholesterol or fiber.

All this has changed with the influx of new information on the importance of these factors in the diet. Over consumption of fat, cholesterol and animal protein; and under consumption of fiber can also be very damaging to a person's health, especially in the long term.

As an aid to planning healthy meals, we recommend you use the "Food Guide Pyramid," shown in Figure 7.1. The pyramid shape shows at a glance the foods that should be the mainstay of your diet and those that should be eaten more sparingly. Following the serving suggestions and guidelines outlined in this food guide will ensure that you not only get enough of the essential nutrients, but that you also incorporate into your meals all the other aspects of a healthy diet—reducing total fat, especially saturated fat, relying less on animal sources for protein needs, and eating adequate amounts of fiber.

Food Guide Pyramid
A Guide to Daily Food Choices

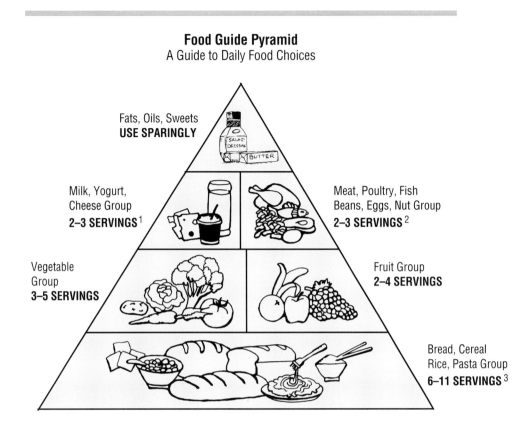

¹ One serving equals 1 cup or 1 ounce cheese. Use skim or low-fat dairy products. Adult men and women over 25 years old require 2 servings/day (except for women who are pregnant, nursing or over 50 years.) The recommendation for children up to 9 years is 2–3 servings/day; for children 9 to 12 years, 3–4 servings/day; for ages 12 to 24 and pregnant women, 3 to 4 servings/day; for nursing mothers, 4 servings per day; and for women over 50 years, 3–5 servings/day.

² In order to minimize saturated fat and cholesterol, eat more beans and less meat. To limit fat to 20% of total calories, eat *a maximum of:*

- 3–4 oz. cooked lean meat, poultry, shrimp, crab or lobster or
- 4–6 oz. cooked fish, clams, scallops and oysters

plus, eat *an average of:*

- 1/2 to 3/4 cup beans per day. (Use nuts sparingly.)

Eggs should be limited to no more than 4 per week from all sources, including baked goods and sauces. If you have elevated cholesterol, it is preferable to use egg substitutes or egg whites, which can be consumed in unlimited quantities.

³ Include at least 2 to 4 servings of whole grain foods.

Figure 7.1 Adapted from: U.S. Department of Agriculture "Food Guide Pyramid"

Meal Planning

Meal planning is critical to improving your diet. It is best to plan one to two weeks at a time, including three meals a day, plus snacks. That way you can see if you are choosing the right amounts each day from the six food groups. It also makes it easier to plan variety into your menus. Eventually you may only need to plan your evening meals if your breakfasts, lunches and snacks consist of fairly similar types of foods.

It is not necessary to immediately incorporate into your diet all the recommended daily servings from each food group. In some cases, it works best to concentrate on one food group at a time, and to gradually work in each one of the suggestions.

Use snacks to improve your diet. For example, if you're not eating enough fruits, vegetables or whole grain foods, choose these for snacks. Frequent snacking can be part of a healthy diet, if done with the right kinds of foods.

Do not overlook your fluid requirements. You should drink eight 8-ounce glasses of liquids per day, not including drinks high in caffeine. It is especially important to drink enough fluids when you increase your fiber intake because fiber attracts water, and thus more is needed to move it through the colon. Inadequate fluids, with or without increased fiber consumption, can cause constipation or mild dehydration.

Meeting Our Protein Needs

Consuming sufficient protein is essential for the body's proper functioning. It is needed to build muscles, tendons, ligaments, skin, hair and nails; to produce enzymes, hormones and antibodies; to maintain proper fluid balance; and to monitor a host of other body functions.

The amount of protein needed is based on age and ideal body weight. Growing children and pregnant women need proportionately more protein because they are experiencing increased growth of new body tissue. If they follow the recommendations in the "Food Guide Pyramid," including the higher dairy requirements, they will be sure to receive adequate protein (even though portion sizes of foods will be smaller for small children).

The Recommended Dietary Allowance (RDA) for protein for an average adult male over 14 years of age is 56 grams a day; for an average female over 18 years of age, it is 44 grams a day. This is based on an "average" ideal body weight of 154 for a male, and 120 for a female.

You can calculate your own protein RDA, based on your ideal body weight (IBW), in two simple steps as shown in Figure 7.2.

How to Calculate Your Protein RDA

Step I: Determine your ideal body weight. (See Weight Table, p.15.)

Step 2: Multiply your IBW by 0.37 to get your protein RDA in grams per day.

Figure 7.2 The two-step process to determine the Recommended Dietary Allowance for protein.

For an example, we will use a 5'6" woman with an ideal body weight of 130 pounds.
Step 1: Ideal body weight = 130 pounds.
Step 2: 130 pounds x 0.37 = 48 grams of protein per day.

As you can see from this example, the protein RDA for a 5'6" woman is 48 grams per day. This quantity of protein is very easy to meet, and most Americans well exceed the RDA. The National Research Council, concerned with the health hazards associated with too much protein, has suggested a *maximum* daily protein consumption of 0.7 grams/pound, based on your IBW. This is approximately double the RDA.

Let's examine the amount of protein in various types of food (Figure 7.3), in order to have a better understanding of our protein sources. Use this chart to help you find combinations of foods to meet your protein needs.

Meeting protein requirements can be accomplished with a variety of different food combinations. It is not absolutely necessary to have 3 to 6 oz. of meat, poultry or fish each day to do this. The RDA for protein also can be met by eating less meat or fish and more beans and grains. When relying on beans as a source of protein, however, be sure to complement them with a grain product, such as bread, pasta, rice or wheat in order to have a complete protein.

More Than Enough Protein

Sometimes we can go overboard with protein consumption. In fact, the average American diet is 50 to 75% over the RDA for protein. Let's look at two typical high protein meals, illustrated in Figure 7.4, to show how easily this can happen. A breakfast of 2 eggs, 3 ounces of ham, a glass of milk and 2 slices of toast contributes 47 grams of protein, enough to meet an entire day's RDA for an average size woman. A lunch of a quarter-pound cheeseburger with a 12-ounce milk shake provides 42 grams of protein—again, almost a full day's recommended amount.

As a healthier alternative, a breakfast of 1 ounce of cereal with 1/2 cup milk, and a piece of toast contributes a more desirable 8 grams of protein. For lunch, a turkey sandwich (lettuce, tomato and 1 ounce of turkey meat), and a glass of milk yields 19 grams of protein. These two meals alone total

Figure 7.3 *The principal sources of protein in the diet.*

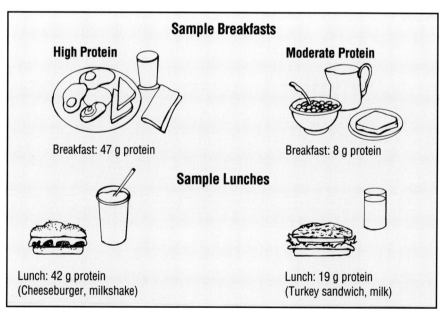

Figure 7.4 *Sample breakfasts and lunches showing high and moderate amounts of protein.*

27 grams of protein. If you have a dinner of 4 ounces of meat, potatoes, vegetable and salad, this would add an additional 38 grams of protein, or a total of 65 grams for the day. As these examples show, it is very easy to meet and often exceed the RDA for protein.

Is Too Much Protein Harmful?

There are no benefits and there may be harm associated with the over consumption of protein (greater than 15% of total calories). In fact, the excess protein is wasted, since it is broken down and either converted to glucose to supply energy for the body, or stored as fat.

High consumption of protein, especially animal protein, is associated with higher rates of obesity, heart disease, cancer and diabetes. Animals fed high protein diets develop enlargement of their livers and kidneys.

Diets too high in protein are often deficient in fruits, vegetables, and whole grain products, resulting in inadequate intakes of certain nutrients. High protein diets also increase the body's excretion of calcium, which means you need more calcium-rich foods to avoid the effects of calcium deficiency—weak bones and teeth. Care should be taken when making daily meal plans to make sure that protein is adequate, but not excessive.

Sample Daily Meal Plans

The following pages provide two weeks of sample meal plans. Preparing these menus should help you keep fat intake to approximately 20% of total calories, and should provide you with adequate amounts of protein, fiber and all the essential vitamins and minerals. Portion sizes will vary depending on caloric needs.

The starred items indicate that the recipes are included in the recipe section of the book. If your time is limited during the week, some of the suggested foods, particularly homemade desserts or muffins, can be made in advance, perhaps on the weekends. You may also save time by buying parts of a meal at the supermarket; for example, baked beans (preferably vegetarian), packaged rice mix or muffins. (Be sure to read the label or inquire about the grams of fat in baked goods. Some are very high.)

The suggested meal plans should give you a good idea of the variety of foods you can and should enjoy, knowing you are following a diet for optimal good health. However, don't limit yourself to these meal plans since there are many other delicious recipes in this book that are healthy and low in fat, and with minimal planning, can provide the balance needed in your diet.

WEEK I

	Sunday	Monday	Tuesday	Wednesday	Thursday	Friday	Saturday
Breakfast	Orange juice Whole grain cereal with milk Coffee/tea	Orange juice *French Toast with whole wheat bread Coffee/tea	Banana Bagel with light cream cheese Coffee/tea	Orange juice All-bran cereal with raisins and skim milk Coffee/tea	Orange juice Scrambled egg substitute Whole wheat toast Coffee/tea	Instant oatmeal Orange Whole wheat toast Coffee/tea	Whole grain cereal with raisins, sliced banana, milk Bagel Coffee/tea
Morning Snack	Apple	*Oatbran Muffin Coffee/tea	Apple	1 oz. pretzels Fruit juice	Low-fat, high-fiber crackers Carbonated drink	Pear	Orange
Lunch	Ham sandwich *Minestrone Soup (canned or home-made) Skim milk	Turkey sandwich on whole wheat Cranberry-Orange Relish Baked beans Skim milk	Ham sandwich on rye *Black Bean Salad Fruit Salad Strawberry shake	*Tuna Pasta Salad French bread Cantaloupe Skim milk	Turkey sandwich on whole wheat Baked Beans Marinated asparagus Skim milk	Tuna Salad (with nonfat mayonnaise) on whole wheat Fruit salad Skim milk	Turkey sandwich on hard roll *Tropical Fruit Slaw Skim milk
Afternoon Snack	Nectarine	Apple	*Oatbran Muffin Coffee/tea	Apple	Banana	Apple	Banana
Dinner	Roast Turkey Breast (leftovers for stir-fry Tues.) *Mashed Potaotes w/ nonfat turkey gravy Cranberry-Orange Relish (canned) *Green Beans Amandine Rolls	*Pasta with Red Clam Sauce Steamed carrots and peas Crusty French bread *Spinach Salad with Honey Mustard Skim milk	*Stir-fry Chicken and Vegetables (substitute turkey) over rice Multi-grain bread *Baked Tomatoes Fig Newtons Skim milk	*Bean Stroganoff Steamed Brussels sprouts French bread Skim milk *Granola Apple Cobbler	*Flank Steak Chile *Bran Muffins (purchased or homemade) Skim milk Canned fruit (in light syrup)	*Stuffed Baked Potato *Tropical Fruit Slaw (make enough for next day) Whole wheat bread or rolls Skim milk	*Marinated Salmon *Mashed Potatoes with Chives Steamed carrots Tossed salad *Chocolate Chip Bundt Cake
Evening Snack	2 large low-salt pretzels Soft drink	Low-fat frozen yogurt	Low-salt pretzels Apple juice	Banana	Cereal with skim milk	Bagel with jam Beverage	*Bran Muffin Skim milk

*Recipes appear in Recipe section of book.

WEEK II

	Sunday	Monday	Tuesday	Wednesday	Thursday	Friday	Saturday
Breakfast	Cantaloupe *Bran Muffin Coffee/tea	Orange juice Oat bran cereal with milk Bagel	Orange juice Cereal combination: All-Bran and Raisin Bran with milk Coffee/tea	Cantaloupe Oat Bran cereal with milk Whole wheat toast Coffee/tea	Grapefruit juice *Oat Bran-Apple Muffin Coffee/tea	Grapefruit Bagel with peanut butter Whole wheat toast Skim milk	Fresh strawberries All-Bran cereal with milk and sliced banana Coffee/tea
Morning Snack	*Bran Muffin Skim milk	Apple Coffee/Tea	*Blueberry muffin	Pear	Banana	Apple Coffee/tea	Pear Coffee/tea
Lunch	Tuna salad (with nonfat mayonnaise) on rye bread Baked beans (vegetarian) Skim milk	Turkey sandwich on whole wheat *Taboule salad or Applesauce Skim milk	Ham sandwich on Kaiser roll Vegetarian baked beans Tossed salad Skim milk	*Stuffed Baked Potato Fruit salad Skim milk	Turkey sandwich on whole wheat Steamed broccoli Applesauce Skim milk	*Lentil Soup French bread Angelfood cake with ice milk Skim milk	*Tuna Stuffed Tomatoes Whole wheat bread Skim milk
Afternoon Snack	Pear Soft drink	*Chocolate Chip Cake Coffee/tea	Banana	Low-fat crackers Soft drink	Bagel with jam Coffee/tea	Tangerine	Bagel Soft drink
Dinner	*Shrimp Jambalaya *Orange Cornbread Tossed salad Chocolate Chip Bundt Cake (leftover) Skim milk	*Beanburgers (mix may be made several days in advance) Slim Waldorf salad Baked tomatoes Fresh strawberries with frozen yogurt Skim milk	*Apple-Date Stuffed Tenderloin *Rice-Mushroom Casserole (or use packaged rice mix) Green beans Cantaloupe Skim milk	*Scallops Florentine over Brown Rice Dinner rolls Sliced tomatoes *Baked Rice Pudding Skim milk	*Vegetable Pasta Stir-Fry French bread Tossed salad Angelfood cake, (purchased) strawberries and vanilla ice milk Skim milk	*Chicken n' Dumplings Fruit Salad Whole wheat bread Vanilla pudding (made with skim milk) with sliced bananas Skim milk	*Light Fried Fish Fillets *Sweet Potato Casserole Steamed broccoli *Custard Pie Skim milk/water
Evening Snack	Sliced banana with skim milk	Pretzels Soft drink	Frozen yogurt	Cold cereal with skim milk	*Baked Rice Pudding	Pretzels Soft drink	Custard pie

*Recipes appear in Recipe section of book.

Vitamins

When Are Vitamins Recommended?

If you are eating a balanced diet, that is, choosing the recommended amounts of foods from each of the food groups, and if you do not have a special medical condition, there is no need to take vitamin supplements to meet your nutritional needs. You would be getting all the vitamins and minerals you need from the foods you eat.

There are certain situations, though, when vitamins are definitely called for. The first is when a doctor prescribes them for a medical reason. For example, during pregnancy they are prescribed because of the increased nutritional needs of the mother and growing baby. Vitamins are also recommended for adults consuming fewer than 1500 calories per day, or for someone eating irregularly for whatever reason. In these cases, the RDA's for vitamins and minerals may not be met with foods alone.

Some people like to take vitamin supplements "just in case" they're not getting enough of certain vitamins and minerals. They give them to their children for the same reason. If you choose the right type of multivitamin, it will not harm you, and may possibly help you. It's important, though, not to rely too heavily on vitamins as a nutrition source, since most vitamin pills supply only 10 to 12 of the more than 40 nutrients you need.

How to Choose the Best Vitamin

In choosing a vitamin supplement, ignore all the advertising hype, and look directly at the list of ingredients with the percentage of the RDAs. Choose one that provides a wide variety of vitamins and minerals in amounts smaller than, equal to, or very close to the RDA. Avoid any variety that provides more than the RDA of vitamins A, D and E, or *any* mineral. Also avoid those that provide more than 10 times the RDA for any other nutrient. Taking megadoses greater than that can cause serious health problems. Remember that the foods you eat also contain vitamins and minerals, so it isn't necessary to receive your entire RDA from a vitamin.

What About Megadoses of Vitamin C?

Dr. Linus Pauling, a Nobel laureate chemist, first popularized the notion of taking megadoses of vitamin C to fight the common cold. In 1970, he published the book, *Vitamin C and the Common Cold*, which sent people out in droves to buy large doses of this vitamin. He recommended taking 1 to 2 grams per day, or 20 to 40 times the RDA.

After pooling data from eight studies, it was shown that taking megadoses of vitamin C produced only 1/10 fewer colds per year, and an average 1/10 of a day shorter duration per cold. The tentative conclusion was that taking high doses of vitamin C had little or no affect on colds for most people. Preliminary studies from the early 1990s, however, show that vitamin C's anti-oxidant properties may be a boost to the immune system in other ways. Supplements of up to 500 milligrams (1/2 gram) appear to be safe for adults.

Toxic Effects of Vitamin C

Taking gram doses of vitamin C on a regular basis can cause toxic effects. It can cause gout in those predisposed to the disease, cause hemolytic anemia in certain ethnic groups, and can interfere with the body's natural process of fighting infections. If tablets are chewed, the ascorbic acid (vitamin C) can damage tooth enamel. It can also lead to kidney stones in some individuals.

Infants born to mothers taking megadoses of vitamin C during pregnancy can experience "rebound scurvy" after birth. They are suddenly cut off from the megadoses and their bodies can't adjust to the sudden reduction in vitamin C. Thus, they experience a severe "deficiency." "Rebound scurvy" may also occur in adults who suddenly stop taking megadoses. Therefore, it is best to reduce the amount of vitamin C gradually, so the body can adjust. These effects do not occur in all individuals, but it is impossible to determine in advance who will be affected.

Vitamins and Minerals Most Frequently Found Deficient

The vitamins and minerals that Americans are most likely to be deficient in are vitamin A, vitamin B6, vitamin C, calcium, iron and magnesium. According to the Nationwide Food Consumption Survey (1978), an average of one-third of Americans from all income levels had food intakes of these nutrients at or below 70% of the RDA. A deficiency is likely to occur when intakes are consistently below the 70% level.

These deficiencies would not occur if everyone ate the recommended servings from the six food groups. The foods most likely to be overlooked in our diet are fruits, vegetables, whole grain products and low-fat dairy products.

Exercise

Exercise is an essential part of a healthy lifestyle. Regular aerobic exercise not only burns calories, but also complements the health benefits of a prudent diet. Diet and exercise work as a team to keep the body at its physical best.

Benefits of Exercise

The health benefits attributed to exercise are numerous. Exercise improves the cardiovascular system by raising HDL or "good" cholesterol and by lowering triglycerides and blood pressure. Exercise also increases bone mass which helps prevent osteoporosis (fragile bones). Regular aerobic exercise is essential to weight reduction, enabling dieters to lose weight more readily and to keep the pounds off. It can also relieve anxiety and stress by releasing certain chemicals called endorphins into the brain. Exercise can also help relieve constipation if done in combination with a diet plan of increased fiber and fluids. With all these benefits, how can anyone choose not to exercise?

Studies have documented the benefits of exercise and the drawbacks of a sedentary life. Researchers at Duke University found that *unfit* people have the same risk of heart disease and stroke as smokers, (2.8 times greater risk) or those 19 years older (3 times greater risk). A study reported in the *Annals of Internal Medicine* found that postmenopausal women who exercised one hour, three times a week, increased their bone mass by 2.6% in one year. On the other hand, sedentary women *lost* an average of 2.4% of bone mass during this same period. Over a number of years, the difference in bone mass between an active and sedentary person could be quite significant.

Long-term exercise can help preserve a youthful mind. Men in their 60's, who have jogged or played racquetball or squash for 20 years or longer, have reaction times that are equal to or better than men in their 20's who are inactive. Reaction time is determined by measuring the length of time it takes to react to a stimulus (such as a buzzing sound) with a response (such as pressing a button).

Exercise has also been shown to help relieve moderate depression. In a study at the University of Wisconsin, it was found that walking and/or running for one hour a day, three times a week, over a 10-week period, worked as well as, or better than, psychotherapy in treating moderate depression.

You're never too old to benefit from exercise. In fact, you can actually increase the size and strength of your muscles even into your nineties. In a study conducted at Tufts-USDA Human Nutrition Research Center on Aging, it was found that a group of men and women who averaged 90 years of age, increased the muscle area of their thighs by 10% through a weight lifting program. Even more significant, they increased the amount of weight they could lift from an average of 17.6 pounds to 44 pounds.

This increase in strength brought some unexpected benefits. They were able to walk faster, take longer strides or just get around more easily.

Kinds of Exercise

The National Heart, Lung and Blood Institute classifies exercise into three distinct types. Type I includes the most vigorous exercises (Figure 7.5). These exercises need to be done for at least 15 minutes per day, three times a week, for adequate conditioning of the heart and lungs.

Type I Exercises

Cross-Country Skiing
Hiking (uphill)
Ice Hockey
Jogging
Jumping Rope
Rowing
Running in Place
Stationary Cycling

Figure 7.5 Type I Exercises. These condition heart and lungs if done for at least 15 minutes per day, three times a week.

Type II exercises are less vigorous, but can condition the heart and lungs if done briskly (Figure 7.6). They should be done vigorously for at least 30 minutes per day, three times a week to get approximately the same conditioning benefits as Type 1 exercises.

Type II Exercises

Bicycling
Downhill Skiing
Basketball
Calisthenics
Field Hockey
Handball
Racquetball
Soccer
Squash
Swimming
Tennis (singles)
Walking

Figure 7.6 Type II Exercises. These can condition the heart and lungs if done vigorously for at least 30 minutes per day, three times a week.

Type III exercises do not condition the heart and lungs, but they are still beneficial in other ways (Figure 7.7). They improve coordination and muscle tone, and can reduce stress.

Figure 7.7 Type III Exercises. These do not condition the heart and lungs, but do improve coordination and muscle tone.

Getting Started—Choosing Your Exercise

Choose an exercise that you enjoy from Type I or II category. If you are doing something you like, the chances are much greater that you will continue it on a long term basis. If you prefer exercising with others, find a friend or group and set up a regular schedule.

The key is to start gradually, pacing yourself according to your level of fitness. Remember that your goal is a minimum of 15 to 30 minutes of vigorous exercise per workout. It is fine to take 3 to 4 months to arrive at that goal.

Are You Exercising Vigorously Enough?

There is a way to tell if you are exercising vigorously enough to benefit your cardiovascular system. This is determined by taking your pulse immediately after exercising. Your pulse, or heart rate, should be 60 to 70% of your maximum heart rate, which is approximately 220 less your age. See Table 7.1 to find the average maximum heart rate and heart rate "target zone" for your age. The "target zone" is the rate your heart should beat immediately following exercise in order to benefit your heart and lungs.

As an example, for a 40-year-old, the chart shows that the average maximum heart rate is 180, and the heart rate "Target Zone" is 108-135 beats per minute. If your heart rate immediately following exercise is below the suggested Target Zone range for your age, exercise a little harder, and if above, exercise with less vigor. After exercising six months or longer, your heart rate can safely go as high as 85% of your maximum heart rate. However, it is not necessary to exercise that hard to stay in good condition.

Should You See a Doctor Before Exercising?

For most people, it is not necessary to see a doctor before beginning an exercise program. The National Institutes of Health recommends

To find your heart rate Target Zone, look for the age category closest to your age and read the line across. For example, if you are 43, the closest age on the chart is 45; your heart rate target zone is 105 to 131 beats per minute.

Age	Heart Rate Target Zone 60-75%	Average Maximum Heart Rate 100%
20 years	120-150 beats per min. (60-75% of 200 beats)	200 beats per minute
25 years	117-146 beats per min.	195
30 years	114-142 beats per min.	190
35 years	111-138 beats per min.	185
40 years	108-135 beats per min.	180
45 years	105-131 beats per min.	175
50 years	102-127 beats per min.	170
55 years	99-123 beats per min.	165
60 years	96-120 beats per min.	160
65 years	93-116 beats per min.	155
70 years	90-113 beats per min.	150

Your maximum heart rate is usually 220 minus your age. However, the above figures are averages and should be used as general guidelines.

To see if you are within your heart rate Target Zone, take your pulse immediately after you stop exercising. Count it for 30 seconds and multiply by two. If your pulse is below your Target Zone, exercise a little harder the next time. If you're above your Target Zone, exercise a little easier. And if it falls within the Target Zone, you're doing fine. Once you're exercising within your Target Zone, you should check your pulse at least once each week during the first 3 months and periodically thereafter.

Source: The National Heart, Lung and Blood Institute, National Institutes of Health

Table 7.1 Use this table to determine your heart rate Target Zone for exercise.

seeing your doctor only if one of the following conditions applies to you:

1) Your doctor said you have heart trouble, a heart murmur, or you have had a heart attack.
2) You frequently have pains or pressure—in the left or midchest area, left neck, shoulder, or arm—during or right after you exercise.
3) You often feel faint or have spells of severe dizziness.
4) You experience extreme breathlessness after mild exertion.
5) Your doctor said your blood pressure was too high and is not under control; or you don't know if your blood pressure is normal.
6) Your doctor said you have bone or joint problems such as arthritis.
7) You are over age 60 and not accustomed to vigorous exercise.
8) Your father, mother, brother, or sister had a heart attack before age 50.

9) You have a medical condition not mentioned here which might need special attention in an exercise program. (For example, insulin-dependent diabetes.)

Special Diet Tips for Athletes

- To replace the fluid lost during exercise, drink two glasses of water for every pound of weight lost while exercising.
- There is no need to drink a "sports drink" to replace electrolytes lost during exercise. Proportionally more water is lost than electrolytes. The next nutritious meal will replace the small amount of electrolytes lost.
- For endurance athletes (exercising vigorously for more than 90 minutes), it is best to take fluid with some calories during performance. Good choices are a 7–10% solution of sugar water (the sugar concentration in a soft drink), apple juice or a banana with water.
- Weight lifters should keep protein intake to no more than 15% of total calories, which is the upper limit recommended for the general public. This is equivalent to approximately 0.7 gram of protein per pound of body weight. For a 150 pound man, this would be a *maximum* of 105 grams of protein per day. (150 pounds x 0.7 grams/pound = 105 grams of protein.)

  (Excess protein, greater than 15% of total calories, does not build larger muscles nor is it stored in muscle tissue. Rather, it is broken down into its components, including urea, which is excreted from the body; and the remainder, which is converted to carbohydrate or stored as fat. Eating too much protein usually means you are not eating enough carbohydrate, the most important energy source for athletes. Carbohydrate is stored in the muscle as glycogen, which is the fuel the body needs during exercise.)

8

Medical Tests For Blood Pressure and Cholesterol—Know Your Numbers

Blood pressure and cholesterol tests help determine the risk for heart disease. Cholesterol tests tell us if excessive artery-clogging fat is circulating in the blood. If so, positive steps can be taken to reduce these levels through diet; and if that is not enough, with the addition of drugs.

Blood pressure measurements indicate whether the heart and blood vessels are being overly stressed while pumping blood throughout the body. If this condition goes unchecked, it can cause enlargement of the heart, weakening of blood vessel walls and can lead to strokes. Changes in diet and lifestyle can reduce blood pressure.

Many of us do not adopt a healthy lifestyle unless a medical test indicates we are at risk. These tests can thus serve as the impetus for positive changes. It makes more sense, though, to adopt a healthy lifestyle regardless of test results, because everyone is at risk to some extent and test results do not tell us everything.

Screening Tests Readily Available

Health care professionals in many communities have provided opportunities to have blood pressure and cholesterol screening tests done at little or no cost. The tests are conducted at shopping malls, drug stores, fairgrounds and other popular locations. If you have an abnormal screening test, or if you think the results are questionable, it would be wise to have the test repeated at your doctor's office. There is no excuse for being unaware of these two very important numbers. It can improve your chances for a longer and healthier life.

Cholesterol Testing

Who Should Be Tested?

All adults over the age of 20 should have their cholesterol checked, according to guidelines of the National Cholesterol Education Program. Children should be tested if there is a family history of heart disease or if one of the parents has high cholesterol. Still, some pediatricians are in favor of screening all school-age children, since some parents do not know their cholesterol levels.

What are Desirable Cholesterol Values?*

A cholesterol screening test measures total blood cholesterol. It can be done as a finger prick test or a vial of blood can be drawn from a vein in your arm. In either case, no fasting is required. Figure 8.1 summarizes the risk classifications based on total cholesterol levels. Values of less than 200 milligrams per deciliter (mg/dl) are "desirable" or low risk. Those between 200 and 239 are "borderline/high risk," and those 240 and above are considered "high risk." This puts over 50% of adult Americans above the desirable level and 25% in the high risk category. If your cholesterol level is below 200, you do not need further testing. You should still follow a prudent diet (less than 30% of calories from fat) to keep it low, and be tested again within five years.

Risk of Heart Disease Based on Total Cholesterol	
Total Cholesterol (mg/dl)	Classification
Less than 200	Desirable (Low risk)
200 - 239	Borderline/High risk
240 and above	High risk

Figure 8.1 Risk of heart disease based on total blood cholesterol.

Cholesterol Values over 200 (mg/dl)

If your cholesterol level is over 200, you should have the test repeated at your doctor's office. The average of the two results is used to make decisions regarding treatment. If the difference in the two values is greater than 30, it is recommended that the test be repeated.

Lipoprotein Analysis

Once your correct value is established, a lipoprotein analysis may be recommended. This is a blood test which measures the HDL or "good"

*The recommendations regarding cholesterol levels are based on the guidelines of the National Cholesterol Education Program's, "Report of the Expert Panel on Detection, Evaluation, and Treatment of High Cholesterol in Adults," October, 1987.

cholesterol, LDL or "bad" cholesterol, and triglycerides. This test should be done if your cholesterol level is above 240; or if it is between 200 and 240, *and* you have obvious signs of heart disease or at least two other heart disease risk factors. A 12-hour fast prior to this test is required. (See Figure 8.2 for the list of risk factors.)

(In February, 1992, an expert panel of the National Heart, Lung, and Blood Institute, recommended that *all* adults have their HDL cholesterol measured as part of standard cholesterol testing. It will probably be just a matter of time before it becomes part of routine cholesterol testing.)

Risk Factors for Heart Disease
(in addition to high cholesterol)

Male gender
Family history of premature heart disease (before age 55)
Cigarette smoking
High blood pressure
Low HDL cholesterol(less than 35 mg/dl)
Diabetes mellitus
Circulatory disorders
Extreme obesity (more than 30% over ideal body weight)

Figure 8.2 Risk factors for heart disease.

A lipoprotein analysis gives a more precise picture of your blood lipids (fats) than total blood cholesterol. By breaking down blood lipids into various components, this test enables your doctor to see the type and degree of cholesterol problem you have. He can then recommend the best treatment for your particular case. You may be at high risk if your LDL cholesterol is too high or your HDL cholesterol is too low.

Desirable LDL Values

The higher your LDL value, the greater your risk for heart disease. There are three classifications of risk based on LDL cholesterol, just as for total cholesterol, as shown in Figure 8.3. The "desirable" level is less than 130; "borderline/high risk" is from 130 to 159; and "high risk" is 160 and above.

Risk of Heart Disease Based on LDL Cholesterol

LDL Cholesterol (mg/dl)	Classification Based On LDL Cholesterol
Less than 130	Desirable (Low risk)
130 to 159	Borderline/high risk
160 and Above	High risk

Figure 8.3 Classification of heart disease risk based on LDL cholesterol.

Decisions regarding dietary or drug treatment will depend not only on the LDL cholesterol level, but also on other risk factors. Those who have definite signs of heart disease *or* two or more other risk factors (Figure 8.2), should reduce LDL cholesterol levels to less than 130. For those who do not have these risk factors, an LDL cholesterol of less than 160 is the goal.

Keep in mind that these goals are *minimal,* and are used to justify the use of drugs if these levels cannot be achieved by diet alone. If lower levels can be achieved, risk is further reduced. Research has shown that for most individuals LDL levels must be lower than 100 in order to reverse atherosclerosis.

Diet modification is the first step in treating high LDL cholesterol. Calories from fat should account for *no more than* 30% of total calories, with *no more than* 10% from saturated fat (Step 1 Diet). If LDL levels are still too high after several months, saturated fat intake should be further reduced to *less than* 7% of total calories (Step 2 Diet). Diet therapy should be maintained for at least six months before drugs are considered, unless LDL levels are extremely high (over 300) and other risk factors are present.

HDL Cholesterol—A Separate Risk Factor

The higher the HDL cholesterol, the lower the risk for heart disease. The function of HDL is to pick up excess cholesterol from the blood stream, vessel walls and tissues, and carry it back to the liver, where it is converted to bile acids and excreted from the body.

Average HDL levels for men are 40 to 50, and for women are 50 to 60. Higher levels have been shown to be protective factors against heart disease. Levels below 35 are a signal of high risk for heart disease. Figure 8.4 lists the risk classifications that correspond with HDL levels.

Risk of Heart Disease Based on HDL Cholesterol	
HDL Cholesterol (mg/dl)	Classification Based On HDL Cholesterol
Above 40	Desirable
35 to 40	Borderline/high risk
Less than 35	High risk

Figure 8.4 Risk of heart disease based on HDL cholesterol.

It is more difficult to raise HDL than lower overall cholesterol. Diet changes do not have much effect. The best ways to increase HDL levels, other than drugs, are to maintain ideal body weight and to participate in regular aerobic exercise, 20 to 30 minutes per day, three to five times per week.

Triglycerides

Triglycerides make up 95% of the lipids (fats) circulating in the body. They travel in the bloodstream in lipoprotein packages, i.e., they are surrounded by protein, just like cholesterol. Triglycerides below 250 (mg/dl) are considered acceptable, although below 150 is desirable. (If cholesterol levels are normal, there is no greater risk for heart disease as long as triglyceride levels are less than 250.) Levels from 250 to 500 are considered moderately elevated, and those above 500 are high.

The role of triglycerides in heart disease is less understood than HDL and LDL cholesterol. Often, an elevated triglyceride level is accompanied by an increase in total cholesterol and LDL cholesterol, and/or a decrease in HDL cholesterol. When two or more of these factors act together, there is an increased risk for heart disease. Most researchers feel, however, that moderately elevated triglycerides alone is not a cause for concern. As a result, most doctors do not advocate treating moderate elevations if the HDL and LDL cholesterol levels are in the desirable range.

William Castelli, renowned director of the Framingham Heart Study, advocates a more aggressive approach. He recommends treatment (first diet for six months, then drugs if needed) if triglycerides are above 150 while HDL is below 40. His research has shown a definite risk factor when even slightly low HDL is combined with triglycerides over 150.

If triglyceride levels are greater than 500, they present a risk not only for heart disease but also for pancreatitis or inflammation of the pancreas. Levels this high call for aggressive diet and drug treatment. Less than 1 person in 1000 has this condition.

Some of the dietary and lifestyle factors that lower triglycerides also have a positive effect on LDL and HDL cholesterol. Reducing saturated fats and losing weight (if overweight) lowers triglycerides as well as LDL cholesterol. Regular, vigorous exercise increases HDL values, while decreasing triglycerides.

There are certain dietary factors that sometimes raise triglycerides but do not appear to increase the risk for heart disease. These include a high carbohydrate diet and *moderate* intakes of alcohol. Neither of these adversely affects cholesterol values. Refer to Figure 8.5 for a summary of the dietary and lifestyle factors that reduce the risk for heart disease.

Cholesterol Ratios

The cholesterol ratio is sometimes used to predict the likelihood of developing heart disease. It is determined by dividing total cholesterol by HDL cholesterol. For example, if your total cholesterol is 180 and your HDL is 50, your cholesterol ratio would be 180/50 or 3.6.

The ideal ratio, which indicates a very low risk for heart disease, is

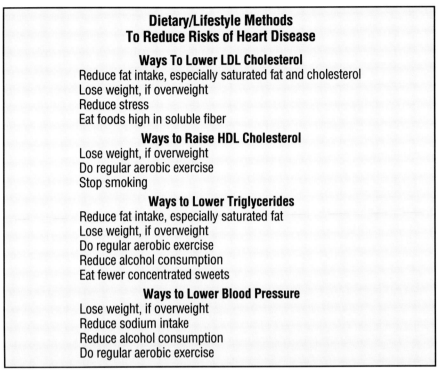

> **Dietary/Lifestyle Methods
> To Reduce Risks of Heart Disease**
>
> **Ways To Lower LDL Cholesterol**
> Reduce fat intake, especially saturated fat and cholesterol
> Lose weight, if overweight
> Reduce stress
> Eat foods high in soluble fiber
>
> **Ways to Raise HDL Cholesterol**
> Lose weight, if overweight
> Do regular aerobic exercise
> Stop smoking
>
> **Ways to Lower Triglycerides**
> Reduce fat intake, especially saturated fat
> Lose weight, if overweight
> Do regular aerobic exercise
> Reduce alcohol consumption
> Eat fewer concentrated sweets
>
> **Ways to Lower Blood Pressure**
> Lose weight, if overweight
> Reduce sodium intake
> Reduce alcohol consumption
> Do regular aerobic exercise

Figure 8.5   A summary of the dietary and lifestyle recommendations to reduce the risk for heart disease.

under 3.5. The ratio which represents an average risk of heart disease for men is 5.0; while for women, it is 4.5. The lower the ratio, the lower the risk. Although the ratio is helpful in predicting the likelihood of CHD, dietary and/or drug treatment is based primarily on the HDL and LDL values.

Cholesterol Levels For Children

We also need to be concerned with the cholesterol levels of children, since heart disease does not begin in middle-aged adults. Rather, the earliest signs of the disease are evident in young children and teens in the form of fatty streaks that line the aorta and coronary arteries. Studies of U.S. soldiers, who died in Korea and Vietnam, showed that many had plaque and a few even had severe blockage of the coronary arteries at a very young age.

Research has shown that cholesterol levels "track" well from childhood into adulthood. In other words, a given measurement tends to keep the same rank as the child gets older. *A child with high cholesterol has an 80% chance of having an elevated level as a young adult.*

Desirable Levels

The National Institutes of Health makes the following recommendations regarding children's cholesterol. If the cholesterol level is below 170, which corresponds with the 75th percentile, it is in the "desirable" range for children. These children should still be encouraged to follow the prudent low-fat diet recommended by the American Heart Association. (This diet consists of *less than* 30% of total calories from fat, of which no more than 10% should be saturated fat. See Chapter 3 to see what constitutes a diet of 30% of calories from fat.)

Children whose cholesterol levels are between 170 and 185 (the 75th and 90th percentile, respectively) should closely follow the low-fat diet recommended by the American Heart Association. The goal is to reduce their level to below 170. They should be retested in a year.

Children who have cholesterol levels from 185 to 200 (90th to 95th percentile) may need to restrict fat intake further (than 30% of total calories). Restricting it to about 20 to 25% of total calories is sometimes necessary to bring cholesterol to the "desirable" level. (See Chapter 3.) Cholesterol levels of 200 in children correspond to values of 260 in an adult.

If cholesterol levels are above 200 (95th percentile), children may have a hereditary form of high cholesterol. These children should closely follow the dietary regimen mentioned previously. Most children respond very well to diet alone. However, if diet produces insufficient response after at least six months, the guidelines (by the National Institutes of Health) suggest that these children "should be considered for treatment" with a cholesterol-lowering drug. Thus far, their use appears to be safe with children. Tests have shown that they have no effect on growth and development. Your pediatrician will make a recommendation on this, taking other risk factors into account.

Parental Approach Is Important

Parents should be careful to use a positive approach in dealing with children whose cholesterol levels are too high. The children should not be made to feel that they have some type of disease or that foods are a form of medicine. The emphasis should be on encouraging all the aspects of a healthy lifestyle and healthy diet. These include regular exercise, maintaining ideal body weight and no smoking. In the long run, this is more important than significantly reducing a moderately elevated cholesterol level.

Overzealous parents can do more harm than good. Some parents may feel that if restricting fat produces good results, that reducing it further will be better. This is not necessarily the case. Restricting fat too much (to less than 20% of total calories) can be harmful to growing children, who need the nutrients and caloric density of at least this much fat. Some very active, slim children may need a little more—25 to 30% of calories from fat.

The Gradual Rise in Cholesterol Levels

Cholesterol levels do not rise during childhood as they tend to do during adult years. In fact, they usually drop slightly following adolescence. In general, not until people reach their 20's does cholesterol begin its upward climb. (See Figures 8.6 and 8.7.)

The increases with age can be greatly reduced if a low-fat diet is adopted and followed from childhood throughout adulthood. The longer a low-fat diet is observed, the greater the reduction in mortality rates from heart disease.

Cholesterol Levels (mg/dl) Change with Age

Percentiles for White Males

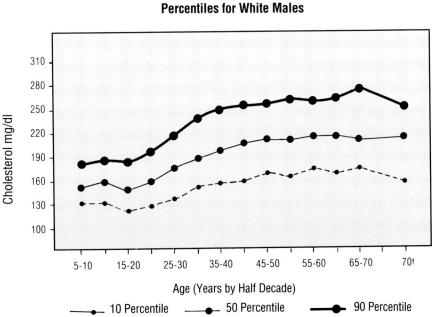

Source: Adapted from the Lipid Research Clinics Population Studies Data Book.

Figure 8.6 How cholesterol levels for white males at the 10th, 50th and 90th percentiles change throughout a lifetime (ages 5 to 70+).

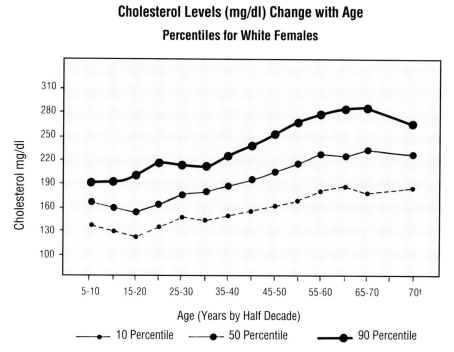

Cholesterol Levels (mg/dl) Change with Age

Percentiles for White Females

Source: Adapted from the Lipid Research Clinics Population Studies Data Book.

Figure 8.7 How cholesterol levels for white females at the 10th, 50th and 90th percentiles change throughout a lifetime (ages 5 to 70+).

Drugs to Treat High Cholesterol Levels

There are a number of drugs on the market to treat high cholesterol. These drugs are recommended *only* when a low-fat diet fails to lower cholesterol adequately. Table 8.1 lists the cholesterol-lowering drugs, with a breakdown of their average costs, effectiveness in decreasing LDL or increasing HDL cholesterol, side effects and special precautions.

Blood Pressure Measurements

High blood pressure is the greatest risk factor for heart disease—even more significant than high cholesterol. It is a major cause of heart failure, kidney failure and stroke. You need to know if your level is high, so you can do whatever is necessary to lower it and reduce the associated health risks. Everyone should have yearly blood pressure checks.

There are still many people who are unaware that they have high blood pressure, but the number is dwindling. Before 1970, only about one-quarter of the estimated 60 million Americans with high blood pressure knew it and only a quarter of these were adequately treated. By

Major Cholesterol-Lowering Drugs

Drugs	Average Cost/mo	Well Tolerated?	Decrease in LDL* Choles.	Effect on HDL* Choles.	Side Effects	Special Precautions
Cholestyramine Questran Cholybar Colestipol Colestid	$75 - 95	Varies	15-30%	slight increase	Upper and lower gastrointestinal (GI) disturbances (constipation, excess gas, stomach acidity).	May alter absorption of other drugs. May increase blood triglyceride levels.
Nicotinic acid, Nicobid, Niacin, Time release niacin	$4 - 8	Varies	15-30%	increase	Flushing, itching, upper GI disturbances (stomach acidity or nausea). Flushing is decreased by pretreatment with aspirin or advil.	Monitor for increased blood uric acid levels, hyperglycemia, and liver abnormalities. Not for use in patients with peptic ulcer liver disease or gouty arthritis.
Lovastatin Mevacor Simvastatin Zocar	$120 - 175	yes	25-45%	increase	Generally well tolerated. Most common side effects include GI disturbances and muscle pain (less than 5% of patients).	Patients should be monitored for changes in liver function. Increased risk of muscle inflammation, if used with niacin or gemfibrozil.
Gemfibrozil Lopid	$65 - 95	yes	5-15%	increase	Infrequent side effects, most common being GI disturbances.	Not for use in patients with gallbladder disease. Increases the effect of blood-thinning drugs. May increase LDL cholesterol in those with high triglyceride levels.
Probucol Lorelco	$105 - 120	yes	10-15%	decrease	Generally well tolerated. Uncommon side effects include diarrhea, gas, nausea or abdominal pain (less than 5% of patients).	Lowers HDL cholesterol. Not recommended for patients with abnormal EKG.

*LDL is the "bad" cholesterol, while HDL is the "good" cholesterol.
Adapted from: National Cholesterol Education Program, *Report of the Expert Panel on Detection, Evaluation and Treatment of High Blood Cholesterol in Adults*, 1989.

Table 8.1 Cholesterol-lowering drugs.

1984, one-half of the hypertensive population were aware of their condition and two-thirds of these received some form of antihypertensive therapy.

What Levels Constitute Hypertension?

For adults, a diagnosis of hypertension is made if the systolic blood pressure (top number) is greater than 140 millimeters of mercury (mm Hg), and/or the diastolic blood pressure (bottom number) is greater than 90. At this level, there is an approximately 50% increase in mortality related to heart disease. Therefore, even modest elevations carry substantial risks. On the other hand, reductions of any amount lower the health risks related to hypertension.

One elevated reading does not necessarily mean you need to be treated for high blood pressure. Instead, a diagnosis is based on the average of *at least* two readings taken on *at least* two different occasions.

Some individuals have a condition called *labile hypertension* in which blood pressure levels climb when they are under stress. They can experience wide fluctuations in their blood pressure, from day to day and even hour to hour. When this is the case, a physician may suggest that they record their blood pressure several times throughout the day, (with a portable blood pressure machine) over a two to four week period; or they may be advised to use a 24-hour recording device to determine blood pressure during normal activities. (A doctor's office can be a stressful environment for some.) Treatment for labile hypertension is based on the average of the home recorded blood pressures.

Hypertension in Children and Adolescents

Children and adolescents can also have hypertension. The National Heart, Lung and Blood Institute considers the following levels to be too high for the various age groups: 116/76 (mm Hg) (three to five years old); 122/78 (six to nine years old); 126/82 (10 to 12 years old); 136/86 (13 to 15 years old; and 142/92 (16 to 18 years old). Your pediatrician can advise you on treatment if your child's level is higher than those listed above.

Recommended Treatment

Diet and Behavior Modification

A low-salt diet (from 1500 to 2400 milligrams of sodium per day) is highly recommended for anyone with hypertension, regardless of whether drugs are required. Eating more potassium-rich foods also may be helpful for some. In addition, certain behavioral changes are encouraged to either eliminate the need for drugs or to increase their effectiveness. These include weight loss (if overweight), regular aerobic exercise, and limiting alcohol consumption.

Diastolic Pressure Is Too High

For those whose diastolic blood pressure (bottom number) is moderately elevated (from 90 to 100), the diet and behavior modification mentioned previously is sometimes all that is needed to bring the level below 90. Those whose diastolic pressure is above 100 almost always require some type of medication.

Generally, drugs are recommended for anyone whose average diastolic pressure remains above 90. The drugs available to treat hypertension include diuretics, beta blockers, angiotensin converting enzyme (ACE) inhibitors, and calcium entry blockers.

The drug of choice depends on the severity of the disease, degree of elevation, and individual side effects. Diuretics are usually the first choice drug for those with moderately elevated blood pressure because they have been proven effective and the side effects are minimal. Beta-blockers are most effective for those who have elevated blood pressure affected by stress. For some, a combination of drugs works best. If you take blood pressure medication and are experiencing unpleasant side effects, discuss this with your doctor. He or she may suggest a different drug or combination of drugs that will work better for you.

Systolic Pressure Is Too High

Treatment of high systolic blood pressure in the absence of high diastolic pressure is still debatable. Although studies have shown an increased risk for heart disease with high systolic pressure, it has not yet been proven that drugs reduce mortality or help in disease prevention.

Still, the overall recommendation is to use conservative drug treatment with a goal of 10% reduction in systolic blood pressure. If drugs produce bothersome side effects, they are usually discontinued.

The thresholds for initiating drug treatment are based on age. The following guidelines suggest who should receive treatment: those under 35 years old who have systolic blood pressure greater than 140; those 35 to 59 years old whose systolic pressure is greater than 150; and those over 65 years old who have systolic pressure over 160.

9

Weight Control

Sixty-two percent of American adults consider themselves over-weight, according to a poll conducted by Weight Watchers, Inc. Actually, 20 to 30% are truly overweight. That is still a high percentage—approximately one-quarter of the adult population.

Why are so many overweight? National food surveys tell us it is not because we consume an inordinately high number of calories. Our ancestors from the early 1900's consumed more calories than we do today and yet fewer of them were overweight. The reason for this is that we get less exercise, and have a higher percentage of fat in our diet; 40% vs. 25–30% for our ancestors. Calories from fat turn into body fat much more efficiently than calories from carbohydrate or protein.

Factors That Influence Body Weight

Fat from Foods

The higher the percentage of fat in the diet, the greater the likelihood of being overweight. There are two reasons for this. The first is that fat calories are converted to body fat more readily than carbohydrate or protein calories. Excess fat from foods is converted to body fat using only 3% of its calories, whereas excess carbohydrate uses 23% of its calories in the process of conversion to body fat. This means fewer of the excess calories from carbohydrate will be converted to and stored as fat. Of course, neither dietary fat nor carbohydrate will be converted to body fat unless *excess* calories, over and above what the body needs to maintain itself, are consumed.

The second reason that higher fat intake means greater weight gain is that it takes more calories to satisfy your appetite or "fill you up" when there is a higher percentage of fat. This is because fat is much more dense than carbohydrate or protein. It contains 9 calories per gram, whereas carbohydrate and protein both contain 4 calories per gram.

To emphasis this point, let's compare the calories in similar quantities of food when 20% of calories come from fat vs. 40% of calories from fat.

The difference in calories is significant. For example, a plateful of food, with 20% of the calories from fat, has 650 calories; while the exact same quantity of food, with 40% of the calories from fat, contains 1050 calories. It is easier to feel satisfied with fewer calories when you can eat a greater volume or quantity of food.

Another example, shown in Figure 9.1, is to compare one cup of fresh strawberries, which has negligible fat, with a Strawberry Snack Pie, where 37% of its calories come from fat. The cup of strawberries has only 45 calories, compared with 340 calories in the snack pie. They have a similar amount of bulk or volume, but the pie has over seven times as many calories. (The concentrated sugar in the snack pie is also a significant contributor to calories.)

On the other hand, you will probably feel hungry again *sooner* after eating the strawberries than the snack pie because fat provides a longer-lasting feeling of satiety (satisfaction and fullness) than carbohydrate or protein because it is digested more slowly. Still, you'll be consuming fewer calories in the long run when eating foods lower in fat, even if you feel the need to snack on low-fat foods between meals.

Fresh Strawberries   **Strawberry Snack Pie**

45 Calories   340 calories

Figure 9.1 A strawberry snack pie, with 37% of its calories from fat, has over seven times as many calories as one cup of fresh strawberries, which has only a trace of fat. Both have approximately the same volume.

Exercise

Exercise is the second factor that affects body weight, since calories are burned during exercise. The more vigorous the exercise, the more calories that are burned in a given period of time. Refer to Figure 9.2 for a comparison of the approximate number of calories burned in various forms of exercise.

Exercise is an aid to weight control in more ways than just burning calories. It enhances the breakdown and loss of body fat, while helping preserve lean muscle tissue. Furthermore, when dieting, the basal metabolic rate slows down, which means the body burns fewer calories while at rest. Exercise while dieting is credited with helping the body return to a normal metabolic rate after dieting has stopped. This is very important in weight maintenance.

Exercise also helps dieters psychologically. Regular exercise encourages an overall feeling of well-being and fitness. This positive feeling helps dieters continue toward dietary goals.

Number of Calories Burned during Exercise	
Activity	Calories per 30 minutes
Domestic Work	90
Walking, 2 1/2 mph	105
Bicycling, 5 1/2 mph	105
Gardening	110
Golf; Lawn mowing, power mower	125
Bowling	135
Walking, 3 3/4 mph	150
Swimming, 1/4 mph	150
Square dancing, Volleyball	175
Roller skating	175
Wood chopping, Hand sawing	200
Tennis	210
Cross country skiing, 10 mph	300
Squash, Handball	300
Jogging, 7 mph (9-minute miles)	300
Bicycling, 13 mph	330
Running, 10 mph (6-minute miles)	450

Figure 9.2 Approximate number of calories burned by a 150-pound person while performing various activities for 30 minutes.

Heredity

The third, and final factor affecting weight is heredity. Recent studies conducted in the late 1980's and early 1990's, show that heredity plays a greater role in weight control than once thought. A Quebec study reported in 1990 that genes determine how the body handles excess calories. Some people's bodies handle the excess calories very inefficiently, converting them to muscle protein rather than body fat. Since it takes nine times as much energy to turn food into muscle as it does to store it as fat, those who turn excess calories into muscle tissue burn up many of their excess calories in the process.

In the Quebec study, 12 pairs of identical twins were hospitalized for 120 days so their diets and physical activity could be closely monitored. For the first 30 days, they were fed the equivalent of their usual diet which maintained their weight during that period. For the next 90 days, each pair of twins was fed 1000 extra calories over their maintenance diet. They were not allowed to do strenuous exercise, but were required to do a specified amount of walking.

The results were surprising to everyone concerned. Within each pair of twins, the weight gain was nearly the same. But there was a great variation from one pair of twins to another. The weight gain of the pairs varied from 9 pounds to 29 pounds.

What this study showed was that some people, because of their genetic makeup, have a greater tendency to put on weight. Of course, *all* who ate excess calories over the three month period did gain weight, but some gained three times as much as others. One can deduce from this study that the reverse is true—it is easier for some people to lose weight or maintain weight than others. Weight control is within everyone's reach, but some will always have to work harder at it than others.

Our Body's Reaction to Dieting

Whenever anyone is dieting, i.e. when calorie intake is restricted to less than what it takes to maintain weight, the body reacts as if it is being starved. To protect itself, the body slows down its metabolism to conserve limited food. What this means is that the body burns fewer calories than usual while at rest. This makes it more difficult, but not impossible, to lose weight.

Weight loss should be gradual, not exceeding one to two pounds per week. (The slower the weight is taken off, the more likely it will stay off. The U.S. Department of Agriculture recommends that dieters lose no more than one pound per week.) When the weight loss is at this rate, approximately 60 to 80% of the weight is lost as fat, and just 20 to 40% as lean body mass. In quick-loss starvation diets, a much greater proportion is lost as lean body mass and fluids. To protect against excess muscle loss, women are encouraged to consume at least 1200 calories per day; and men, a minimum of 1500 calories per day.

After dieting for a period of time, many dieters complain of reaching a plateau, where they cannot seem to lose more weight. When weight is lost, 10 to 20 pounds for example, less food is needed to maintain the lower weight. It takes fewer calories to maintain 140 pounds than 160 pounds. If additional weight loss is desired, either calories need to be restricted further or exercise increased.

Once the desired weight is reached by a gradual method of weight loss in combination with regular exercise, the metabolic rate increases to a rate normal for the new weight. The new metabolic rate is generally within 10% of the original metabolic rate. Still former dieters must eat less than they did previously to maintain the lower weight.

What It Takes to Gain/Lose Weight

To gain a pound of weight, you must consume an excess of approximately 3500 calories. That means 3500 calories over and above what you need to maintain your weight. One piece of pecan pie (495 calories) will not do it.

The reverse is true if you are trying to lose weight. If your goal is to lose a pound a week, you must eliminate about 3500 calories over a week's time, either through exercise or calorie reduction. This averages out to 500 fewer calories per day. You can either eat 500 fewer calories, exercise enough to burn 500 calories, or a combination of both, which is preferable. For weight loss of one to two pounds per week, you will need to eliminate 500 to 1000 calories per day.

Types of Diets

Medically Supervised Liquid Diets

These diets are characterized by extreme calorie restriction; usually no more than 420 to 800 calories per day. For the first two to three months, nutritional needs are met by a liquid formula only, which contains protein, vitamins and minerals. After the liquid diet phase, solid food is gradually reintroduced. The expected weight loss while on liquid diets is 3–5 pounds per week. The more popular medically supervised liquid diets are Optifast, Medifast and Health Management Resources (HMR).

All of these programs are fairly expensive, ranging from about $1000 to $3500, and they last anywhere from 6 to 18 months. All are available only through hospitals and clinics, and most require that participants be at least 50 pounds, or 20% over their ideal body weight. The dropout rate is high—usually about 40 to 50%.

There are a number of serious drawbacks to rapid weight loss diets. The most obvious is that dieters who lose weight this quickly will most likely not *keep* the weight off. Based on studies of liquid diet programs at university medical centers, it is estimated that no more than 10% keep the weight off a year or two after completing the program. What makes subsequent weight gain nearly inevitable is that fat cells can not shrink fast enough, nor metabolism readjust adequately when weight loss is this rapid. The body tries to make up for the deficiencies it experienced by putting weight back on with only a minimal amount of calories—perhaps only 1200 to 1500 calories a day. This makes it extremely difficult to keep pounds off when solid foods are reintroduced.

Another drawback is that proportionally more lean muscle mass and less fat is lost with liquid diets. *The body is capable of losing no more than one to two pounds of fat per week.* Any pounds lost over and above this are muscle and water. Consequently, not much more, and sometimes even less fat is lost with this type of diet than with a conventional low-calorie diet.

Unpleasant side effects usually occur as the body responds to starvation diets. First, to conserve calories, the body temperature drops, causing a "chilly" feeling. Second, the body cuts back its blood supply to the tiny vessels near the skin's surface, which creates rough, dry skin. Third, exercise becomes difficult as the result of being in a weakened state. It is often met by dizziness and/or cramps.

The medical rationale for these diet programs is that these patients have not been able to lose weight using more conventional methods and that their obesity is increasing their risks for heart disease, high blood pressure, stroke and diabetes. Even though it does not work for many, i.e. not many succeed in *keeping* the pounds off, it does work for some. Starvation or liquid diets should be diets of last resort.

Over-the-Counter Liquid Diets

Some self-prescribed liquid diet products are available at the grocery stores and drug stores and require no professional supervision. Slender by Carnation encourages you to use only their product, with no supplements of real food. If you drink four servings per day, as recommended, you will consume 880 calories. It claims to contain 100% of the RDA for protein, vitamins and minerals.

Another product, Ultra Slim Fast comes in powdered form to be mixed with 8 ounces of milk, water or fruit juice. The instructions recommend three servings per day—at breakfast, lunch and an afternoon snack—plus a regular meal at dinner. The three servings of liquid formula contain 660 calories plus 12 grams of fiber.

These diets are characterized by a yo-yo form of weight loss, i.e., rapid weight loss followed by quick weight gain when off the liquid diet. (See "Medically Supervised Liquid Diets," above.) This tendency is slightly lessened if there is at least one regular meal per day. A major concern with unsupervised liquid diets is that dietary deficiencies can occur. Also, without proper medical supervision, the heart and gallbladder can be adversely affected if pounds are shed too quickly.

Real Food Diets with Required Special Products

Two popular diet programs that require special products are Jenny Craig and Nutri/System. Both stress nutrition education and behavior modification, and encourage regular aerobic exercise. Their weight loss goal is 1 to 2 pounds per week. They require the use of pre-packaged meals during the weight loss period. The use of these foods is essentially their way of choosing low-fat foods and monitoring calorie intake for you.

These diets are beneficial for those who do not want to count calories or make their own food choices. On the other hand, it would be very difficult for those who must eat out frequently. In the beginning of a diet program, pre-packaged meals may be helpful in educating dieters on food selection and recommended portion sizes.

There are two main disadvantages to using this type of diet plan. One is that their foods are more expensive than buying similar types at the grocery store. The cost of the pre-packaged meals is $60 to $70 per week, not including the fresh produce and skim milk you buy on your own. Another disadvantage is that eventually when your weight-loss goal is reached, you will be required to select your own foods, and this may be difficult if you have not had to do it all along.

Both programs continue for one year after the weight loss goal is reached to help with the maintenance diet. Educating clients on how to make healthy food choices on their own is the goal during this phase.

Real Food Diets Without Special Products

The strengths of these programs lie in their educational efforts to teach dieters how to make the right food choices on their own without the use of special products. If good eating habits are learned and implemented by the dieter during the period of weight loss, it should be easier to adjust to a maintenance diet once the goal has been reached. Three diet programs that offer this approach are Diet Workshop, Weight Loss Clinic, and Weight Watchers.

Diet Workshop and Weight Watchers educate their clients on food selection, exercise, etc. through weekly group meetings headed by trained "graduates" of their programs. Weight Loss Clinic encourages short (5 to 10 minutes) one-on-one meetings with staff members, as often as the client desires, Monday through Friday. Staff members may be nurses, dietitians or company-trained counselors.

Weight loss recommendations from these programs are similar. Diet Workshop recommends a weight loss of 1 1/2 to 2 pounds/week; Weight Watchers, 1 to 2 pounds/week; and Weight Loss Clinic, 2 to 3 pounds/week. Maintenance phases vary from 4 weeks to 6 months. Both Diet Workshop and Weight Watchers offer free lifetime memberships for those who maintain their losses.

The costs of Diet Workshop and Weight Watchers are similar. Both have modest initial membership fees plus weekly charges until maintenance. Weight Loss Clinic is a more expensive program. Prices vary slightly in different locations, so check the prices in your area.

Tips on Choosing the Best Diet Plan for You

All diet programs have advantages and disadvantages, and some people have more success with one type than another. No matter what method you use to lose weight, however, to keep it off involves a *lifelong commitment* to making wise, low-fat food choices on a regular basis and incorporating an exercise program into your lifestyle.

The following is a list of points to consider in choosing a diet plan:

1) Can you create your own diet plan without relying on a special program? Many people are able to lose weight successfully on their own by reducing percentage of fat, reducing portion sizes, and exercising regularly. Now that you know what constitutes healthy low-fat food choices, you too will have a good chance at success.

2) Can you live with the diet plan indefinitely? Some programs are set up in the very beginning so that you can continue with them indefinitely. Obviously, you cannot live with a liquid diet or pre-packaged meals forever; but perhaps the maintenance phase of some of these diet programs could be continued indefinitely.

3) Do you need special crutches to aid in proper food selection and portion control (prepackaged meals and snacks); or, with proper education, can you make the right choices on your own?

4) Is the program individualized to take into account different rates of metabolism and caloric needs?

5) Does the program put you in touch with health professionals, such as physicians, dietitians or nurses? If not, ask your physician if the program is reputable. Some programs have been developed by health professionals and have well trained staffs who are knowledgeable about nutrition, behavior modification and the importance of exercise.

6) Is the recommended rate of weight loss the generally acceptable 1 to 2 pounds per week?

7) What percentage of the program's clients reach their goal weight and maintain it for at least one year? Generally, these numbers are not well documented, but it is still worth asking.

8) Will the maintenance plan fit your needs? Is it long enough and is the educational component adequate?

9) Can you afford the program? There is a wide variation in costs of different types of programs. The more expensive are not necessarily better.

10

Helpful Hints for Special Situations

Eating in Restaraunts

If you are a typical American, you eat out at least one meal in three, and by the year 2000, half of your food expenditures will go to the restaurant industry. For those who dine out frequently, it is imperative to make healthy food choices when you do. Otherwise, the tendency is to eat too much fat, cholesterol and sodium; and not enough calcium, fiber, fruits and vegetables. Gone are the days when you could justify abandoning your diet for the special occasions when you would eat out. For most people, eating out is no longer reserved just for special occasions.

Contrary to popular thinking, you can combine good taste with healthy food choices when eating out. Today there is a greater selection of low-fat menu items than ever before because of the increased demand for it by American consumers. In some cases, lower fat choices are marked with the American Heart Association symbol to designate that they are "heart healthy." This makes the selection process easier, but you must be careful not to add excess fat in the form of salad dressings, butter, sour cream or bacon bits. This could bring the meal well over the guidelines of the American Heart Association.

If you are unsure about how the food is prepared, do not be afraid to ask. You can also request that it be prepared a certain way, or that the sauce be on the side. Most restaurants are happy to oblige you if it is possible, since they want to have happy customers who will return. Also, inquire if substitutions are permissible, such as a vegetable or fruit, instead of hash browns or French fries. (Refer to the chart of Menu Terminology, Figure 10.1, to become familiar with the composition of sauces, various methods of food preparation, etc.)

If you are at a buffet where most of the fare is laden with mayonnaise and high-fat sauces, don't be discouraged. Take small portions of these foods, or omit them entirely, and fill up on breads and fruits, which are almost always available. When traveling by air, you can contact the airlines at least 24 hours in advance to order a low-fat, low-cholesterol or vegetarian meal.

Menu Terminology

Au gratin — a thick, creamy cheese sauce usually mixed with sliced potatoes or other vegetables and baked in an oven until a light brown crust is formed.

Bearnaise Sauce — a creamy sauce for beef or fish made with egg yolks, butter, vinegar, white wine and spices.

Bechamel Sauce — a white sauce made of cream, butter, flour, etc.

Blackened — a method of cooking meat, fish or poultry which was popularized as a form of Cajun (highly spiced) cooking. The food to be blackened is usually first dipped in oil, then covered by hot Cajun spices, and pan-fried at a very high temperature, thus "blackening" the fish or meat on the outside, while preserving the interior juices.

Bordelaise Sauce — a brown sauce flavored with red wine and shallots.

Bouillabaisse — a chowder made with several kinds of fish and shellfish, vegetables, seasonings, etc.

Braised — meat or poultry cooked slowly in a covered utensil in a small amount of liquid or in steam.

Creamed — as in creamed potatoes or creamed peas. Generally, a sauce made with flour, butter and cream or whole milk, that accompanies a vegetable.

Fricasseed — a method of cooking meat whereby it is cut into small pieces, stewed or fried, and served in a sauce of its own gravy.

Hollandaise Sauce — a creamy sauce, usually for fish or vegetables, made of butter, egg yolks, lemon juice, etc.

Poached — to cook in a boiling or simmering liquid. Fish or eggs are the foods most often cooked this way.

Ratatouille — a French appetizer or side dish containing eggplant, tomatoes, onions, green pepper and seasonings. It may be served hot or cold.

Sautéed — fried quickly, usually in a small amount of fat, although in some cases, greater amounts of fat are used.

Scalloped — to bake in a casserole with a milk or cream sauce and usually with bread crumbs.

Figure 10.1 Definitions of terms that commonly appear on restaurant menus.

Best Choices When Eating Out

The following suggestions should make it easier to choose healthy meals when eating out. The suggestions are far from complete, but should serve as a helpful guide.

Breakfast
* Egg whites or egg substitutes (no yolks), scrambled or in omelet form without cheese
* Bread, toast, English muffins, bagels (with thin scraping of cream cheese, margarine, and/or jams and jellies)
* Waffles or pancakes with syrup (preferably no butter, and little or no margarine)
* Cereal, cooked or cold, with low-fat or skim milk
* Fruits and fruit juices
* Low-fat cottage cheese

Lunch
* Soups—broth based or bean, including lentil, minestrone, split pea (avoid creamed soups)
* Sandwiches—plain turkey, chicken or tuna (without heavy mayonnaise); with mustard or small amount of mayonnaise. Add vegetables as desired.
* Salads—Choose from an assortment of greens and add plain or marinated vegetables when at a salad bar. Top with vinegar, lemon juice or a low-calorie salad dressing. Avoid or limit salads mixed with mayonnaise, including chicken salad, potato salad and macaroni salad. If salad comes with meal, ask for salad dressing on the side. (Limit or avoid bacon, egg, and cheese.)
* Small hamburger (no mayonnaise, cheese, or special sauce)
* Fresh fruit salad
* Baked potato, topped with low-fat cottage cheese, plain yogurt, baked beans or nonfat sour cream.
* Vegetarian chili, chicken fajita, bean burrito (Limit cheese and sour cream.)

Dinner—Appetizers
* Shrimp or crabmeat with seafood cocktail sauce
* Steamed shellfish including clams and mussels, served plain, with seafood cocktail sauce, or in broth (no butter or cheese sauces)
* Vegetables, fresh or marinated (preferably in vinegar with no oil—if oil is used, let most of oil drip off.)
* Fresh fruit

Dinner—Entrees
* Fish, shellfish, chicken, or turkey prepared with *little* or no fat—baked, grilled, blackened*, poached, steamed, roasted or stir-fried.
* Lean beef, pork tenderloin or lean ham. (Ideally, portions should be limited to 4 ounces.) Best beef choices include stir-fry dishes, shish kabobs, round steak and filet mignon, all prepared with little or no added fat.
* Create your own vegetarian entree by combining several side dishes of grains and vegetables.
* If you order a large portion of meat (7 ounces or more), split it with a companion, or take half of it home to eat later. Order an extra side dish of fruit, vegetables, rice, etc., prepared with little or no fat.
* Entrees made with wine or tomato sauces are better than those made with cream sauces.

Dinner—Side Dishes
* Fresh garden salads with low-fat dressings on the side. (Limit mayonnaise-based salads, including cole slaw, most pasta salads, and potato salad.)
* Baked potato topped with low-fat cottage cheese or plain low-fat yogurt and chives. Limit butter or sour cream to a teaspoon.
* Bring your own Butter Buds, or a similar powdered non-fat butter product, to use on a baked potato or steamed vegetables.
* Vegetables, with little or no fat. (Omit those with cheese or cream sauces.)
* Whole wheat and rye breads are preferable, but all plain breads are fine. (Avoid croissants and pre-buttered rolls or garlic bread.)

Dinner—Desserts
* Fresh fruit
* Sherbet, fruit ices, gelatin, sorbet, meringue shells with fruit, or angel food cake.
* The fillings in fruit pies are generally low in fat, but pie crusts are very high in fat. Cut down on fat by not eating the pie crust.

Ethnic Restaurants
Since America is the great "melting pot," we are blessed with a wide variety of ethnic restaurants. Many of the foods available to us are as authentic as that of the home country. These restaurants provide us with an endless choice of foods, many with names we cannot even pronounce.

*Blackened foods should be ordered only occasionally, because this cooking method encourages the formation of HAs, a carcinogen formed when meats and fish are charred at very high temperatures. (See page 131 for additional information on HAs.)

The following provides a sampling of some of the best and worst food choices (from a health standpoint) available at these restaurants.

These suggestions, of course, make up only a small portion of all the foods that are available. When dining out, if in doubt, be sure and ask how the food is prepared, the ingredients in a particular sauce, and/or approximately how much fat (butter, margarine, or cooking oil) is used in the preparation. Bon appetit!

Ethnic Restaurants Eating Hints

Chinese and Indochinese

These foods are characterized by large amounts of vegetables and grains, primarily rice, and limited portions of animal protein—a good start toward healthful eating. Choose dishes prepared by boiling, steaming, sauteing or stir-frying.

Avoid crispy chow mein noodles because they are high in fat; and all deep-fried foods, including batter-dipped meats or seafood, egg rolls and fried won tons. Choose white rice over fried rice.

If you wish to limit sodium, request that your food be prepared without monosodium glutamate (MSG) or soy sauce. You may want to add a small amount of soy sauce at the table for flavor. For an alternative flavor, you could request that your dish be prepared using fresh minced ginger and garlic. Soups are best avoided when limiting sodium.

Thai and Vietnamese cooking are generally low in fat, while full of interesting flavors.

Italian

Pasta is the cornerstone of many Italian dishes. High in complex carbohydrates, it comes in all shapes and sizes and can be used with a variety of sauces and fillings. The type of sauce and/or filling used will determine whether the pasta dish is high or low in fat. Those low in fat include pasta with red clam sauce; pasta with a marinara sauce (tomato-based), plain or with shrimp, chicken pieces (not breaded), or vegetables. Pasta primavera, which consists of fresh vegetables with pasta, is another good choice, provided it is not laden with butter and cream.

Chicken Marsala is cooked in a wine-based sauce, and is generally low in fat. Other healthy options include simply prepared chicken, shellfish and fish dishes; and thick crusted pizzas with a limited amount of cheese, covered with a variety of vegetables, Canadian bacon, or shrimp.

Some of the highest fat Italian foods to avoid are pizzas with pepperoni or sausage, lasagna, and breaded veal and chicken dishes topped with cheese. High fat sauces are those that contain ground beef or sausage, lots of cheese, or large quantities of butter or cream.

French

French restaurants can pose a real challenge because of their rich, high-fat sauces. Still, there are entrees that can be enjoyed without a guilty conscience, including those with a wine sauce, such as coq au vin (chicken with wine), or bouillabaisse, a fish chowder. Other good choices are steamed mussels; fish en papillote (fish baked in paper to preserve natural juices and seasonings); and ratatouille, a mixture of eggplant, tomatoes and other vegetables. The French also have many simple vegetable dishes and some fat-free desserts—sorbets and pears in wine.

Foods to avoid are French onion soup, because of its high sodium and high fat (from the cheese), quiche Lorraine, duck a l'orange, and those that contain hollandaise, bearnaise, or bechamel sauces.

Greek

Some good choices at Greek restaurants are plaki (fish cooked with tomatoes, onions, and garlic), meat and vegetable shish kabobs, taboule (parsley-wheat salad), rice pilaf and couscous (steamed, finely cracked wheat). To reduce the fat and sodium in Greek salads, omit or limit the olives and feta cheese, and request that the dressing be served on the side.

Most foods made with lamb or phyllo dough are high in fat, so it is best to avoid them, as well as all deep-fried foods. Eggplant is low in fat but when made into babaganoosh, an appetizer, it too is very high in fat.

Japanese

A variety of Japanese dishes are prepared with a minimal amount of fat. To begin with, one of the staples of Japanese cooking is steamed rice. Low-fat accompaniments for the rice include steamed fish, sushi (raw fish), and yakimono (broiled) fish and chicken. Other good choices are chicken or fish teriyaki, and tofu (soybean curd) dishes. Request that foods be broiled without fat.

Dishes that should be bypassed are tempura and other deep-fried foods, such as tonkatsu (deep-fried pork), katsudon (deep-fried pork, onion, and poached egg), and torikatsu (deep-fried chicken). To limit sodium, ask that salt, MSG and/or soy sauce be omitted or used sparingly.

Mexican and Southwestern

These highly spiced meals are often a good source of fiber because whole grains and beans are important components of Mexican dishes. Choose corn over flour tortillas (made with lard), and make sure that they are baked, not fried. Poultry or shellfish and vegetables, cooked with little or no extra fat, provide good fillers for the tortillas. Baked tortillas without meat or cheese fillings would also be healthy choices.

Other wholesome meals include rice and beans, either plain or with onions, tomatoes and spices; bean, chicken or seafood burritos; and enchiladas.

Refried beans are usually cooked in a small amount of lard, so do not eat large quantities of them. Rice is preferable. Be mindful that sour cream, cheese and avocado, which often accompany Mexican dishes, are very high in fat.

Indian and the Far East

Because of their preference for yogurt-based sauces and dals (legume dishes), these restaurants have many healthy, highly spiced varieties to choose from. In addition to the dals, other good choices are biryanis and pilafs (rice-based dishes), vegetable curries and tandoori chicken or fish. Baked breads are good, but avoid fried breads. Sometimes ghee (clarified butter) is used in the preparation of entrees. You can request that it not be used. Also, stay away from curries made with coconut milk, and all lamb dishes, since they are high in saturated fat.

Vegetarian

Although vegetarian dishes do not have meat, this does not necessarily mean that they are low in fat. Some vegetarian entrees are prepared with a large quantity of oil, high-fat dairy products, eggs, nuts and/or seeds. Still, vegetarian restaurants usually feature a variety of whole grain products, vegetables, and bean dishes—all very good. It would be best to request that they limit or omit butter, margarine, sour cream, cheese, cooking oil and/or eggs. Also request that only a sprinkling of nuts and seeds be used.

These suggestions are not all inclusive, but hopefully will be helpful to you the next time you eat in an ethnic restaurant. As you can see, there are still many interesting entrees to choose from when following a healthy low-fat diet. If, on rare occasion, you plan to splurge and eat a high-fat meal, be sure to pay especially close attention to eating low-fat meals several days before and after to make up for it.

Fast Food Restaurants

Fast food restaurants are here to stay. Children love them; they make eating out affordable for the whole family; and since they are quick and predictable, they are often the perfect answer to eating while traveling. Even though these restaurants have a notorious reputation for serving unhealthy foods, high in fat and sodium, that need not be the case if you choose foods carefully. Eating a modest amount of fat is possible if you know what to order, what "special" sauces to eliminate, etc. Restricting sodium is more difficult to do.

In response to the consumer's desire for healthier, lower fat foods, new choices have been added to fast food menus. Some of the newcomers to the scene are grilled (not deep-fried) chicken breast sandwiches and a variety of salads. If you omit the mayonnaise, these chicken sandwiches generally contain one to two teaspoons (5 to 10 grams) of fat. With the mayonnaise, the total fat jumps to between 3 and 4 teaspoons. If you want to use a condiment, use catsup or mustard instead, which have no fat. Another choice offered by most fast food franchises is a small burger, most of which contain just 2 teaspoons (10 grams) of fat. If you want to reduce the sodium, you can ask for the burger without pickles.

Caution: Salad Dressings and Deep-Fried Foods

Watch out for salads! They can serve as a healthy low-fat entree, only if they are *not* covered with a packet of high-fat salad dressing, which can add as many as 350 calories, and 25 to 40 grams of fat. Most salad dressing packets contain 4 tablespoons of dressing, while the calorie and fat content listed on the outside label are for a 1-tablespoon serving. The light dressings are much lower in fat. Taco salads, including the shell, are generally the highest fat salads, with Taco Bell's version packing in 61 grams of fat and 905 calories!

Do not be fooled into thinking that foods deep-fried in "heart-healthy" vegetable oils are good for you. Too much fat is never good, no matter what kind of fat it is. A large order of French fries has from 4 to 5 teaspoons (17 to 22 grams) of fat.

Some fast food restaurants, such as McDonalds, have taken the guesswork out of their food composition. They now provide consumers with a printout of the nutrient contents of all their foods, including quantities of fat, cholesterol, sodium, etc. When this information is not provided, the best way to cut down on fat at fast food establishments is to avoid the major fat culprits—deep-fried foods, cheese, mayonnaise and most special sauces. Figure 10.2 shows how much fat can be eliminated from a fast food item just by removing a major fat contributor. (Also refer to Appendix A, page 395, for more complete nutrient information on fast foods.)

Picnics and Outdoor Grilling

Outdoor grilling has become a popular American pastime, suitable for a most elegant meal or a simple outdoor picnic. It makes cooking an adventure in which the whole family, and even guests, can participate. In addition, it opens up a whole new world of interesting flavors through the use of marinades, sauces, etc.

Adjusting the Fat Downward

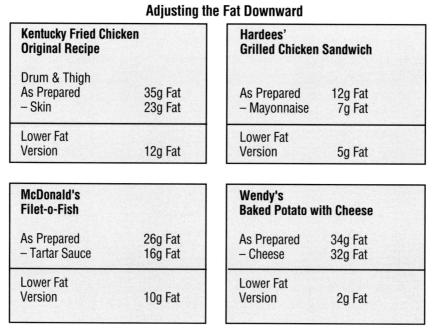

Kentucky Fried Chicken Original Recipe		
Drum & Thigh		
As Prepared	35g Fat	
– Skin	23g Fat	
Lower Fat Version	12g Fat	

Hardees' Grilled Chicken Sandwich	
As Prepared	12g Fat
– Mayonnaise	7g Fat
Lower Fat Version	5g Fat

McDonald's Filet-o-Fish	
As Prepared	26g Fat
– Tartar Sauce	16g Fat
Lower Fat Version	10g Fat

Wendy's Baked Potato with Cheese	
As Prepared	34g Fat
– Cheese	32g Fat
Lower Fat Version	2g Fat

Figure 10.2 These examples show how you can drastically reduce the fat in fast foods by simply removing one of the high-fat components. Low-fat condiments, such as low-calorie salad dressings or catsup can be used to add flavor in place of the cheese or high-fat sauces.

When cooking outdoors, be mindful of more than just creating outstanding entrees enhanced by a charcoal or mesquite flavor. Also consider which foods are best for grilling from a health standpoint, and the safest ways to grill foods. Grilled meats and fish will be discussed first, followed by side dishes that accompany an outdoor meal.

Meats and Fish—Grill with Care

Care should be taken when grilling meat or fish to reduce the carcinogens that can form when fat is burned. These carcinogens, called PAHs (polycyclic aromatic hydrocarbons), are formed when fat drips onto a flame or heating element. The PAHs travel upward with the smoke and are deposited on the grilled meat. They are also present in charred foods. Grilled meats are the principle source of PAHs in the diet.

The best way to prevent PAHs from forming is to keep fat from dripping onto the heat source. Below is a list of safe grilling tips, which should reduce the number of PAHs. It is impossible to tell how great a threat they pose, but most experts feel that those who grill frequently, i.e. several times a week, should take care to follow the precautions. If you grill once a week, your risk is probably insignificant.

Safe Grilling Tips

* Select the leanest cuts of meat.

* Trim all visible fat from meat before grilling. This will help prevent flare-ups from dripping fat.

* Choose fish or chicken over beef and pork, since they are generally lower in fat. (Lean beef and pork are still appropriate on occasion.)

* Avoid eating charred parts of meat.

* If you grill frequently (several times a week), consider precooking (microwaving or parboiling) the meat so it is not on the grill as long. Grill immediately after precooking.

* To keep fat from dripping onto the coals and producing smoke, place aluminum foil on top of grate and place food directly on the foil, turning up the sides slightly to contain the meat juices; or put a metal drip pan beneath the food to be grilled.

* Baste with barbecue sauce or marinate in low-fat salad dressings, or other marinades low in fat.

* Serve food from the grill on a clean platter, not one that has raw, possibly contaminated, meat juices on it.

* Grill vegetables with little or no added fat.

* Mesquite produces more PAHs than hardwood because it is a softwood and burns at a higher temperature. Therefore, you may want to limit its use.

* Clean the grill after each use.

Good Choices for Outdoor Grilling

* Shish kabobs with vegetables. Use lean beef, chicken or fish and serve over a bed of long grain and wild rice.

* Marinated chicken breast, grilled. Serve on a bun with lettuce, tomato and condiments of choice.

* Grilled pork tenderloin. Baste with honey mustard. Serve with a rice casserole and fruit salad.

* Barbecued chicken. Remove skin before grilling, place chicken pieces on aluminum foil, and brush with barbecue sauce.

* Grilled seafood of any type.

Care should also be taken when broiling or pan-frying meats to limit the formation of a different carcinogen, HAs (heterocyclic amines). They are formed by the burning of amino acids and other substances in meats. Their numbers can be reduced by cooking more slowly, rather than at very high temperatures.

Side Dishes for Picnics

Some of the customary side dishes and snack foods served at picnics are fairly high in fat—potato chips have 8 grams of fat for 10 medium-size chips; potato salad has from 7 to 13 grams of fat per one-cup serving. Many fruit or vegetable salads with mayonnaise, heavy cream, or sour cream have 3 or more teaspoons of fat (15 grams) per serving. If your goal is to keep fat intake to within 7 to 9 teaspoons (35 to 45 grams) of fat per day, you need to limit most of these higher fat side dishes, especially if your picnic meal includes a meat dish.

Another concern about side dishes at picnics is that they not be allowed to stand at room temperature or outdoors for too long before being eaten. In hot weather (85 degrees F and above), food should not sit out over an hour; at room temperature, perishable foods should not be left out over 2 hours. To prevent bacteria from multiplying and causing illness, hot foods should stay at 150 degrees F or higher and cold foods at 45 degrees F or lower. (Refrigerator temperature should be 40 degrees F or lower.) Leftovers should be refrigerated promptly. The foods at greatest risk for bacterial multiplication are meats, gravies, cream sauces, eggs, dairy products, mayonnaise and custards.

When planning your next picnic, you may want to choose your side dishes from the list provided in Figure 10.3. Those marked with an * appear in the recipe section of this book. All have less than one teaspoon of fat per serving.

Suggested Side Dishes To Accompany Grilled Foods

- Baked potato with nonfat sour cream or yogurt, chives and 1 teaspoon tub margarine (optional)
- Corn on the cob served with Butter Buds (powdered nonfat butter flavor) or margarine (less than one teaspoon).
- Rice-Mushroom Casserole*
- New Potato Salad*
- Tropical Fruit Slaw*
- Fresh fruit salad
- Congealed salads with fruits or vegetables (without sour cream or cream cheese)
- Vegetarian baked beans
- Creamy Cucumber Salad*
- Marinated Vegetable Salad*
- Taboule*
- Slim Waldorf Salad*

*Recipes appear in recipe section.

Figure 10.3 Low-fat side dishes to accompany a picnic meal.

Nutritious Snacks

Creating healthy snacks that are tasty and easy to prepare can be lots of fun. If you have young children, they will love helping you. Just use your imagination in trying different combinations of foods. One example is a banana yogurt shake. Use a food processor to blend a banana with low-fat frozen yogurt, adding both nutrients and flavor to the yogurt. The banana actually makes the shake taste thick and "creamy."

Another choice popular with children is a fresh or canned pear half, filled with a dab of peanut butter. If using canned pears, it is best to buy the pears in light syrup, to avoid too many empty calories from sugar. Lightly sweetened cold cereals, plain or with fruit, also make excellent snacks. Figure 10.4 provides a list of healthy snacks, which require little or no preparation time.

Quick Healthy Snacks

* Pretzels, preferably low-salt
* Graham crackers
* Frozen yogurt, nonfat or low-fat
* Fresh fruit
* Dried fruit—raisins, prunes, or apricots
* Canned fruit in light syrup, with or without low-fat cottage cheese
* Jello with fruit
* Prepackaged instant hot cereals
* Ice milk, plain or topped with fruit
* Cold cereals served with skim milk (with whole milk for children under two years old.)
* Bagel, plain or raisin, topped with light scraping of margarine, peanut butter, or jelly

---

Figure 10.4 A sampling of healthy snacks which require minimal preparation time.

Food Storage and Safety

Each year, approximately 7 million Americans suffer from foodborne illnesses, also called food poisoning. Some are not aware of the cause of their affliction, thinking they have the flu or some other ailment. An estimated 85% of these food poisonings are avoidable, if people would just handle foods properly. The following includes some helpful hints from the U.S. Department of Agriculture to reduce the risk of food poisoning:

Buying and Storing Foods

- If food is stamped with a "use-by" date, eat it before that date.
- When you buy refrigerated foods, make sure they are cold to the

touch; frozen foods should be rock solid; and canned goods should be free of dents, cracks or bulging lids.

   - The refrigerator should run at 40 degrees F; the freezer at 0 degrees F. Generally you should keep your refrigerator as cold as possible without freezing your milk or lettuce.

   - Freeze fresh meat, poultry or fish immediately if you can't use it within a few days.

   - Put packages of raw meat, poultry or fish on a plate in the refrigerator so their juices will not drip on other food. Also, when preparing meats or fish, keep raw juices from coming into contact with ready-to-eat foods, since these juices often contain bacteria.

Preparing Foods

   - Use plastic cutting boards rather than wooden ones where bacteria can hide in the grooves.

   - Do not thaw food on the kitchen counter, but rather in the refrigerator or in the microwave.

   - Marinate foods in the refrigerator, rather than the kitchen counter. (You can safely marinate foods on the kitchen counter if the marinating time is 30 minutes or less.) Reserve a portion of the marinade for a dip or basting sauce that hasn't had raw meat in it. Do not re-use the marinade used on raw meat unless it's been boiled.

   - Cook red meat to 160 degrees F, and poultry to 180 degrees F. Use a meat thermometer when in doubt to make sure that it's cooked all the way through. It takes thorough cooking to kill harmful bacteria, so you're taking chances when you eat meat, poultry, or fish that are raw or only partly cooked. Hamburger that is red in the middle, plus rare and medium-rare steaks, are undercooked from a safety standpoint. Poultry juices should run clear and the flesh should not be pink. Fish should be cooked until it flakes with a fork.

   - Use a clean plate for serving cooked foods. Be especially careful *not* to re-use a plate that had raw meat on it.

   - Cook eggs until the yolk and white are firm, not runny. Scramble eggs to a firm texture. Don't use recipes in which eggs remain raw or only partially cooked. Salmonella, a bacteria that causes food poisoning, can grow inside fresh, unbroken eggs. (Commercial egg substitutes do not carry a risk of Salmonella, because they are pasteurized.)

   - When microwaving food, use only microwave-safe containers. Cover foods with a lid or plastic wrap, vented, and do not allow plastic wrap to touch the food. Observe the standing time called for in the recipe, because during this time the food finishes cooking. Insert a temperature probe or meat thermometer in several spots to check that food is done.

Serving Foods and Handling Leftovers

- When you serve food, never leave it out over 2 hours. In hot weather (85 degrees F and above), food should never sit out over 1 hour. If these time limits are exceeded, throw the food out. Even reheating it to high temperatures (165 degrees F) will not destroy the disease-causing toxins that may have formed.

- With poultry or other stuffed meats, remove stuffing and refrigerate it in separate containers.

- If reheating leftovers, bring sauces, soups and gravy to a boil, and heat other leftovers thoroughly to 165 degrees F.

- Discard moldy foods, because poisons in molds are often present under the surface of the foods. Exception: Hard cheeses and firm fruits and vegetables with visible mold can be safely used provided a large area around the mold is removed.

- Never taste food that looks or smells strange to see if you can use it. Just throw it out.

- Refer to the Cold Storage chart to see how long food can be stored in the refrigerator or freezer at optimum quality.

Cold Storage

These SHORT but safe time limits will help keep refrigerated food from spoiling or becoming dangerous to eat. These time limits will keep frozen food at top quality.

Product	Refrigerator (40°F)	Freezer (0°F)
Eggs		
Fresh, in shell	3 weeks	Don't freeze
Raw yolks, whites	2-4 days	1 year
Hardcooked	1 week	Don't freeze well
Liquid pasteurized eggs or		
egg substitutes, opened	3 days	Don't freeze
unopened	10 days	1 year
Mayonnaise, commercial		
Refrigerate after opening	2 months	Don't freeze
TV Dinners, Frozen Casseroles		
Keep frozen until ready to serve		3-4 months
Deli Products		
Store-prepared (or homemade) egg,		
chicken, tuna, ham, macaroni salads	3-5 days	These products
Pre-stuffed pork & lamb chops,		don't freeze well
chicken breasts stuffed with dressing	1 day	
Store-cooked convenience meals	1-2 days	

Product	Refrigerator (40°F)	Freezer (0°F)
Soups & Stews		
Vegetable or meat-added	3-4 days	2-3 months
Hamburger, Ground & Stew Meats		
Hamburger & stew meats	1-2 days	3-4 months
Ground turkey, veal, pork, lamb		
& mixtures of them	1-2 days	3-4 months
Hotdogs & Lunch Meats		
Hotdogs, opened package	1 week	
unopened package	2 weeks	In freezer wrap,
Lunch meats, opened	3-5 days	1-2 months
unopened	2 weeks	
Fresh Meat		
Steaks, beef	3-5 days	6-12 months
Chops, pork	3-5 days	4-6 months
Chops, lamb	3-5 days	6-9 months
Roasts, beef	3-5 days	6-12 months
Roasts, lamb	3-5 days	6-9 months
Roasts, pork & veal	3-5 days	4-6 months
Variety meats—Tongue, brain,		
kidneys, liver, heart, chitterlings	1-2 days	3-4 months
Meat Leftovers		
Cooked meat and meat dishes	3-4 days	2-3 months
Gravy and meat broth	1-2 days	2-3 months
Fresh Poultry		
Chicken or turkey, whole	1-2 days	1 year
Chicken or turkey pieces	1-2 days	9 months
Giblets	1-2 days	3-4 months
Cooked Poultry, Leftover		
Fried chicken	3-4 days	4 months
Cooked poultry dishes	3-4 days	4-6 months
Pieces, plain	3-4 days	4 months
Pieces covered with broth, gravy	1-2 days	6 months
Chicken nuggets, patties	1-2 days	1-3 months

Source: U.S. Department of Agriculture, Food Safety and Inspection Service, Home and Garden Bulletin No. 248.

Common Diet Misconceptions Clarified

Myth: Children should be discouraged from drinking chocolate-flavored milk because it is a poor source of calcium and contains unhealthy amounts of sugar.

Fact: Chocolate milk is actually a good source of calcium for children, especially if they wouldn't otherwise choose milk. Low-fat chocolate milk (1% fat) is a healthier alternative than whole milk. They both have approximately the same number of calories (about 150 for an 8-ounce cup), but whole milk has much more fat. It has 8 grams of fat compared with only 3 grams in 1% fat chocolate milk. Generally, chocolate milk contains at least 90% of the calcium of white milk.

Myth: Snacking is an unhealthy habit.

Fact: To the contrary, snacking can be a very healthy practice as long as it is done in moderation with the right foods. Refer to Table 10-2 for a list of healthy snack choices. Snacking in mid-afternoon may prevent binging at mealtime because of feeling starved.

Myth: Cured meats, like other meats, can be frozen in order to preserve them for use at a later time.

Fact: Do not freeze cured meats. It adversely affects the taste and texture of the meat, and the seasonings in the meat quicken its rancidity while frozen.

Myth: Even moderate amounts of caffeine are harmful to most people and should be avoided.

Fact: Moderate use of caffeine, i.e. the equivalent of two to four cups of coffee per day, is not harmful for most people. Studies from the 1970s showing that it increased the risk for heart disease, cancer, fertility problems, ulcers and fibrocystic breast changes have all been discredited. However, it is recommended that you limit consumption if it makes you jittery, or if you have certain health conditions. These include: irregular heartbeats or recent heart attack, peptic ulcer, heartburn, high blood pressure, insomnia, anxiety disorders, or if you are pregnant or nursing.

Myth: Luncheon meat that is 80% fat free is lean meat.

Fact: Any luncheon meat that is 80% fat free is actually high in fat. What 80% fat free means is that 20% of the total weight of the meat is fat and 80% is carbohydrate, protein and water. Since water has weight but no calories, and since fat contains more calories per gram than carbohydrate and protein, 80% fat free is misleading. Meat that is 80% fat free contains approximately 67% of its calories from fat. Truly lean luncheon meat is generally 95 to 98% fat free.

Myth: You should eat extra protein if you want to build up muscles through weightlifting.

Fact: Protein is needed to build muscle, but even serious weight lifters should not exceed the recommended upper limit of protein consumption, which is 15% of total calories. (See page 90.) The body can use only so much protein, and the excess cannot be stored as muscle. Instead, it is converted to fat and carbohydrate and the by-products are eliminated in the urine. Too much protein can cause health problems including dehydration and kidney damage.

Part II

The Cookbook

Introduction to Recipes

Important nutrition information is included with each recipe. They have been analyzed, per serving, for: calories, protein, total fat, saturated fat, cholesterol, fiber, sodium, and percentage of calories from fat. The serving sizes given are quite generous—larger than in most low-fat or diet cookbooks.

Optional ingredients are omitted from the nutrition analysis. When the serving size is listed as a range, such as "4 to 6 servings," the figure in the middle, in this case 5 servings, is used for the analysis. When an amount is not specified, such as salt and pepper to taste, the ingredients are not figured into the analysis. If a choice of ingredients is given, i.e., low-fat or nonfat, the first ingredient mentioned is used.

The recipe analysis used Food Processor II software program.* In cases where a recipe ingredient was missing from the program, Bowes and Church's *Food Values of Portions Commonly Used*, 15th Edition, or nutrition information from food labels was used instead.

In certain recipe categories, particularly salads and vegetables, the percentage of calories from fat is often higher than in other food categories. Do not be overly concerned when this is the case, *if* the grams of fat per serving is low. Because the calories from the vegetables themselves are so low, a small amount of added fat, has a greater effect on the percentage of calories from fat.

A number of recipes call for "defatted" broth, either chicken or beef. This indicates that the visible fat should be skimmed off the top. The fat can be removed more easily if the broth is first cooled in the refrigerator, but this is not essential.

If you are carefully watching the amount of sodium in your diet, be sure to consider all the foods that will be eaten with the meal. For example, the sodium content of a casserole dish can be higher than for a side dish, since a casserole of meat, starches and vegetables is almost a complete meal in itself. On the other hand, with a side dish, you will probably eat three or four other foods with the meal, which will significantly increase the amount of sodium.

The Preparation Time and Cooking Time have been provided so you can tell at a glance approximately how much time is involved in preparing

* From ESHA Research, P.O. Box 13028, Salem, Oregon 97309

a particular dish. The Preparation Time is the time you spend actively preparing the dish. It includes sauteing time, if you need to be closely observing or frequently stirring a food while it is cooking.

Cooking time is the time the food takes to cook while you are not actively working on the food, i.e. if the food is baking in the oven or simmering on the stove.

The approximate time it takes from beginning of preparation to when the food is ready for the table is the Preparation Time plus Cooking Time. Marinating time is also included when foods are marinated, and is usually given as a range.

The following is a summary of the recommended consumption levels of certain key nutrients:

Protein—the Recommended Dietary Allowance (RDA) for an average adult male over 14-years-old is 56 grams a day; for an average female (not pregnant) over 18, it is 44 grams a day. (To calculate your own RDA for protein (in grams), you multiply your ideal body weight in pounds by 0.37. See page 90 in text.)

Fat—the American Heart Association recommends that fat consumption be limited to less than 30% of total calories. More recent studies have shown that reducing fat to 20 to 25% of total calories is both practical and more effective in reducing the incidence of obesity, cancer and heart disease.

Cholesterol—the American Heart Association recommends less than 300 mg per day in the Step-One Diet; and less than 200 mg per day in the Step-Two Diet. (Keep in mind, these are *not target* but *ceiling* recommendations. Lowering intake below the ceiling levels has been shown to be more beneficial in reducing cholesterol values in some individuals.)

Fiber—the recommended level is 20 to 30 grams per day.

Sodium—the recommended level is less than 2400 milligrams per day.

Menus For Entertaining

*Starred recipes may be found in this book.

Sunday Brunch Buffet

Beverages
Hot Cranberry Punch*, Bloody Mary

◆

Buffet
Crustless Spinach Quiche*
Baked Apple-Date Delight*
Mini-Ham Biscuits
Fresh Fruit Salad
Slim Waldorf Salad*

◆

Breads
Lemon Tea Bread*
Date-Nut Bread*
Blueberry Muffins*

◆

Desserts
Peaches in Wine*
Frosted Apple Cookies*
Coffee, Tea

Ladies' Summer Luncheon

Beverage
Fruit–Flavored Carbonated Punch

◆

Entree
Curry Chicken Salad*
Spinach Salad with Honey Mustard Dressing*
Carrot Bran Muffins*

◆

Dessert
Lemon Custard Delight*
Coffee, Tea

Bridge Club Luncheon

Beverage
Hot Mulled Cider*

◆

Entree
Chicken-Seafood Artichoke Casserole*
Green Bean–Mushroom Salad*
Bran Muffins*
Cornbread Muffins*

◆

Dessert
Mock Cherry Cheesecake*
Coffee/Tea

Candlelight Dinner

Oysters Rockefeller*
Taboule* with Melba Rounds

◆

Entree
Pork Medallions with Mushroom Sauce*
Wild Rice Baked Casserole*
Baked Apple-Date Delight*
Mandarin Salad*
Dinner Rolls

◆

Dessert
Brownie Baked Alaska*
Coffee, Espresso

Hearty Seafood Supper

Appetizers
Tuna Vegetable Dip* with Crackers
Spinach Quiche Appetizer*

◆

Entree
Stuffed Flounder*
Saffron Rice*
Steamed Baby Carrots
Swiss-Style Garden Salad*
Dinner Rolls, Date-Nut Bread*

◆

Dessert
Ice Cream Cake Roll*
With Blueberry Sauce*
Coffee, Espresso

Traditional Turkey Dinner

Appetizers
Tangy Shrimp*
Artichoke Relish with Pita Chips*

◆

Entree
Baked Turkey Breast
Mashed Potatoes with Nonfat Turkey Gravy*
Sweet Potato Casserole*
Spinach–Artichoke Casserole*
Fresh Cranberry Molded Salad*
Dinner Rolls, Banana Nut Bread*

◆

Dessert
Steamed Date–Nut Pudding with Brandy Sauce*
Coffee, Espresso

Dinner At Eight

Appetizers
Shrimp Cocktail
Hummous* with Pumpernickel Rounds

♦

Soup
Salmon Bisque*

♦

Entree
Pork Marengo with "Eggless" Egg Noodles*
Baked Tomatoes with Spinach*
Mandarin Salad*
Dinner Rolls, Bran Mini-Muffins*

♦

Dessert
Strawberry Russe*
Coffee, Espresso

Friday Night Fish Dinner

Appetizers
Spinach Quiche Appetizer*
Tuna Vegetable Dip with Melba Rounds*

◆

Entree
Marinated Salmon*
Mashed Potatoes with Chives*
Green Beans Amandine*
Spinach Salad with Honey Mustard Dressing*
Dinner Rolls, French Bread

◆

Dessert
Chocolate Chip Bundt Cake*
Coffee, Espresso

Gourmet Club Dinner Party

Appetizers
*Crab Canapes**
Marinated Vegetables

◆

Entree
*Orange Roughy with Mushroom Sauce**
*Herbed Red Potatoes**
*Sesame Broccoli**
*Fresh Cranberry Molded Salad**
Dinner Rolls, Bran Mini-Muffins

◆

Dessert
*Frozen Yogurt Charlotte**
Coffee, Tea

New Orleans Dinner

Appetizers
Escargots*
Tuna Canapes*

◆

Soup
Seafood Gumbo* with Garlic Toast*

◆

Entree
Shrimp Creole*
Scrumptious Asparagus*
Celestial Salad*
Dinner Rolls, Cornbread Mini-muffins

◆

Dessert
New Orleans Bread Pudding topped with Hard Sauce*
Coffee

Labor Day Picnic

Appetizers
*Fresh Fruit Platter with Yogurt Dip**
Crabmeat Vegetable Dip with Crackers*

◆

Entree
*Grilled Breast of Chicken Sandwich**
*New Potato Salad**
*Marinated Vegetable Salad**
*Carolyn's Baked Beans**
*Banana Nut Bread**

◆

Dessert
*Strawberry Shortcake**
*Lemon Glazed Spice Bars**
Coffee, Iced Tea

Summer Picnic At Home

Appetizers
Stuffed Cherry Tomatoes*
Artichoke Relish* with Party Rye

◆

Entree
Barbecued Shredded Turkey Breast*
Served on Hard Rolls
"Sour Cream" Potato Salad*
Black Bean Salad*
Slim Waldorf Salad*
Tomatoes with Chopped Herbs*

◆

Dessert
Carrot Cake with Cream Cheese Frosting*
Low-fat Lemon Bars*
Coffee/Tea

Appetizers & Beverages

MARINATED CHICKEN KABOBS

For 1 kabob:
Calories...... 68
Protein (g)... 11
Fat (g)....... 1.7
Sat. Fat (g).. 0.4
Choles. (mg).. 27
Fiber (g)..... 0.4
Sodium (mg)... NA
%Cal-Fat...... 22%

4 boneless chicken breasts
1/4 cup Lite soy sauce
1/4 cup prepared barbecue sauce
2 tablespoons lemon juice
1/4 teaspoon ground ginger
1/4 teaspoon garlic powder
2 large green peppers, cut into 1-inch pieces
2 large red peppers, cut into 1-inch pieces
18 6-inch wooden skewers
Vegetable cooking spray

Cut chicken breasts into 1-inch pieces; place in a medium-size bowl or plastic container.

Combine next five ingredients in a small bowl. Stir briskly with a wire whisk. Pour over chicken. Cover and refrigerate at least 2 hours, stirring occasionally to marinate evenly. Do not marinate longer than 8 hours.

Meanwhile, cut red and green peppers into 1-inch pieces.

Remove chicken from marinade, reserving marinade. Place chicken and peppers on skewers in this order: red pepper, green pepper, two pieces of chicken, green pepper and red pepper.

Spray grill with cooking spray. Place kabobs on grill approximately 6 inches from medium-hot coals. Spoon 2 to 4 tablespoons marinade over top. Grill for 15 to 20 minutes or until done, turning as needed; or, kabobs may be broiled in an oven, 6 inches from broiler, for approximately same length of time.

Yield: 12 to 16 kabobs.

This appetizer is ideal for a cocktail party with heavy hors d'oeuvres. The red and green peppers make it very colorful.

Preparation Time: 30 minutes

Cooking Time: 20 minutes

MARINATED SHRIMP WITH SNOW PEAS

1/4 cup olive oil
3 tablespoons wine vinegar
2 tablespoons Dijon mustard
1 tablespoon finely chopped parsley
1 teaspoon finely chopped ginger
1 clove garlic, minced
1 tablespoon chopped fresh dill
Pinch salt, pepper, sugar
2 pounds large fresh shrimp, cooked and cleaned
1/2 pound fresh snow peas, or 10 ounces frozen
Curly leaf lettuce or Romaine
Parsley and thin lemon slices for garnish

For 2 appetizers:
Calories...... 99
Protein (g)... 16
Fat (g)....... 2
Sat. Fat (g).. 0.7
Choles. (mg).. 88
Fiber (g)..... 1.2
Sodium (mg)... 157
%Cal-Fat...... 18%

Blend together oil, vinegar, mustard, parsley, ginger, garlic, dill, salt, pepper and sugar. Mix well and pour over shrimp. Refrigerate at least four hours and up to two days, stirring occasionally.

Cut off tops of snow peas. If peas are fresh, parboil for 30 seconds and plunge immediately into cold water to retain their bright color. Drain. If peas are frozen, thaw and drain. Halve the peas lengthwise and wrap half around each shrimp. Secure with toothpicks and arrange on the lettuce. Garnish with parsley and lemon slices, twisted.

Yield: about 30–40 appetizers.

Preparation Time: 1 hour

Marinating Time: 4 hours to 2 days

TANGY SHRIMP

For 6 shrimp:
Calories...... 97
Protein (g)... 16
Fat (g)....... 2
Sat. Fat (g).. 0.6
Choles. (mg).. 147
Fiber (g)..... 0.6
Sodium (mg)... 187
%Cal-Fat...... 19%

1/8 cup olive oil
2 cloves garlic, minced
1 tablespoon Dijon mustard
6 tablespoons lemon juice
2 tablespoons red wine vinegar
1 tablespoon chopped fresh dill
Dash of cayenne pepper
1 medium red onion, thinly sliced
1 green pepper, cut into 1/4-inch strips
2 tablespoons chopped pimiento
1 tablespoon chopped parsley
1 1/2 to 2 pounds cooked medium shrimp
   (60 to 70 shrimp)

In a medium-size bowl, combine oil, garlic, mustard, lemon juice, vinegar, dill and cayenne. Mix well. Add onion slices, green pepper, pimiento, parsley and shrimp, tossing until well coated. Refrigerate, covered, for 1 to 4 hours.

Place shrimp mixture in a serving bowl. Serve with toothpicks.

Yield: 60 to 70 shrimp, enough for 8 to 12 people

Preparation Time: 25 minutes

Marinating time: 1–4 hours

SPINACH QUICHE APPETIZER

8 egg substitutes (2 cups)
1 12-ounce can evaporated skim milk
1/2 teaspoon salt
1/8 teaspoon cayenne pepper
1/2 teaspoon ground nutmeg
2 teaspoons olive oil
1/4 cup chopped onion
2 10-ounce packages frozen chopped spinach, thawed
  and drained (squeezed dry)
1 cup (4 ounces) shredded Swiss or Cheddar cheese
2 tablespoons flour

For 4 appetizers:
Calories...... 59
Protein (g)... 6
Fat (g)....... 2.5
Sat. Fat (g).. 1.1
Choles. (mg).. 5
Fiber (g)..... 0.7
Sodium (mg)... 129
%Cal-Fat...... 37%

Preheat oven to 350 degrees.

Combine egg substitutes, milk, salt, pepper and nutmeg in large mixing bowl. Beat slightly. Set aside.

Heat olive oil in medium-size saucepan. Add onion and saute until onion becomes translucent. Mix thawed and drained spinach with onion mixture. Add to egg mixture.

Toss grated cheese with flour.

Spray 10 x 15-inch jelly roll pan with vegetable cooking spray. Sprinkle cheese evenly over bottom of pan. Pour egg mixture over top.

Bake at 350 degrees for 35 to 40 minutes. Cool slightly and cut into 1 1/4-inch squares.

Yield: 96 appetizers

The dark green color of this appetizer is especially attractive on a light colored serving dish. Garnish with fresh sprigs of parsley, or with holly around the Christmas holidays.

Preparation Time: 25 minutes

Cooking Time: 40 minutes

TUNA (OR CRAB) CANAPES

For 1 appetizer:
Calories...... 43
Protein (g)... 4
Fat (g)....... 0.8
Sat. Fat (g).. 0.4
Choles. (mg).. 3
Fiber (g)..... 0.5
Sodium (mg)... 151
%Cal-Fat...... 16%

**1 6 1/2-ounce can tuna in spring water,
      drained and flaked**
1/2 cup nonfat mayonnaise
1 tablespoon finely chopped pimiento
**2 tablespoons finely chopped green onion,
      including tops**
1/2 cup Parmesan cheese, divided
**24 small pumpernickel bread rounds, or 6
pumpernickel slices, quartered**

In a medium-size mixing bowl, combine tuna, mayonnaise, pimiento, green onion and 3/8 cup (6 tablespoons) Parmesan cheese. Mix thoroughly.

Spread on bread rounds or bread slices, quartered. Sprinkle with remaining 2 tablespoons Parmesan cheese. Place on a baking sheet and broil 5 inches from heat for 4 to 5 minutes, or until slightly browned. Serve hot.

Yield: 24 appetizers

To make Crab Canapes, substitute 8 ounces backfin crabmeat for the tuna. Be sure to carefully check and remove any shell fragments that may be present in crabmeat. Follow remaining recipe instructions as indicated above.

Preparation Time: 25 minutes

Cooking Time: 5 minutes

OYSTERS ROCKEFELLER

10 ounces fresh spinach
2 green onions, including tops
3 sprigs of parsley
1/4 head iceberg lettuce
1/2 cup dry breadcrumbs
2 tablespoons Anisette liqueur (licorice-flavored)
1 tablespoon Worcestershire sauce
Dash Tabasco sauce
Salt to taste
1 tablespoon tub margarine, melted
3 dozen oysters, packed in own liquid
36 slices Party Pumpernickel (1 8-ounce loaf)
6 tablespoons Parmesan cheese

For 1 appetizer:
Calories...... 47
Protein (g)... 3
Fat (g)....... 1.2
Sat. Fat (g).. 0.4
Choles. (mg).. 11
Fiber (g)..... 1.3
Sodium (mg)... 94
%Cal-Fat...... 25%

Wash spinach and remove tough stems. Grind spinach, onions, parsley and lettuce in a food processor.

Place spinach mixture in a large mixing bowl. Add breadcrumbs, Anisette, Worcestershire sauce, Tabasco and salt (if desired). Stir to mix. Return to food processor and puree. Set aside and refrigerate until ready to assemble. (The spinach paste may be made a day ahead.)

Cook oysters: Bring them to a boil in their own liquid. As soon as the liquid comes to a boil, remove from heat. Let oysters stand in hot liquid until ready to assemble.

Preheat broiler to medium setting. Melt margarine in microwave. Rinse oysters.

To assemble: Place small pumpernickel slices on cookie sheet. Top with oyster. Place rounded teaspoon of spinach mixture over each oyster and drizzle with margarine. Sprinkle with Parmesan cheese. Place under broiler 10 to 20 minutes, or until tops begin to brown slightly.

Yield: 36 appetizers

Preparation time: 30-35 minutes

Cooking time: 10-20 minutes

SALMON TERIYAKI APPETIZER

1 3-pound salmon fillet
1/4 cup Lite soy sauce
1/2 cup Chablis wine
1/2 teaspoon paprika
3 teaspoons sugar
3 lemons and parsley for garnish

Prepare marinade by combining soy sauce, wine, paprika, and sugar. Place fish in a shallow container and pour marinade over. Marinate for 30 minutes at room temperature, or 1 to 2 hours in refrigerator.

Meanwhile, set oven control to broil.

Spray broiler rack with vegetable cooking spray. Remove salmon from marinade and place on rack. Spoon 3 tablespoons of marinade over top of fish. Broil approximately 6 inches from heat, skin side down for 10 to 15 minutes, or until fish flakes easily with a fork.

Place salmon fillet on an oval platter, skin side down. Cut into 1-inch squares, leaving skin intact. Garnish with lemon halves with serrated tops and parsley. Serve with toothpicks or cocktail forks.

Yield: Approximately 72 1-inch pieces.

Preparation time: 15 minutes

Cooking time: 15 minutes

Marinating time: 30 minutes to 2 hours

FRESH FRUIT PLATTER WITH YOGURT DIP

1 honeydew melon (shell halves reserved for garnish)
1 or 2 fresh pineapples with tops
2 other fruits in season (strawberries, cantaloupe, grapes,
  watermelon or kiwi fruit)
1 head Romaine lettuce

Yogurt dip:
2 cups nonfat or low-fat plain yogurt
1/4 cup brown sugar, firmly packed
1/4 teaspoon cinnamon

*For 1/2 cup fruit and
2 tablespoons dip:*
Calories...... 64
Protein (g)... 2
Fat (g)....... 0.2
Sat. Fat (g).. 0
Choles. (mg).. <1
Fiber (g)..... 1.3
Sodium (mg)... 27
%Cal-Fat...... 5%

Cut up fruit into bite-size pieces. Save honeydew shells and pineapple tops (with leaves) for garnish. Cover and refrigerate fruit until ready to assemble tray.

Make yogurt dip by adding brown sugar and cinnamon to yogurt. Mix thoroughly. Set aside until ready to serve.

To serve, line 16 x 20-inch tray with Romaine leaves. Arrange fruit and yogurt dip on tray. Yogurt may be served in hollowed out honeydew shell with serrated top, or small bowl. Serve with toothpicks.

For garnish on tray: Serrate top edge of melon shell(s). Place shell in center of tray or place one at each end of tray. Place pineapple top(s) with leaves inside melon shell(s).

Vary quantity of fruit depending on number of guests and other foods served. A 16 x 20-inch tray filled with fruit will be adequate for 20 to 35 guests. Have additional fruit to replenish tray if serving more guests.

Preparation time: 45 minutes

ESCARGOTS (SNAILS)

1 can (18 count) extra-large snails
1 tablespoon tub margarine
1 1/2 tablespoons flour
1 cup clear chicken broth
1 tablespoon powdered butter flavoring
1 teaspoon minced garlic
2 teaspoons chopped green onion tops
18 snail shells, real or artificial
2 tablespoons grated Parmesan cheese
2 tablespoons fresh minced parsley
1/2 loaf French baguette, sliced thin (optional)

Preheat oven to 500 degrees. Drain liquid from can of snails. Rinse and set aside.

In a medium-size skillet, heat margarine over moderate heat. Add flour, stirring with a fork until well blended. Add chicken broth and cook, stirring constantly, until mixture comes to a boil and thickens.

Stir in powdered butter flavoring, garlic, and green onion tops. Simmer for 3 minutes, uncovered, over medium-low heat. Place one snail in each snail shell.

Place in snail pan or shallow muffin tins, open side up. Spoon 1 to 2 teaspoons chicken broth mixture into each shell. Sprinkle Parmesan cheese over top of each opening.

Bake, uncovered, in a 500 degree oven for 5 minutes, or until cheese is lightly browned and liquid is bubbly.

Remove from oven and cool 5 minutes. Sprinkle minced parsley over top of each opening. Serve immediately. Use cocktail forks to remove snails. If desired, serve on thin slice of French baguette (long narrow French bread).

Yield: 18 appetizers

Preparation time: 20 minutes

Cooking time: 5 minutes

STUFFED ARTICHOKE HEARTS

1 14-ounce can artichoke hearts, packed in water
1/2 cup dry bread crumbs
1/4 teaspoon garlic powder
1/4 teaspoon paprika
1/4 teaspoon Tabasco sauce
Dash of dried parsley
Dash of oregano
1/3 cup artichoke liquid
1/4 cup Parmesan cheese, divided

Drain artichoke hearts, reserving liquid. Cut into quarters, lengthwise. Remove centers leaving several layers of leaves to form a shell.

In a medium-size bowl, place artichoke centers. Mash with a fork. Add bread crumbs, garlic powder, paprika, Tabasco sauce, parsley, oregano, artichoke liquid and 2 tablespoons Parmesan cheese. Mix well.

Stuff mixture into shells and sprinkle with remaining Parmesan cheese. Toast quickly under broiler, about 3 to 5 minutes.

Yield: Makes 20 to 24 bite-sized pieces.

Preparation Time: 35 minutes

For 2 appetizers:
Calories...... 44
Protein (g)... 3
Fat (g)....... 1
Sat. Fat (g).. 0.5
Choles. (mg).. 2
Fiber (g)..... 2.9
Sodium (mg)... 95
%Cal-Fat...... 20%

STUFFED CHERRY TOMATOES

24 cherry tomatoes
3/4 cup hummous (Recipe, page 173)
3 sprigs parsley, finely chopped

Cut tops off cherry tomatoes and scoop out pulp. Fill cavity with hummous, using either a teaspoon or a pastry tube. Sprinkle top with fresh, finely chopped parsley. Chill until ready to serve.

Yield: 24 individual appetizers.

Preparation time: 40 minutes

For 2 appetizers:
Calories...... 27
Protein (g)... 1
Fat (g)....... 0.7
Sat. Fat (g).. 0.1
Choles. (mg).. 0
Fiber (g)..... 1
Sodium (mg)... 38
%Cal-Fat...... 25%

ARTICHOKE RELISH

**2 14-ounce cans artichoke hearts, drained and
  chopped
1 4-ounce jar diced pimiento, drained
4 green onions, thinly sliced
4 tablespoons freshly grated Parmesan cheese
2 cloves of garlic, minced
4 tablespoons lemon juice
2 tablespoons olive oil
1 teaspoon dried whole thyme
1/4 teaspoon pepper
2 tablespoons chopped fresh parsley**

Drain artichoke hearts and chop coarsely in food processor. In medium bowl, combine artichokes with remaining ingredients, except parsley. Mix well.

Cover and refrigerate 4 hours or overnight. Sprinkle relish with parsley before serving. Serve with Toasted Pita Chips (Recipe, page 173) or Melba rounds.

Yield: 3 cups of relish; enough for 10 to 14 persons.

Leftover relish tastes great on a slice of bread, or as part of a sandwich. It can also be served as a side dish for lunch.

Preparation Time: 25 minutes

TUNA VEGETABLE DIP

1 9 1/4-ounce can tuna fish packed in water, drained
1/2 cup Lite mayonnaise
1/2 cup nonfat mayonnaise
1 cup nonfat "sour cream"
1 small onion, chopped
1 1.4-ounce package Knorr vegetable soup mix
1 8-ounce can water chestnuts (chopped)
5 ounces chopped spinach (1/2 10-ounce package frozen chopped spinach)
1 loaf unsliced round or oval bread, or low-fat crackers

Drain can of tuna fish. Place in medium bowl, breaking up chunks of tuna. Add remaining ingredients, except bread, and mix well. Chill at least two hours before serving.

Serve in hollowed out loaf of bread or with low-fat crackers.

To serve in bread loaf, slice off top 1/3 of loaf. Hollow out lower 2/3 by pulling out pieces of bread until shell of loaf remains. Fill with dip. Serve with bread removed from loaf, torn into bite-size pieces.

Yield: 2 1/2 cups dip.

To make Crabmeat Vegetable Dip, substitute 8 ounces backfin crabmeat for the tuna. Be sure to carefully look through the crabmeat to remove any shell fragments that may be present.

Preparation time: 25 minutes

TABOULE

Per 2 tablespoons:
Calories...... 23
Protein (g)... 1
Fat (g)....... 0.1
Sat. Fat (g).. 0
Choles. (mg).. 0
Fiber (g)..... 1.4
Sodium (mg)... 34
%Cal-Fat...... 2%

1 cup fine or medium-grade bulgur
Water
1 cup chopped fresh parsley (about 1/2 bunch)
1 tablespoon minced fresh dill or 1 teaspoon dill weed
1/2 cup chopped green onions, including tops
2 medium tomatoes, diced
1 medium cucumber, peeled, deseeded, chopped
1/2 cup no-oil Italian dressing
Juice of 1/2 lemon
Freshly ground pepper to taste
Romaine lettuce leaves
Garnish: black olives, tomato wedges, parsley sprigs

Place bulgur in large mixing bowl. Add water to cover and let stand about 1 hour or until bulgur has doubled in size and most of the liquid is absorbed. Drain well and squeeze dry.

Add parsley, dill, green onions, tomatoes and cucumber. Toss gently.

Add Italian dressing, lemon juice and pepper and toss until well mixed. Refrigerate.

Serve with small pita wedges or melba rounds.

Yield: 3 1/2 cups Taboule

Taboule, which can also be served as a salad, makes a delicious, low-calorie topping for crackers.

Preparation time: 30 minutes
(plus 1 hour to soak bulgur)

BEAN DIP

1 4-ounce can chopped green chilies, drained
1/2 cup tomato sauce
4 green onions, chopped
1/2 teaspoon ground cumin
1/2 teaspoon Tabasco sauce
1 clove garlic, minced
1 16-ounce can black-eyed peas, drained, (Reserve 2
   tablespoons liquid)

For 2 tablespoons:
Calories...... 33
Protein (g)... 2
Fat (g)....... 0.3
Sat. Fat (g).. 0.1
Choles. (mg).. 0
Fiber (g)..... 2
Sodium (mg)... 152
%Cal-Fat...... 7%

Combine first six ingredients in a saucepan and cook until onions are tender.

Place can of black-eyed peas and reserved liquid in a food processor and process to a slightly lumpy paste. Transfer to a medium bowl and add ingredients from saucepan. Mix until well blended. Serve hot or cold with bread rounds, melba rounds or toasted pita chips. (Recipe, page 173.)

Yield: Makes 1 1/2 cups.

This dip also makes a delicious warm burrito filling. To prepare, heat bean dip in saucepan and spoon onto warmed flour tortilla and roll up. Or, if using a microwave, spoon filling onto tortilla and microwave on medium for 1 1/2 minutes.

Preparation time: 20 minutes

Cooking time: 10 minutes

HUMMOUS

For 2 tablespoons:
Calories...... 44
Protein (g)... 2
Fat (g)....... 1.4
Sat. Fat (g).. 0.2
Choles. (mg).. 0
Fiber (g)..... 1.5
Sodium (mg)... 72
%Cal-Fat...... 27%

2 cups cooked garbanzo beans (one 16-ounce can,
   or 3/4 cup raw garbanzos, cooked)
3 tablespoons garbanzo cooking liquid or juice from can
3 tablespoons sesame seeds or tahini (sesame seed oil)
2 tablespoons lemon juice
2 cloves garlic, minced
1/2 teaspoon cumin
1/4 teaspoon salt (optional)
Pinch pepper

Drain garbanzo beans, reserving 3 tablespoons liquid. Combine all ingredients, including the reserved liquid, in a food processor. Process continuously for one to two minutes, until light and fluffy.

Yield: 2 cups

Excellent as a spread on pita bread or low-fat crackers. Fat content is much lower than a cheese spread.

Preparation time: 15 minutes

TOASTED PITA CHIPS

For 6 pita chips:
Calories...... 82
Protein (g)... 3
Fat (g)....... 0.4
Sat. Fat (g).. 0.1
Choles. (mg).. 0
Fiber (g)..... 0.5
Sodium (mg)... 169
%Cal-Fat...... 5%

6 slices pita bread, whole wheat or plain

Cut pita bread into 12 pie-shaped wedges using sharp knife or kitchen shears. Arrange in a single layer on a cookie sheet.
Bake at 350 degrees until crisp and slightly browned (about 10 minutes). Cool completely. Store in an airtight container.

Yield: Makes 72 pita chips.

Preparation time: 5 minutes

Cooking time: 10 minutes

HOT CRANBERRY PUNCH

9 cups cranberry juice cocktail
9 cups unsweetened pineapple juice
4 1/2 cups water
1 cup brown sugar
4 1/2 teaspoons whole cloves
4 cinnamon sticks, broken
1/4 teaspoon salt

In 30-cup percolator coffee maker, place fruit juices, water and brown sugar. In percolator basket, place cloves, cinnamon sticks and salt. Turn on coffee maker, perk and serve.

Yield: 22 8-ounce cups hot punch

A delicious and quick hot drink to serve during the winter months, especially appropriate around the Christmas holidays.

Preparation time: 15 minutes

Cooking Time: 35 minutes (to perk)

For an 8 ounce cup:
Calories...... 153
Protein (g)... <1
Fat (g)....... 0
Sat. Fat (g).. 0
Choles. (mg).. 0
Fiber (g)..... 0.6
Sodium (mg)... 32
%Cal-Fat...... 1%

HOT MULLED CIDER

1 quart apple cider
2 cups cranberry juice
5 whole cloves
4 sticks cinnamon

Combine all ingredients in a large sauce pan. Bring to a boil and simmer, covered, 1 hour. Remove cloves and cinnamon sticks. Serve in coffee mugs.

Yield: 6 1-cup servings

Preparation time: 10 minutes

Cooking time: 1 hour

Per serving:
Calories...... 118
Protein (g)... <1
Fat (g)....... 0.2
Sat. Fat (g).. 0.1
Choles. (mg).. 0
Fiber (g)..... 0.4
Sodium (mg)... 6
%Cal-Fat...... 2%

BANANA YOGURT SHAKE

Per serving:
Calories...... 292
Protein (g)... 9
Fat (g)....... 5.6
Sat. Fat (g).. 0.1
Choles. (mg).. 13
Fiber (g)..... 0.9
Sodium (mg)... 106
%Cal-Fat...... 17%

2 cups low-fat vanilla frozen yogurt
1 banana

Place frozen yogurt and banana in food processor. Process until smooth.

Yield: 2 8-ounce shakes

This makes a great low-fat after school snack that children love. The banana provides important nutrients and lends a "creamy" texture to the shake. Other flavors of yogurt may be substituted.

Preparation Time: 5 minutes

CHRISTMAS WASSAIL

Per serving:
Calories...... 272
Protein (g)... 1
Fat (g)....... 0.5
Sat. Fat (g).. 0.1
Choles. (mg).. 0
Fiber (g)..... 0.6
Sodium (mg)... 9.7
%Cal-Fat...... 2%

2 quarts apple cider
4 cups orange juice
Juice of 2 lemons
3/4 cup honey
4 sticks cinnamon
2 tablespoons whole cloves
2 tablespoons whole allspice
1 teaspoon grated nutmeg

Combine all ingredients in large sauce pan. Heat to boiling and simmer for 10 minutes. Strain out spices.
Serve in a punch bowl decorated with holly or other Christmas greens, or pour from a pitcher.

Yield: 12 8-ounce servings

Preparation time: 15 minutes

Cooking time: 20 minutes

LIGHT HOLIDAY EGGNOG

1 teaspoon canola oil
4 egg substitutes (1 cup)
1/4 cup granulated sugar
2 pints ice milk or fat-free ice cream, softened
1 teaspoon ground nutmeg, or to taste
Rum or brandy to taste (optional)

In large mixing bowl, combine canola oil, egg substitutes and sugar. Beat with wire whisk for 2 to 3 minutes. Add softened ice milk or fat-free ice cream and nutmeg. Stir with wire whisk until smooth.

This eggnog may be served immediately, with or without alcohol; or it may be refrigerated and served later. It will keep several days in the refrigerator. If you prefer a less thick eggnog, thin it by adding skim milk.

Yield: 6 servings

Preparation time: 10 minutes
(if ice cream is already softened)

For a 4-ounce serving (using ice milk):
Calories...... 198
Protein (g)... 9
Fat (g)....... 6
Sat. Fat (g).. 2.7
Choles. (mg).. 13
Fiber (g)..... 0
Sodium (mg)... 144
%Cal-Fat...... 27%

(With fat-free ice cream: 2 g fat/serving)

HOT CHOCOLATE MIX

1 25.6-ounce box instant dry milk
1/4 cup Hershey's cocoa powder
1 6-ounce box 10x powdered sugar
1 16-ounce container chocolate-flavored Nestle's Quik

Mix all ingredients together in a large mixing bowl. Pour into jars or containers to store.

To make hot chocolate, place 1/4 cup hot chocolate mix into coffee mug. Pour boiling water over. Stir until all lumps disappear.

Yield: 30 cups hot chocolate

Preparation time: 10 minutes

For an 8-ounce cup:
Calories...... 162
Protein (g)... 9
Fat (g)....... 0.8
Sat. Fat (g).. 0.5
Choles. (mg).. 4
Fiber (g)..... 0.2
Sodium (mg)... 171
%Cal-Fat...... 4%

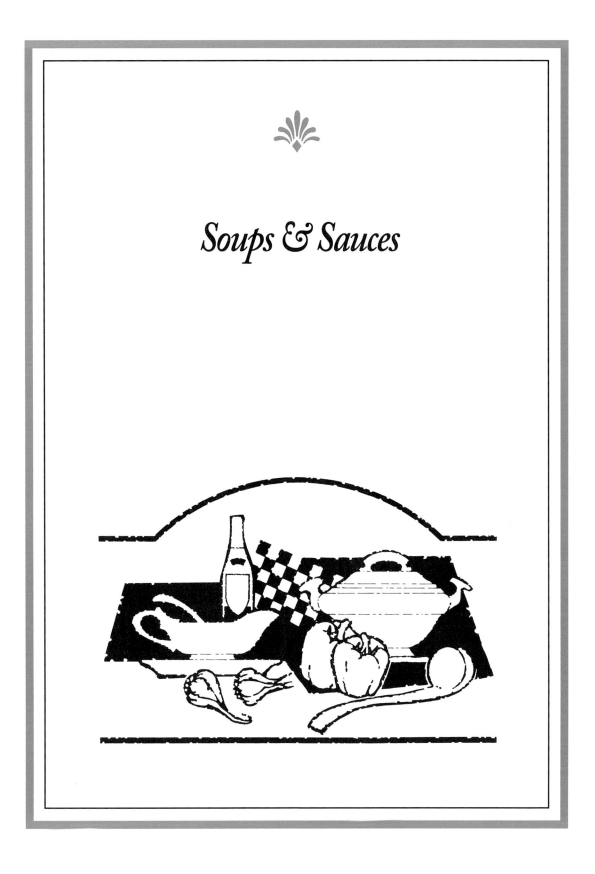

Soups & Sauces

SEAFOOD GUMBO

Per serving:
Calories...... 545
Protein (g)... 39
Fat (g)....... 7.5
Sat. Fat (g).. 1.7
Choles. (mg).. 192
Fiber (g)..... 3.3
Sodium (mg)... 754
%Cal-Fat...... 13%

2 tablespoons tub margarine
2 tablespoons flour
1/2 cup chopped green onions or leeks
1 green pepper, chopped
1/2 cup chopped celery
3 cloves garlic, minced
2 cups okra (fresh or frozen), sliced crosswise
2 14 1/2-ounce cans clear chicken broth, defatted or
    from own stock, (divided)
1 cup water
1/4 cup flour
1 10-ounce can tomato puree
1/2 pound lump crabmeat
2 tablespoons Worcestershire sauce
2 tablespoons brown sugar
1/4 teaspoon thyme
1/2 teaspoon paprika
1/4 teaspoon cayenne, or to taste
2 bay leaves
1 1/2 pounds raw shrimp, peeled and deveined
1 pint oysters with juice
6 to 8 cups prepared rice, white or brown
Salt and freshly ground pepper to taste

Heat margarine in large soup kettle. Add 2 tablespoons flour and stir constantly until roux (flour and oil mixture) turns dark brown. Add green onions, green pepper, celery and garlic. Saute 5 minutes. Add okra and saute an additional 5 minutes. Stir frequently to avoid sticking or burning.

With a wire whisk, mix 1/4 cup flour into 1/2 cup chicken broth. Add to kettle along with remaining chicken broth and water. Add tomato puree and mix well.

Add crabmeat, Worcestershire sauce, brown sugar, thyme paprika, cayenne, and bay leaves. Simmer 1 hour, covered.

Add shrimp and oysters with juice. Simmer until edges of oysters begin to curl, about 10 minutes.

Serve over rice in large soup bowls.

Yield: 8 servings

Preparation time: 30 minutes

Cooking time: 70 minutes

BOUILLABAISSE (FISH STEW)

1 tablespoon olive oil
1 medium onion, chopped
2 cloves garlic, minced
1 leak, chopped finely
4 ounces fresh mushrooms, sliced
1 28-ounce can whole tomatoes, chopped
1/2 cup bottled clam juice
1 1/2 cups dry white wine
1 tablespoon fresh basil, or 1 teaspoon dried
1 bay leaf
Pinch saffron (optional)
2 tablespoons chopped fresh parsley
Salt and pepper to taste (optional)
1 small lobster tail, cut into pieces
1/2 pound raw shrimp, shelled and deveined
1/2 pound scallops
1/2 pound mussels, well scrubbed and debearded
1 pound red snapper, cod, or whitefish, cut into bite-size
    pieces

Per serving:
Calories...... 307
Protein (g)... 40
Fat (g)....... 5.3
Sat. Fat (g).. 0.8
Choles. (mg).. 140
Fiber (g)..... 2.3
Sodium (mg)... 611
%Cal-Fat...... 13%

In large soup kettle, heat olive oil. Add onion, garlic, leek, and mushrooms and saute for five minutes, or until onion is translucent.

Add chopped tomatoes, clam juice, white wine, basil, bay leaf, saffron, parsley, salt and pepper. Bring to a boil and simmer 20 minutes.

Add lobster, shrimp, scallops, mussels, and red snapper and simmer an additional 15 minutes. Remove bay leaf. Serve immediately in large soup bowls.

Serve with Garlic Crustinos (Recipe, page 354), or French bread.

Yield: 6 large servings

Traditionally, bouillabaisse, a fish stew, is made with whatever fish is available. Therefore other fish or shellfish, in similar quantities, may be substituted for those given in this recipe.

Preparation time: 30 minutes

Cooking time: 15 minutes

LINGUINE CHICKEN SOUP

1 pound boneless chicken breasts, skinned
2 cups clear chicken broth, defatted (canned or from
  stock)
2 small onions, sliced and separated into rings
4 carrots, sliced into julienne strips
1/2 cup celery, chopped
12 ounces mushrooms, sliced
1/4 cup fresh parsley, chopped finely
3/4 teaspoon dried tarragon
16 ounces linguine
1/2 cup minced green onions or chives
Grated Parmesan cheese
Freshly ground pepper, to taste
Salt, to taste (optional)

Cut up chicken into strips 1/2-inch by 1 1/2-inches.

In large soup kettle, heat chicken broth over medium heat. Add chicken strips and onions. Bring to a boil and simmer, covered, 8 to 10 minutes.

Add carrots, celery, mushrooms, parsley and tarragon to soup kettle. Return to a boil and simmer, covered, an additional 8 to 10 minutes, or until vegetables are tender.

Meanwhile, cook linguine according to package directions. Drain. Add to soup mixture, after vegetables are fully cooked. Add minced green onions.

Serve in large soup bowls. Sprinkle with Parmesan cheese and freshly ground pepper. Salt to taste, if desired.

Yield: 6 main-dish servings

This soup with its generous amount of "noodles" resembles an oriental soup and can serve as the entree of a hearty evening meal.

Preparation time: 20 minutes

Cooking time: 10–15 minutes

NEW ENGLAND CLAM CHOWDER

3 6 1/2-ounce cans chopped clams, including liquid
1 tablespoon tub margarine
1/2 cup chopped onion
1/2 cup liquid from clams
1 1/2 cups water
4 cups diced potatoes
2 cups skim milk, divided
1/4 cup flour
1 cup canned evaporated skim milk
1 teaspoon salt
1/4 teaspoon pepper

Per 1-cup serving:
Calories...... 116
Protein (g)... 12
Fat (g)....... 2
Sat. Fat (g).. 0.4
Choles. (mg).. 21
Fiber (g)..... 1
Sodium (mg)... 373
%Cal-Fat...... 15%

Drain clams, reserving liquid.

In heavy soup kettle, melt margarine. Add onion and saute until it becomes translucent. Add clams, 1/2 cup liquid from clams, water and potatoes. Bring to a boil, reduce heat, and simmer for 20 to 30 minutes, or until potatoes are soft.

Mix flour with 1/2 cup skim milk until smooth. Add flour mixture, remaining 1 1/2 cups skim milk, evaporated milk, salt and pepper to soup kettle. Heat just to a boil, stirring occasionally. Serve immediately.

Yield: Makes 10 1-cup servings, or 4 large main course servings

Preparation time: 25 minutes

Cooking time: 30 minutes

OYSTER STEW

Per Serving:
Calories...... 186
Protein (g)... 15
Fat (g)....... 3.7
Sat. Fat (g).. 0.9
Choles. (mg).. 49
Fiber (g)..... 1
Sodium (mg)... 446
%Cal-Fat...... 18%

3 medium potatoes, peeled and diced
1/4 cup finely chopped onion
2 teaspoons margarine
1 pint shucked oysters, with liquid
1 12-ounce can evaporated skim milk
1 teaspoon seasoned salt
Dash of cayenne pepper, or to taste
1 teaspoon Worcestershire sauce
1/4 cup plus 1 tablespoon flour
2 1/2 cups skim milk
Salt to taste
2 tablespoons fresh chopped parsley
Oyster crackers (optional)

Place diced potatoes in large saucepan with just enough water to cover top of potatoes. Bring to a boil and simmer 15 minutes or until potatoes are tender.

Meanwhile, in medium saucepan, saute onion in margarine until onion becomes translucent. Add oysters and liquid. Bring to a boil and simmer 10 minutes or until the edges of oysters curl.

As soon as potatoes are tender, drain water. Add oyster mixture, evaporated milk, seasoned salt, cayenne pepper, and Worcestershire sauce. Set aside.

In small bowl, mix flour with skim milk until all lumps disappear. Add to potato mixture. Salt to taste. Heat stew, stirring frequently, until it comes to a boil and thickens slightly. Sprinkle with chopped parsley. Serve immediately. Serve with oyster crackers, if desired.

Yield: 6 10-ounce servings

Preparation time: 20 minutes

Cooking time: 20–25 minutes

LENTIL SOUP

2 cups dry lentils
7 cups water
1 1/2 teaspoons minced garlic
4 medium carrots, chopped
3 stalks celery, chopped
1 medium onion, chopped
16 ounces tomato sauce
1 fresh tomato chopped
2 tablespoons white wine vinegar
1 tablespoon Lite soy sauce
1 1/2 tablespoons brown sugar
1 1/2 teaspoons dried basil
1/4 teaspoon black pepper
Juice of 1/2 lemon
Parmesan cheese (optional)

Per serving:
Calories...... 198
Protein (g)... 14
Fat (g)....... 0.7
Sat. Fat (g).. 0.1
Choles. (mg).. 0
Fiber (g)..... 7.8
Sodium (mg)... 402
%Cal-Fat...... 3%

Rinse lentils; drain and place in soup kettle. Add water, garlic, carrots, celery and onion. Cover and simmer 1 1/2 hours.

Add remaining ingredients and simmer, covered, 30 minutes longer. If soup is too thick, add additional water. Sprinkle with Parmesan cheese, if desired.

Yield: 8 to 10 servings.

Leftover soup tastes great over pasta or freezes well.

Preparation time: 25 minutes

Cooking time: 2 hours

MINESTRONE SOUP

1 20-ounce package dried 15-bean mixture
11 cups water
1 large onion, chopped
3 carrots, chopped
2 cloves of garlic, minced
1 28-ounce can tomatoes, chopped
3 chicken bouillon cubes
2 teaspoons basil
1 tablespoon olive oil (optional)
Pepper to taste
Juice of 1/2 lemon
8 ounces dumpling pasta

Soak minestrone bean mix overnight or at least 2 to 3 hours in enough water to cover beans. Drain.

In a large kettle, put beans, 11 cups water, and remaining ingredients except pasta. Cook over medium heat for 3 hours or until beans are tender.

Shortly before serving, add pasta to soup and boil 10 to 15 minutes longer, until pasta is ready. If soup gets too thick, add more water as needed.

Serve immediately. If desired, sprinkle with Parmesan cheese.

Yield: Makes 16 one-cup servings, or 8 2-cup servings.

Soaking beans is not essential, but is recommended. If soaking is omitted, increase cooking time slightly.

Preparation time: 20 minutes

Cooking time: 3 hours, 15 minutes

SOUTHWESTERN-STYLE BEAN SOUP

1 15 1/2-ounce can navy beans or Northern beans,
   rinsed and drained
1 15 1/2-ounce can kidney beans, rinsed and drained
1 15 1/2-ounce can pinto beans, rinsed and drained
1 15-ounce can clear chicken broth, defatted
1 cup water
3 fresh tomatoes, chopped coarsely
1 10-ounce pkg. frozen whole kernel corn, thawed
2 medium carrots, sliced
1 large onion, chopped
1 8-ounce can tomato sauce
1/4 teaspoon minced garlic
1/4 teaspoon Tabasco sauce
1 to 2 teaspoons chili powder

Combine all ingredients in a 4-quart heavy saucepan. Bring to a boil. Reduce heat, cover, and simmer for 45 minutes or longer. Serve with corn bread.

Yield: 4 to 6 servings

Preparation time: 20 minutes

Cooking time: 45 minutes

Per serving:
Calories...... 437
Protein (g)... 25
Fat (g)....... 2.9
Sat. Fat (g).. 0.6
Choles. (mg).. 0
Fiber (g)..... 12
Sodium (mg)... 850
%Cal-Fat...... 6%

LOUISIANA-STYLE RED BEAN SOUP

Per serving:
Calories...... 280
Protein (g)... 14
Fat (g)....... 3.3
Sat. Fat (g).. 0.5
Choles. (mg).. 0
Fiber (g)..... 4
Sodium (mg)... 672
%Cal-Fat...... 11%

2 teaspoons olive oil
1 large onion, chopped
1 large green pepper, chopped finely
2 cloves garlic, minced
1 large stalk celery, chopped
2 15-ounce cans red kidney beans, drained and rinsed
1 14-ounce can clear chicken broth, defatted
1 16-ounce can "no salt added" tomatoes, chopped
2 cups water
1/2 cup long grain rice, uncooked
1/2 teaspoon thyme
1/4 teaspoon cumin
1 teaspoon paprika
1 tablespoon red wine vinegar
Tabasco sauce to taste (1/4 to 1/2 teaspoon)
Salt to taste

Heat olive oil in heavy soup kettle and saute onion, green pepper, garlic and celery, until vegetables are tender, but not brown.

Add remaining ingredients. Bring to a boil, and simmer 30 minutes or until rice is tender.

Yield: 4 to 6 servings

Delicious with toasted French bread and a green salad.

Preparation time: 20 minutes

Cooking time: 30 minutes

SPLIT PEA SOUP

1 pound dried split green peas
4 cups water
2 14 1/2-ounce cans clear chicken broth, defatted
1 clove garlic, crushed
3/4 cup diced carrot
1/2 cup diced celery
3/4 cup diced onion
1 1/2 ounces chopped low-fat boiled ham (2 sandwich slices)
1/2 teaspoon dried thyme
1 bay leaf
Freshly ground black pepper (optional)
Garnish with fresh thyme (optional)

Per serving:
Calories...... 263
Protein (g)... 20
Fat (g)....... 1.9
Sat. Fat (g).. 0.4
Choles. (mg).. 4
Fiber (g)..... 10
Sodium (mg)... 510
%Cal-Fat......6%

Rinse peas under cold water to remove any foreign particles.

Place all the ingredients except the pepper and fresh thyme in a large soup kettle. Bring to a boil and simmer, covered, for 2 1/2 to 3 hours. Serve hot.

Sprinkle freshly ground black pepper over individual bowls of soup, and garnish with sprigs of fresh thyme, if desired.

Yield: 6 to 8 servings

Preparation time: 15 minutes

Cooking time: 3–4 hours

SALMON BISQUE

Per serving:
Calories...... 177
Protein (g)... 14
Fat (g)....... 2.5
Sat. Fat (g).. 0.5
Choles. (mg).. 16
Fiber (g)..... 1
Sodium (mg)... 544
%Cal-Fat...... 13%

2 14 1/2-ounce cans clear chicken broth, defatted
8 ounces fresh salmon
1/2 cup chopped celery
2 tablespoons chives, finely chopped
1 6-ounce can tomato paste
3/8 cup sherry (6 tablespoons)
2 12-ounce cans evaporated skim milk
1/2 cup flour
1/4 teaspoon pepper
1 teaspoon seasoned salt (optional)

In 4-quart saucepan, pour defatted chicken broth. Add salmon, celery, and chives. Bring to a boil, reduce heat and simmer, covered, for 10 minutes. Carefully remove salmon from broth with a spatula. Set aside.

Add tomato paste and sherry to saucepan, mixing well with a wire whisk. Bring to a boil and simmer an additional 20 minutes.

Meanwhile, remove skin from salmon and mash into small pieces with a fork.

In medium-size bowl, stir flour and evaporated milk with a wire whisk until all lumps disappear. Add milk mixture, salmon, pepper and seasoned salt to saucepan. Heat just until bisque comes to a boil and thickens.* Remove from heat and serve.

Yield: 8 to 9 1-cup servings

Do not boil more than a few minutes after adding the milk mixture to avoid curdling.

Preparation time: 20 minutes

Cooking time: 25 minutes

CREAM OF BROCCOLI SOUP

1 bunch broccoli, divided
2 medium onions, chopped
1 cup chopped celery
1 carrot, chopped
2 14 1/2-ounce cans clear chicken broth, defatted
1/2 teaspoon minced garlic
1 cup water
1/2 cup flour
2 12-ounce cans evaporated skim milk
1/2 teaspoon thyme
1/4 teaspoon black pepper
Chopped scallions (optional)
Parmesan cheese (optional)

Per serving:
Calories...... 186
Protein (g)... 16
Fat (g)....... 1.6
Sat. Fat (g).. 0.4
Choles. (mg).. 3
Fiber (g)..... 3
Sodium (mg)... 492
%Cal-Fat...... 7%

Thinly slice 2 cups of broccoli flowerets. Set aside. Coarsely chop remaining broccoli (including stems), onions, celery, and carrot.

Place chicken broth in 4-quart heavy saucepan. Add chopped vegetables (except for 2 cups flowerets), minced garlic and water. Bring to a boil and simmer until vegetables are tender (about 30 minutes).

Puree broth mixture in food processor until smooth. Return to saucepan.

In a medium-size mixing bowl, add flour to evaporated skim milk, mixing with wire whisk until smooth. Add to pureed mixture. Add flowerets, thyme and pepper. Bring to a boil over medium heat, stirring frequently. Simmer until flowerets are tender.

Pour into soup bowls. Sprinkle with scallions or Parmesan cheese, if desired.

Yield: 8 servings

Preparation time: 25 minutes

Cooking time: 40 minutes

CREAM OF CARROT SOUP

Per serving:
Calories...... 150
Protein (g)... 6
Fat (g)....... 2
Sat. Fat (g).. 0.5
Choles. (mg).. <1
Fiber (g)..... 7
Sodium (mg)... 398
%Cal-Fat...... 13%

2 pounds carrots, peeled and thinly sliced
1 1/2 cups chopped onion
1 cup sliced celery
1 14 1/2-ounce can clear chicken broth, defatted
1 1/2 cups water
2 teaspoons tub margarine
1 teaspoon freshly grated ginger root
1 5-ounce can evaporated skim milk
1 tablespoon sherry
Garnish with sprigs of fresh rosemary (optional)

Combine sliced carrots, onion, celery, chicken broth, and water in large saucepan. Bring to a boil. Cover and simmer 20 minutes, or until carrots are tender. Let cool slightly. Drain carrots, reserving liquid.

Meanwhile, in small frypan, saute ginger root in margarine for 3 minutes. Add to drained carrot mixture.

In a food processor or blender, puree drained carrots until smooth, gradually adding all the reserved liquid during the processing. Return to soup kettle. Whisk in evaporated milk. Heat slowly until soup almost comes to a boil. Just before serving, stir in sherry.

Garnish with sprigs of fresh rosemary.

Yield: 4 to 6 servings

Preparation time: 25 minutes

Cooking time: 15 minutes

EGG & LEMON SOUP

10 cups defatted chicken or turkey broth
1 small onion, halved
4 cloves garlic, crushed
2 sprigs parsley
2 celery stalks with leaves
1 bay leaf
1 cup orzo (pasta)
Salt to taste
1/4 teaspoon pepper
4 egg substitutes (1 cup)
Juice of 2 lemons (6 tablespoons) or to taste
Freshly ground pepper (optional)

Per serving:
Calories...... 158
Protein (g)... 12
Fat (g)....... 2.9
Sat. Fat (g).. 0.7
Choles. (mg).. <1
Fiber (g)..... 1.3
Sodium (mg)... NA
%Cal-Fat...... 17%

Combine broth, onion, garlic, parsley, celery, and bay leaf in soup kettle or large saucepan. Bring to a boil. Strain broth into a bowl. Return broth to kettle and discard vegetables.

Add orzo, salt, and pepper to broth. Bring to a boil. Reduce heat and simmer, covered, for 10 to 15 minutes or until orzo is soft.

Place egg substitutes and lemon juice in a food processor. Process until smooth. Add about 1 cup soup to egg mixture in food processor. Blend until frothy. Add another 1 cup soup to mixture in food processor. Process until smooth.

Add egg/lemon mixture to soup in kettle. Serve immediately. (If you need to heat up the soup after adding the lemon juice mixture, be very careful not to overheat it because curdling can occur. The soup will curdle just before reaching the boiling point.) Sprinkle with freshly ground pepper, if desired.

Yield: 8 to 10 servings.

To limit sodium, use unsalted broth from your own stock, or use 5 cups canned chicken broth and 5 cups water.

Preparation time: 30 minutes

Cooking time: 10 minutes

GAZPACHO SOUP

2 cups tomato sauce (no salt added)
2 cups tomato juice
1 small onion, finely chopped
2 cups fresh tomatoes, diced
1 cup minced green pepper
2 tablespoons fresh parsley, finely chopped
1 diced cucumber
1 teaspoon honey
1 clove garlic crushed
Juice of 1/2 lemon
Juice of 1 lime
2 tablespoons wine vinegar
1 teaspoon tarragon
1 teaspoon basil
Dash of ground cumin
1/4 teaspoon Tabasco sauce (or to taste)
Pepper to taste
1 tablespoon olive oil (optional)

Combine all ingredients. Chill for at least 2 hours. This soup can be pureed, if desired.

Yield: 8 one-cup servings

A refreshing crunchy cold soup ideal for lunch or a light supper during the summer. A crusty French bread or corn bread would be a perfect accompaniment.

Preparation time: 20 minutes

Chill 2 hours before serving

CABBAGE VEGETABLE SOUP

2 medium potatoes, cubed
1 16-ounce can chick peas, drained
4 cups cabbage, chopped
4 carrots, sliced 1/8-inch thick
2 14 1/2-ounce cans clear chicken broth, defatted
3 cups water
16-ounce can "no salt added" canned tomatoes, chopped
1/4 teaspoon celery seed
1/4 teaspoon black pepper
1/2 teaspoon basil
1 tablespoon fresh parsley, chopped
Salt to taste

Per serving:
Calories...... 121
Protein (g)... 7
Fat (g)....... 1.9
Sat. Fat (g).. 0.3
Choles. (mg).. 0
Fiber (g)..... 5.5
Sodium (mg)... 386
%Cal-Fat...... 13%

Prepare vegetables as indicated above. Drain chick peas and skim fat from top of chicken broth. Combine all ingredients in large soup kettle. Bring to a boil and simmer 1 hour. Serve immediately.

Yield: 10 one-cup servings, or 6 12-ounce servings.

Preparation time: 20 minutes

Cooking time: 1 hour

TUNA FISH SAUCE

1 3 1/2-ounce can white albacore tuna, packed in water
2 anchovy fillets
1 tablespoon brine from jar of capers
2 cloves garlic, minced
3/4 cup nonfat mayonnaise
Lemon juice to taste (about 1 teaspoon)
2 tablespoons capers (optional)

For 1 tablespoon:
Calories...... 19
Protein (g)... 2
Fat (g)....... 0
Sat. Fat (g).. 0
Choles. (mg).. 2
Fiber (g)..... 0
Sodium (mg)... 183
%Cal-Fat...... 4%

Drain tuna. Combine tuna and remaining ingredients, except capers, in a food processor. Blend 2 to 3 minutes, or until sauce is smooth. Stir in capers, if desired.

Spread sauce generously over cooked and chilled chicken breasts or thin-sliced veal. Serve immediately or refrigerate for up to three days.

Yield: 1 cup sauce

This sauce is a favorite delicacy in Northern Italy. Now, with the availability of nonfat mayonnaise, it can be made nearly fat-free. The sauce, served with chilled chicken or veal, is ideal for lunch or before the main course at dinner. It is also delicious spread on crackers or bread.

Preparation time: 15 minutes

BORDELAISE SAUCE

For 1/4 cup sauce:
Calories...... 30
Protein (g)... 1
Fat (g)....... 1.1
Sat. Fat (g).. 0.3
Choles. (mg).. 0
Fiber (g)..... 0.2
Sodium (mg)... 165
%Cal-Fat...... 9%

3/4 cup sliced fresh mushrooms
2 tablespoons finely chopped chives or green onions
1 tablespoon tub margarine
1/4 cup all-purpose flour
1 14 1/2-ounce can clear beef broth, defatted
1 teaspoon dried tarragon, crushed
1 tablespoon lemon juice
3 tablespoons dry red wine
Dash cayenne pepper (to taste)

In large non-stick skillet, saute mushrooms and chives in margarine until mushrooms turn dark in color.

Meanwhile, remove fat from top of canned beef broth. Pour into mixing bowl. Add flour and mix with wire whisk until well blended.

Add broth mixture to mushrooms in skillet. Bring to a boil, stirring occasionally. Add remaining ingredients. Simmer 5 to 10 minutes. Serve over pork or beef.

Yield: 2 1/4 cups

Preparation time: 20 minutes

Cooking time: 10 minutes

WHITE SAUCE

2 tablespoons all-purpose flour
1 cup skim milk
1/4 teaspoon salt
1/8 teaspoon white pepper

In small bowl, combine flour and milk, mixing with a wire whisk until all lumps disappear.

Place small skillet over medium heat. Add flour/milk mixture. Add salt and pepper. Heat until sauce comes to a boil and thickens.

Yield: 1 cup sauce

For thicker sauce, increase flour to 1/4 cup; for thinner sauce, decrease flour to 1 tablespoon.

Preparation time: 10 minutes

For 1/4 cup sauce:
Calories...... 36
Protein (g)... 3
Fat (g)....... 0.2
Sat. Fat (g).. 0
Choles. (mg).. 1
Fiber (g)..... 0
Sodium (mg)... 165
%Cal-Fat...... 4%

TARTAR SAUCE

1/2 cup nonfat mayonnaise
1 tablespoon finely chopped dill pickle
1 teaspoon finely chopped chives
1/2 teaspoon finely chopped pimiento
1 teaspoon fresh parsley, finely chopped

Combine all ingredients, mixing well. Chill at least 2 hours. Serve with fish.

Yield: 1/2 cup sauce.

Preparation time: 10 minutes

Chill 2 hours before serving

For 1 tablespoon:
Calories...... 13
Protein (g)... 0
Fat (g)....... 0
Sat. Fat (g).. 0
Choles. (mg).. 0
Fiber (g)..... 0
Sodium (mg)... 216
%Cal-Fat...... 0%

Salads & Salad Dressings

CHICKEN SALAD IN PINEAPPLE BOATS

Per serving:
Calories...... 269
Protein (g)... 31
Fat (g)....... 8.6
Sat. Fat (g).. 1.8
Choles. (mg).. 83
Fiber (g)..... 1.5
Sodium (mg)... 265
%Cal-Fat...... 28%

2 whole fresh pineapples with tops
2 1/2 cups cooked chicken breast, cubed (1 lb.)
1 cup cubed pineapple
1 cup seedless grapes, halved
1/2 cup diced celery
3/4 cup nonfat or low-fat plain yogurt
1/4 cup light mayonnaise
1/4 teaspoon salt
1/8 cup toasted slivered almonds
8 fresh strawberries for garnish (optional)

Make pineapple boats by first slicing whole pineapples, including decorative crown, lengthwise. Cut out pineapple fruit, reserving shell and crown. Cut pineapple into bite-size pieces. Set aside.

In a large mixing bowl, combine cubed chicken, pineapple, grapes and celery. Toss.

In a small bowl, combine yogurt, mayonnaise and salt. Add to chicken mixture, tossing to coat well. Chill.

To serve chicken salad, fill pineapple boats; or, if fresh pineapple is not available, arrange lettuce on plate, top with pineapple slice, followed by chicken salad. Garnish plate with fresh strawberries.

Yield: 4 servings.

This dish is ideal for a refreshing spring luncheon or a light summer meal. Leftover turkey breast may be substituted for the chicken breast.

**Preparation time: 20–25 minutes
(provided chicken is precooked)**

CURRY CHICKEN SALAD

2 cups diced cooked chicken (5 chicken breast halves)
1 1/2 cups cooked white rice
3/4 cup coarsely chopped celery
1 cup raisins
2 tablespoons slivered almonds or chopped pecans
2 tablespoons finely chopped onion
1/2 cup nonfat plain yogurt
1/4 cup light mayonnaise
1 1/2 teaspoons curry powder
1/2 teaspoon salt
1 tablespoon lemon juice
2 tablespoons sugar

Per serving:
Calories...... 285
Protein (g)... 17
Fat (g)....... 5.9
Sat. Fat (g).. 1.1
Choles. (mg).. 38
Fiber (g)..... 2.3
Sodium (mg)... 289
%Cal-Fat...... 18%

Lightly toss together the chicken, rice, celery, raisins, almonds and onion.

Make dressing of yogurt, mayonnaise, curry powder, salt, lemon juice and sugar. Add dressing to chicken-rice mixture and toss until well mixed. Chill thoroughly.

Serve over pieces of Romaine lettuce. Garnish with additional almonds and/or lemon slices.

Yield: 6 servings

This dish is ideal for a ladies' luncheon, served with cornbread muffins, cantaloupe slices and a light dessert.

**Preparation time: 20–25 minutes
(provided chicken and rice are precooked)**

GRILLED CHICKEN SALAD

Per serving:
Calories...... 270
Protein (g)... 37
Fat (g)....... 7.6
Sat. Fat (g).. 1.9
Choles. (mg).. 96
Fiber (g)..... 3
Sodium (mg)... NA
%Cal-Fat...... 25%

1 pound boneless chicken breast
1/4 to 1/2 cup no-oil Italian salad dressing
4 large carrots, peeled and sliced thin
1 large onion, sliced thin
1 bunch fresh parsley, chopped coarsely

Quick Low-fat Vinaigrette dressing:
5 tablespoons no-oil Italian dressing
1 tablespoon olive oil
3 tablespoons Balsamic vinegar

Marinate chicken breasts in no-oil Italian salad dressing at least 2 hours. Cook on preheated grill 8 to 10 minutes per side, or until chicken is no longer pink inside. Chop into bite-size pieces.

While chicken is on grill, slice carrots and onion, and chop parsley. Set aside.

To assemble salad, place chicken pieces in bottom of 9 x 9-inch baking dish. While chicken is still warm, top with layer of sliced carrots, followed by layer of sliced onions. Sprinkle parsley over top.

Pour vinaigrette dressing evenly over top of salad. Serve within 30 minutes, or refrigerate and serve later.

Yield: 4 servings

This is a quick and easy salad - perfect for an evening meal after a busy day. Serve with your favorite bread and a fruit for dessert.

Marinating time: 2 hours

Cooking time: 15–20 minutes

Preparation time: 15–20 minutes

POACHED SALMON SALAD

1 head Romaine lettuce
1 yellow pepper, cut into thin strips
1 green pepper, cut into thin strips
1 red pepper, cut into thin strips
1 carrot, sliced julienne
1/4 cup crunchy sprout mix (bean sprouts)
4 ounces Farmer's cheese
12 ounces salmon filet, poached
Salad dressing of choice (low-fat or nonfat)

Per serving:
Calories...... 213
Protein (g)... 30
Fat (g)....... 6.8
Sat. Fat (g).. 1.3
Choles. (mg).. 44
Fiber (g)..... 2.5
Sodium (mg)... 65
%Cal-Fat...... 28%

Follow instructions for poached salmon (Recipe, page 289). Chill.

Wash Romaine and break into bite-size pieces. Place in very large salad bowl. Cut up peppers and carrot and place over top. Sprinkle sprout mix over top. Set aside until ready to serve.

To serve, divide salad equally onto four dinner plates. Top with 1 ounce chunk Farmer's cheese and 3 ounces salmon. Drizzle dressing of choice over top.

Yield: 4 servings

A main dish salad with a spectacle of color that is great for lunch or for dinner on a hot summer day. Serve with a choice breads - French, multi-grain and/or muffins.

Preparation time: 20 minutes

Cooking time: 15 minutes to poach salmon

TUNA PASTA SALAD

Per serving:
Calories...... 286
Protein (g)... 25
Fat (g)....... 4.8
Sat. Fat (g).. 1.3
Choles. (mg).. 37
Fiber (g)..... 3
Sodium (mg)... 525
%Cal-Fat...... 15%

8 ounces pasta spirals
1/2 cup sliced green onions
1 green pepper, chopped
1 cup seedless cucumber, sliced and quartered
1 cup cherry tomatoes, halved
1 13-ounce can tuna, packed in water, drained
1/4 cup black olives, halved

Salad Dressing:
1 tablespoon olive oil
2 tablespoons white wine vinegar
2 tablespoons lemon juice
1/4 cup no-oil Italian dressing
1/4 cup Parmesan cheese
1/4 cup fresh parsley, chopped
1/4 teaspoon salt
1/4 teaspoon pepper
1/2 teaspoon garlic powder

Prepare pasta according to package directions. Drain and immediately pour cold water over. While pasta is cooking, prepare vegetables.

In a 4 or 5-quart casserole, combine pasta, green onions, green pepper, cucumber, cherry tomatoes, tuna and olives. Mix well.

Make dressing by combining all ingredients in small mixing bowl. Beat with wire whisk. Pour over pasta mixture and mix until thoroughly blended.

Cover and refrigerate at least 8 hours before serving.

Yield: 6 servings

To add extra zip, you may want to add additional no-oil Italian dressing, to taste. Also, to save time, 1/2 cup no-oil Italian dressing, plus 1/4 cup Parmesan cheese may be used as the salad dressing for this pasta salad.

Preparation time: 25 minutes

SCALLOP ANTIPASTO SALAD

1 1/2 pounds small red potatoes, unpeeled
1/4 cup red wine vinegar (preferably Balsamic vinegar)
1 tablespoon olive oil
3 tablespoons chopped red onion
3 tablespoons chopped fresh parsley
1/2 teaspoon Dijon mustard
1/4 teaspoon dill leaves
1/8 teaspoon salt
1/4 teaspoon fresh ground black pepper
1 pound bay scallops
1/2 teaspoon garlic powder
1/2 cup chopped celery
1/4 cup sliced black olives
1 cup snow peas, cut in half lengthwise

Per serving:
Calories...... 305
Protein (g)... 26
Fat (g)....... 5.5
Sat. Fat (g).. 0.7
Choles. (mg).. 38
Fiber (g)..... 8.5
Sodium (mg)... 377
%Cal-Fat...... 16%

Cook potatoes in boiling water until tender, about 20 minutes. Cut into quarters and place in large bowl. Cool.

Combine vinegar, olive oil, onion, parsley, mustard, dill leaves, salt and pepper. Mix well. Pour over cooled potatoes.

Rinse scallops. Place in a single layer in shallow oven-proof dish. Sprinkle with 1/4 teaspoon garlic powder. Broil on top shelf of oven until lightly browned, about 5 minutes. Toss scallops. Sprinkle with remaining 1/4 teaspoon garlic powder. Broil 5 additional minutes.

Pour scallops with juice over potato mixture. Add celery, olives and snow peas. Toss gently.

Yield: 4 servings

Delicious served with baked apples and French bread.

(For added crispness, soak snow peas in cold water in refrigerator for 1 hour. Drain. Snap in half.)

Preparation time: 30–40 minutes

TUNA STUFFED TOMATOES

Per serving:
Calories...... 172
Protein (g)... 28
Fat (g)....... 1.5
Sat. Fat (g).. 0.8
Choles. (mg).. 54
Fiber (g)..... 2.4
Sodium (mg)... 519
%Cal-Fat...... 8%

1 12 1/2-ounce can tuna fish, in spring water
2 baby dill pickles, finely chopped
1/4 cup finely chopped onion
1/2 cup chopped celery
1/4 to 1/2 cup nonfat mayonnaise
4 large tomatoes
2 tablespoons chopped parsley

Drain water from tuna fish. Place in large bowl. Add remaining ingredients except tomatoes and parsley. Set aside.

Cut off upper 1/3 of tomato. Scrape out pulp. Add tomato pulp to tuna mixture and stir until well blended. Fill tomatoes with tuna salad. Sprinkle with parsley flakes.

Yield: 4 servings

Preparation time: 15–20 minutes

SWISS-STYLE GARDEN SALAD

Per serving:
Calories...... 129
Protein (g)... 5
Fat (g)....... 1
Sat. Fat (g).. 0.2
Choles. (mg).. 0
Fiber (g)..... 4.7
Sodium (mg)... 26
%Cal-Fat...... 9%

2 small cucumbers, peeled, cut in half lengthwise,
  deseeded, and sliced 1/4-inch thick
2 medium carrots, finely shredded
1 11-ounce can "no salt added" corn, drained
1 bunch leaf lettuce, torn into bite-size pieces
Salad dressing of choice (low-fat or nonfat)

Prepare vegetables as indicated above. In 4 large individual salad bowls, place equal portions of sliced cucumbers, shredded carrots, and corn, placing each in separate sections of bowl. Top with leaf lettuce. Pour salad dressing over top.

Yield: 4 large salads

Preparation time: 15–20 minutes

BLACK BEAN SALAD

1 pound dried black beans*
1 1/2 teaspoons salt
1 teaspoon cumin
2 cups corn, fresh or frozen
1 green pepper, coarsely chopped
1 red bell pepper, coarsely chopped
1 medium purple onion, finely chopped
Dressing:
1/4 cup Balsamic vinegar,
1 teaspoon dried cilantro
1 teaspoon cumin
1/2 teaspoon coriander
Freshly ground pepper to taste
2 tablespoons olive oil

Per serving:
Calories...... 236
Protein (g)... 12
Fat (g)....... 4.4
Sat. Fat (g).. 0.7
Choles. (mg).. 0
Fiber (g)..... 11.6
Sodium (mg)... 415
%Cal-Fat...... 16%

Wash beans, removing any debris. Put into large pot with 8 cups cold water and soak overnight.

To cook beans, first drain beans in colander and rinse thoroughly. Return to pot. Add three cups cold water, salt and cumin. Bring to a boil, reduce heat and simmer just until tender, about 45 minutes. Remove from heat and let cool. Drain off any excess liquid.

Meanwhile, cook corn until tender. Cool.

After beans are cooled, add corn, chopped green pepper, red pepper, and onion. Toss together lightly.

To make dressing, combine vinegar, cilantro, cumin, coriander and pepper in a jar or container with a lid. Shake well to mix. Add olive oil. Shake again and pour over bean salad. Toss to combine well.

Chill for several hours or overnight. If refrigerated, salad stays fresh for at least three days.

Yield: 8 large salads

Four cups canned black beans may be substituted for 1 pound dried beans. Be sure to drain and rinse if using canned beans, and do not add additional salt.

Preparation time: 25 minutes

Cooking time: 45–60 minutes (to cook beans)

GARBANZO-TOMATO SALAD

Per serving:
Calories...... 129
Protein (g)... 6
Fat (g)....... 2.5
Sat. Fat (g).. 0.3
Choles. (mg).. 0
Fiber (g)..... 5.6
Sodium (mg)... 317
%Cal-Fat...... 17%

1 pound cherry tomatoes, washed and dried
1 15 1/2-ounce can garbanzo beans, rinsed and drained
1 cup chopped celery
1/4 cup sliced green olives

Dressing:
3 tablespoons no-oil Italian dressing
2 tablespoons fresh lemon juice
2 teaspoons honey mustard
1/4 teaspoon salt
1/4 teaspoon freshly ground black pepper
1/4 cup chopped fresh parsley

Cut tomatoes into quarters. Place in large mixing bowl. Add beans, chopped celery and sliced olives.

To make dressing, whisk together Italian dressing, lemon juice, mustard, salt and pepper. Stir in parsley. Pour over garbanzo bean mixture. Mix well, making sure beans and vegetables are well coated. Let flavors marinate at least 2 hours before serving.

This salad may be made a day ahead of time.

Yield: 6 to 8 servings

Three medium-size tomatoes, chopped, may be substituted for the cherry tomatoes.

Preparation time: 20–25 minutes

MANDARIN SALAD

1/4 cup sliced almonds
5 teaspoons sugar
1 head Romaine lettuce
1/2 head Boston lettuce
3 slices red onion, rings separated
1 cup chopped celery
1 11-ounce can mandarin oranges, drained

Salad Dressing:
2 tablespoons olive oil
1/4 cup wine vinegar
1/4 cup sugar
2 tablespoons chopped fresh parsley
1/2 teaspoon salt
Freshly ground pepper to taste
Dash of Tabasco sauce

Per serving:
Calories...... 108
Protein (g)... 1
Fat (g)....... 5.3
Sat. Fat (g).. 0.5
Choles. (mg).. 0
Fiber (g)..... 1.5
Sodium (mg)... 151
%Cal-Fat...... 43%

Cook almonds and sugar in a small saucepan over medium heat, stirring constantly until sugar is dissolved and almonds are coated. Watch very carefully since the sugar can turn brown and burn. Cool to room temperature. Store in an airtight container to maintain freshness.

Make dressing by mixing all ingredients together. Chill until ready to serve.

Wash Romaine and Boston lettuce and tear into bite-size pieces. Add sliced onion and chopped celery. Just before serving, add sugared almonds and mandarin oranges. Pour dressing over and toss to coat greens evenly.

Yield: 8 servings

Preparation time: 30–35 minutes

CELESTIAL SALAD

Per serving:
Calories...... 95
Protein (g)... 1
Fat (g)....... 3
Sat. Fat (g).. 0.6
Choles. (mg).. 0
Fiber (g)..... 2
Sodium (mg)... 8
%Cal-Fat...... 32%

1 head Romaine lettuce
1 11-ounce can mandarin oranges (drained)
1 cup seedless grapes (halved)
1/2 cup chopped green onions
1/2 cup sliced mushrooms
1/4 cup sliced toasted almonds (optional)

Salad Dressing:
2 tablespoons olive or canola oil
1/4 cup sugar
1 teaspoon celery seeds
2 tablespoons chopped parsley
2 tablespoons red wine vinegar
1/4 cup orange juice
1/2 teaspoon dry mustard

Wash Romaine lettuce and tear into bite-size pieces. Add remaining salad ingredients, and 1/2 of the almonds, if using almonds.

To make dressing, combine all ingredients in a jar with a tight fitting lid. Shake well. Just before serving, pour over greens. Toss lightly. Sprinkle remaining almonds over top, if desired.

Yield: 8 servings

A sweet salad that is a perfect complement to a spicy or highly seasoned main dish. Spinach greens may be substituted for the Romaine, or a combination of Romaine and spinach may be used.

Preparation time: 20–25 minutes

SPINACH SALAD WITH HONEY MUSTARD DRESSING

10 to 12 ounces raw spinach
1/2 red onion, sliced thin
1 cup fresh mushrooms, sliced thin

Dressing:
1/4 cup honey
1 tablespoon Dijon mustard
1 tablespoon canola oil
2 tablespoons white wine
1/2 teaspoon Worcestershire sauce
2 teaspoons poppy seeds (optional)

Per serving:
Calories...... 91
Protein (g)... 3
Fat (g)....... 2.7
Sat. Fat (g).. 0.2
Choles. (mg).. 0
Fiber (g)..... 3
Sodium (mg)... 100
%Cal-Fat...... 24%

Wash spinach greens in cold water. Cut away the tough stems and discard. Drain leaves, wrap in paper towels, and place in plastic bag. Chill in refrigerator until ready to assemble salad.

Tear spinach leaves into bite-size pieces and place in large salad bowl. Top with sliced mushrooms and onion rings.

Make dressing by combining all ingredients in small bowl. Mix well with wire whisk. Pour over salad and toss.

Yield: 6 servings

This spinach salad may also be assembled on individual salad plates with the honey mustard dressing drizzled over top.

Preparation time: 25–30 minutes

PARSLEY-WHEAT SALAD (TABOULE)

Per serving:
Calories...... 137
Protein (g)... 5
Fat (g)....... 0.4
Sat. Fat (g).. 0
Choles. (mg).. 1
Fiber (g)..... 8.6
Sodium (mg)... 205
%Cal-Fat...... 2%

1 cup fine or medium-grade bulgur
Water
1 cup finely chopped fresh parsley (about 1/2 bunch)
1 tablespoon minced fresh dill or 1 teaspoon dried
1/2 cup chopped green onions, including tops
2 medium tomatoes, diced
1 medium cucumber, peeled, deseeded, chopped
1/2 cup no-oil Italian dressing
Juice of 1/2 lemon
Freshly ground pepper to taste
Romaine lettuce leaves
Garnish: black olives, tomato wedges, parsley sprigs

Place bulgur in large mixing bowl. Add water to cover and let stand about 1 hour or until bulgur has doubled in size and most of the liquid is absorbed. Drain well and squeeze dry.

Add parsley, dill, green onions, tomatoes and cucumber. Toss gently.

Add Italian dressing, lemon juice and pepper and toss until well mixed. Refrigerate.

To serve, line a salad bowl with Romaine leaves and mound salad on top; or make individual servings by placing single piece of Romaine lettuce on plate and placing a scoop of salad on top. Garnish with olives, tomato wedges and parsley sprigs.

Yield: 4 to 6 servings

A delicious low-calorie version of Taboule, which is high in fiber with whole grain nutrients.

Preparation time: 30 minutes
(plus 1 hour to soak bulgur)

MARINATED VEGETABLE SALAD

8 ounces broccoli flowerets (about 1 large stalk)
8 ounces cauliflower flowerets (about 1/2 head)
1 cup cherry tomatoes, halved
1 zucchini squash, sliced 1/8-inch thick
1/2 cup crunchy sprouts
1/2 to 3/4 cup no-oil Italian dressing

Per serving:
Calories...... 37
Protein (g)... 3
Fat (g)....... 0.4
Sat. Fat (g).. 0.1
Choles. (mg).. 0
Fiber (g)..... 3.2
Sodium (mg)... 301
%Cal-Fat...... 8%

Bring about 8 cups water to a boil in large saucepan.

Meanwhile, cut up broccoli and cauliflower flowerets into bite-size pieces. Blanch vegetables by dropping into boiling water. When water returns to a second boil, drain vegetables immediately, and immerse in cold water to prevent further cooking.

Cut tomatoes in half and slice zucchini.

In a large bowl, combine all vegetables. Pour crunchy sprouts over top and mix together. Pour Italian dressing over all, and mix well, coating all vegetables.

For best results, let vegetables marinate at least four hours or overnight before serving.

Yield: 6 large servings

A colorful, nutritious, very low-fat dish which is a great accompaniment to a summer picnic meal.

Preparation time: 20–25 minutes

GREEN BEAN-MUSHROOM SALAD

Per serving:
Calories...... 64
Protein (g)... 2
Fat (g)....... 3.4
Sat. Fat (g).. 0.5
Choles. (mg).. 0
Fiber (g)..... 3
Sodium (mg)... 174
%Cal-Fat...... 43%

1 pound fresh green beans
1 small red onion, sliced and rings separated
3/4 cup sliced mushrooms
12 black olives
Boston Bib or Romaine lettuce

Balsamic Vinegar Dressing:
2 tablespoons water
2 tablespoons Balsamic vinegar
1 tablespoon olive oil
1/4 teaspoon salt
Dash black pepper
1 tablespoon fresh parsley or basil, chopped

Prepare Balsamic Vinegar dressing by combining all ingredients. Set aside.

To prepare string beans, cut off tops. Bring water to a boil in medium saucepan. Add beans and boil for eight minutes. Drain. Immediately immerse in ice water. Drain again. Pat dry and set aside.

Meanwhile slice red onion and separate rings. Wash mushrooms and slice.

Put beans, onion rings, and mushrooms into large plastic container with an airtight lid. Pour dressing over. Marinate 1 to 2 hours. Occasionally turn over container to thoroughly cover vegetables with dressing.

Arrange lettuce leaves on salad plates. Carefully remove vegetables from marinade and place on lettuce leaves. Pour remaining dressing over individual salads. Garnish with black olives.

Yield: 6 servings

Preparation time: 30 minutes

Marinating time: 1 hour

NEW POTATO SALAD

1 1/2 pounds new potatoes, unpeeled
2 ribs celery, chopped
1 bunch chopped green onions, including tops
1 carrot shredded
1/2 cup nonfat mayonnaise
2 tablespoons nonfat Catalina dressing
2 tablespoons skim milk
2 tablespoons dill pickle juice
Salt and pepper to taste

Per serving:
Calories...... 124
Protein (g)... 4
Fat (g)....... 0.2
Sat. Fat (g).. 0.1
Choles. (mg).. 0
Fiber (g)..... 5.4
Sodium (mg)... 500
%Cal-Fat...... 2%

Place potatoes and enough water to cover them in medium-size saucepan. Bring to a boil. Simmer 25 minutes or until potatoes are tender. Drain and cool.

After potatoes are cooled, cut into bite-size pieces and put into large bowl. Add chopped celery, green onions and shredded carrot.

In small bowl, mix together mayonnaise, Catalina, skim milk and pickle juice. Add salt and pepper if desired. Pour over potato mixture and stir carefully until potatoes are evenly coated.

Yield: 6 servings

Preparation time: 20–25 minutes

Cooking time: 25 minutes (to cook potatoes)

"SOUR CREAM" POTATO SALAD

Per serving:
Calories...... 105
Protein (g)... 1
Fat (g)....... 3.5
Sat. Fat (g).. 0.7
Choles. (mg).. 0
Fiber (g)..... 1.7
Sodium (mg)... 367
%Cal-Fat...... 30%

4 medium-size potatoes
1/2 cup chopped celery
3/4 cup chopped onions
1/4 cup chopped parsley
1/4 cup bread and butter pickles, finely chopped
1 cup nonfat sour cream
1/4 cup light mayonnaise
1 teaspoon seasoned salt
1/4 teaspoon pepper
1 1/2 tablespoons fresh dillweed or 1 1/2 teaspoons dried
3/4 teaspoon horseradish
3 tablespoons juice from bread and butter pickles
2 tablespoons skim milk

Boil potatoes, unpeeled, until soft, but slightly firm. Cool. Peel potatoes and cut into 1/2-inch cubes.

In large bowl, combine chopped potatoes, celery, onions, parsley and pickles.

Combine remaining ingredients in medium-size bowl. Add to potatoes and mix well. For best results, cover and refrigerate at least 4 hours before serving.

Yield: 6 servings

Preparation time: 25–30 minutes

Cooking time: 30 minutes (to cook potatoes)

SLIM WALDORF SALAD

3 apples, cored, cut into bite-size pieces
1/2 cup chopped celery
1/4 cup raisins
1/4 cup walnuts, coarsely chopped (optional)
1 cup vanilla low-fat yogurt

In medium-size bowl, combine apples, celery, raisins and walnuts. Stir in yogurt until well mixed.

Yield: 4 to 6 servings.

Omit walnuts if trying to reduce calories and fat.

Preparation time: 15–20 minutes

Per serving:
Calories...... 140
Protein (g)... 3
Fat (g)....... 1
Sat. Fat (g).. 0.5
Choles. (mg).. 2
Fiber (g)..... 3.4
Sodium (mg)... 41
%Cal-Fat...... 6%

TROPICAL FRUIT SLAW

2 medium oranges, peeled
1 medium banana, sliced
2 tablespoons orange juice
1 8-ounce can pineapple chunks, drained
3 cups finely shredded cabbage
1 cup thinly sliced celery
1 8-ounce carton low-fat lemon yogurt
2 tablespoons slivered almonds (optional)

Section oranges. Toss banana slices in orange juice and drain. In a large bowl combine fruits, cabbage and celery.
Add yogurt and toss lightly to coat. Cover and serve immediately or refrigerate for up to 3 hours before serving.
If desired, sprinkle with almonds.

Yield: 8 to 10 servings.

Preparation time: 20–25 minutes

Per serving:
Calories...... 67
Protein (g)... 2.2
Fat (g)....... 0.6
Sat. Fat (g).. 0.3
Choles. (mg).. 2
Fiber (g)..... 2
Sodium (mg)... 34
%Cal-Fat...... 7%

CREAMY CUCUMBER SALAD

4 cups sliced cucumbers
1/2 teaspoon salt
1 tablespoon chopped onion
1/2 cup plain nonfat yogurt
2 tablespoons sugar

Wash cucumbers and cut into slices about 1/8-inch thick. Place in large bowl and sprinkle with salt. Let soak for one hour. Rinse salt from cucumbers and drain well. Add chopped onion.

In small bowl, combine yogurt and sugar. Pour over cucumbers and mix well. Salad tastes best if refrigerated at least one hour before serving.

Yield: 8 servings

Preparation time: 15 minutes

Soaking time: 1 hour

Per serving:
Calories...... 40
Protein (g)... 2
Fat (g)....... 0.2
Sat. Fat (g).. 0.1
Choles. (mg).. 0
Fiber (g)..... 1.5
Sodium (mg)... 147
%Cal-Fat...... 5%

LEMON-TAHINI SALAD DRESSING

1/3 cup sesame tahini
1/4 cup lemon juice
2 or 3 cloves garlic, minced
1/4 cup cold water
1/4 teaspoon salt
1/4 teaspoon pepper

Combine all ingredients in food processor. Blend until well mixed. Serve immediately, or if thicker dressing is desired, let it set overnight.

Yield: 3/4 cup salad dressing, enough for 6 to 8 servings.

Preparation time: 15 minutes

Per 1 tablespoon serving:
Calories...... 43
Protein (g)... 1
Fat (g)....... 3.8
Sat. Fat (g).. 0.5
Choles. (mg).. 0
Fiber (g)..... 0.7
Sodium (mg)... 47
%Cal-Fat...... 73%

FRESH CRANBERRY MOLDED SALAD

1 package whole cranberries
4 apples, chopped with peelings
3/4 cup sugar
1 6-ounce package lemon jello
1 1/2 cups boiling water
1 1/2 cups cold water
3/4 cup celery, chopped
1/2 cup walnuts, chopped

Per serving:
Calories...... 87
Protein (g)... 2
Fat (g)....... 1.4
Sat. Fat (g).. 0.1
Choles. (mg).. 0
Fiber (g)..... 2
Sodium (mg)... 42
%Cal-Fat...... 14%

Coarsely chop cranberries in food processor. Place in large mixing bowl. Core apples, cut into quarters, and chop in food processor. Add to cranberries. Add sugar. Set aside for 2 to 3 hours or overnight.

Pour package of jello into large bowl. Add 1 1/2 cups boiling water and stir until completely dissolved. Add 1 1/2 cups cold water.

Place in refrigerator until jello begins to thicken or set. Add cranberry mixture, celery and walnuts.

Spray a 6 1/2 to 8-cup jello mold with vegetable cooking spray. Pour jello into mold. Refrigerate until jello is firm, about 2 to 4 hours.

To serve, loosen edges and unmold jello onto a platter covered with lettuce leaves.

Yield: 16 servings

Jello salad may be made a day before it is served. It can also be made in a 9 x 9-inch square pan and cut into squares and served on lettuce leaves.

Preparation time: 20–25 minutes

CRANBERRY FRUIT SALAD

Per serving:
Calories...... 147
Protein (g)... 2
Fat (g)....... 0
Sat. Fat (g).. 0
Choles. (mg).. 0
Fiber (g)..... 1.5
Sodium (mg)... 76
%Cal-Fat...... 1%

With walnuts:
Fat (g)....... 2.3
%Cal-Fat...... 12%

2 3-ounce packages lemon-flavored gelatin
2 cups boiling water
1 cup cold water
1 8-ounce can crushed pineapple, in its own juice
1 16-ounce can whole berry cranberry sauce
1 cup chopped celery
1/4 cup chopped walnuts (optional)

Dissolve gelatin in boiling water. Add cold water, crushed pineapple (including juice), and cranberry sauce. Mix until well blended. Chill until partially set. Fold in celery and walnuts.

Spray a 6-cup ring mold with vegetable cooking spray. Pour jello into mold. Chill until firm. Loosen edges of jello and unmold on crisp greens.

Yield: 8 to 10 servings

Preparation time: 15–20 minutes

ORANGE MANDARIN RING

Per serving:
Calories...... 93
Protein (g)... 2
Fat (g)....... 1.2
Sat. Fat (g).. 0.l
Choles. (mg).. 0
Fiber (g)..... 1
Sodium (mg)... 34
%Cal-Fat...... 12%

1 6-ounce package orange jello
2 cups boiling water
1 20-ounce can crushed pineapple, with juice
1 11-ounce can mandarin oranges, drained
1/2 cup orange juice
1/4 cup chopped walnuts

Dissolve orange jello in 2 cups boiling water. Stir in crushed pineapple (with juice), mandarin oranges (drained), and orange juice. Chill until partially set. Stir in chopped walnuts.

Spray a 6 1/2-cup ring mold with vegetable cooking spray. Pour jello mixture into mold. Chill until firm. Loosen edges and unmold on crisp greens.

Yield: 12 to 16 servings

Preparation time: 15–20 minutes

GRAPEFRUIT SALAD

3 envelopes unflavored gelatin
3/4 cup cold water
1/4 cup orange juice
3/4 cup sugar
1 cup boiling water
3 large pink grapefruits, peeled and cut into sections
1 14-ounce can crushed pineapple, in its own juice
   (reserve juice)
1/4 cup slivered almonds

Per serving:
Calories...... 150
Protein (g)... 4
Fat (g)....... 2
Sat. Fat (g).. 0.2
Choles. (mg).. 0
Fiber (g)..... 2.2
Sodium (mg)... 5
%Cal-Fat...... 12%

Combine cold water and orange juice in small bowl. Soften gelatin in cold water mixture. Dissolve sugar in boiling water. In large bowl, combine gelatin and sugar water. Refrigerate until partially set.

Meanwhile, prepare grapefruits by peeling, breaking into sections, and removing filaments. Cut each section in half. Fold grapefruit sections, pineapple with juice, and almonds into gelatin-sugar mixture. Pour into an 8-inch square baking dish or a 6-cup mold. Refrigerate until set, about 3 hours.

Unmold over lettuce or cut into 2 1/2-inch squares and serve over single leaf of lettuce.

Yield: Makes 9 servings.

Preparation time: 35 minutes

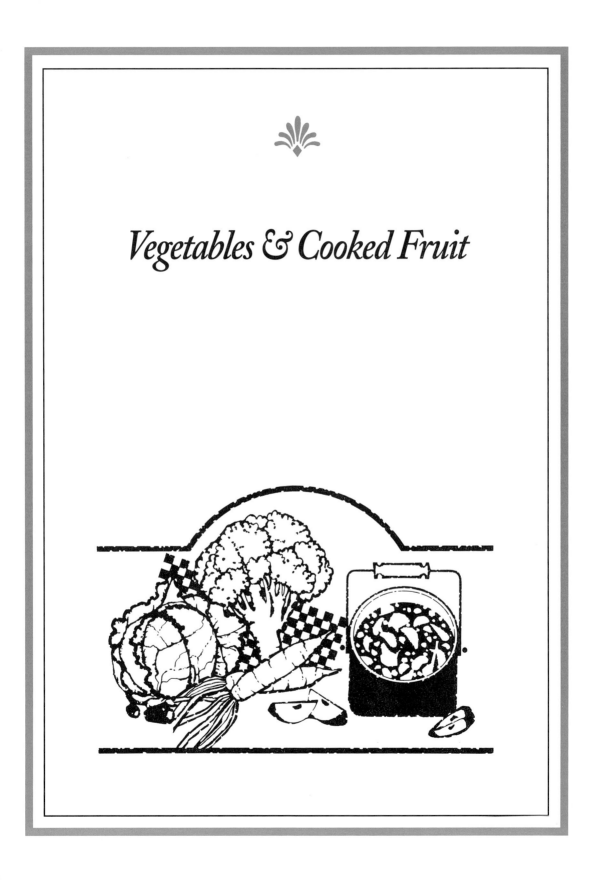

Vegetables & Cooked Fruit

BAKED TOMATOES WITH SPINACH

Per serving:
Calories...... 82
Protein (g)... 7
Fat (g)....... 1.8
Sat. Fat (g).. 0.7
Choles. (mg).. 4
Fiber (g)..... 2
Sodium (mg)... 190
%Cal-Fat...... 18%

3 green onions, chopped, including tops
1 teaspoon tub margarine
1 10-ounce package frozen chopped spinach
1/2 cup bread crumbs
2 egg substitutes (1/2 cup)
1/4 teaspoon salt
1/2 teaspoon thyme
1/4 teaspoon black pepper
1/4 cup grated Parmesan cheese, divided
4 large sun-ripened tomatoes

Preheat oven to 350 degrees.

Sauté onions in margarine, until tender. Thaw spinach and drain. Lightly squeeze out excess water.

Combine spinach, onions, bread crumbs, egg substitutes, salt, thyme, pepper and 2 tablespoons Parmesan cheese in a large mixing bowl. Mix until well blended.

Cut each tomato into 2 thick slices and cut out top stem. Arrange slices, cut side up, on a non-stick baking dish and top with mounds of spinach mixture. Sprinkle with remaining Parmesan cheese.

Bake at 350 degrees for 20 to 30 minutes or until tomato is slightly soft.

Yield: 8 servings.

Preparation time: 20 minutes

Cooking time: 20-30 minutes

BAKED TOMATOES

3 fresh tomatoes
2 tablespoons bread crumbs, plain or seasoned
1 tablespoon Parmesan cheese
Chopped fresh parsley
Parsley sprigs for garnish

Cut tomatoes in half and cut out top stem. Place cut side up in a baking dish, and sprinkle with bread crumbs, Parmesan cheese and parsley.

Bake at 350 degrees for 20 minutes or until slightly soft and heated through. Garnish serving dish with fresh parsley sprigs.

Yield: 6 servings.

Preparation time: 5-10 minutes

Cooking time: 20 minutes

Per serving:
Calories...... 32
Protein (g)... 1
Fat (g)....... 0.7
Sat. Fat (g).. 0.2
Choles. (mg).. 0
Fiber (g)..... 1.5
Sodium (mg)... 40
%Cal-Fat...... 17%

TOMATOES WITH CHOPPED HERBS

3 tomatoes, sliced
1 tablespoon chopped fresh parsley
1 tablespoon chopped fresh basil
Freshly ground black pepper

Slice tomatoes and arrange on platter. Sprinkle with herbs and pepper. Serve chilled or at room temperature.

Yield: 6 servings

Preparation time: 5 minutes

Per serving:
Calories...... 14
Protein (g)... 1
Fat (g)....... 0.1
Sat. Fat (g).. 0
Choles. (mg).. 0
Fiber (g)..... 1
Sodium (mg)... 6
%Cal-Fat...... 12%

STEAMED VEGETABLE MEDLEY

Per serving:
Calories...... 78
Protein (g)... 2
Fat (g)....... 0.3
Sat. Fat (g).. 0
Choles. (mg).. 0
Fiber (g)..... 4.8
Sodium (mg)... 26
%Cal-Fat...... 3%

3 large carrots
1 large potato
1/2 pound fresh green beans
3 leeks or bunch green onions
1 14 1/2-ounce can clear chicken broth, defatted
Butter Buds (powdered butter flavor without fat)
Fresh parsley for garnish

Prepare vegetables: Peel carrots, cut into 3-inch lengths, cut again in half lengthwise; peel potato, cut into strips approximately the size of carrots; cut ends from green beans; cut the roots off leeks, cut each leek into 3-inch lengths, and wash thoroughly (or do the same with green onions).

Arrange vegetables on steamer rack placed in a large kettle. Pour broth over vegetables. Cover kettle with lid, and place on stove. Bring to a boil, reduce heat, and steam slowly about 20 minutes, or until vegetables are tender.

Arrange vegetables on a single platter, sprinkle immediately with Butter Buds and minced parsley. Garnish with sprigs of parsley.

Yield: 4 or 5 servings

Other vegetables may be used in place of those given in this recipe, including rutabagas, turnips, or broccoli. Cut into approximately equal size pieces, and try to include an assortment of colors to create an eye-appealing dish.

Preparation time: 20 minutes

Cooking time: 25 minutes

excellent

MASHED POTATOES WITH CHIVES

4 large potatoes, peeled and cut into chunks
3/4 cup skim milk, heated
3 tablespoons dry non-fat milk powder
1 tablespoon tub margarine
1 tablespoon powdered butter flavoring (no fat)
1/2 teaspoon seasoned salt
1/4 teaspoon black pepper
1 tablespoon chopped chives or green onions
2 tablespoons finely chopped fresh parsley
1/4 cup Parmesan cheese

Per serving:
Calories...... 96
Protein (g)... 4
Fat (g)....... 2.1
Sat. Fat (g).. 0.9
Choles. (mg).. 3
Fiber (g)..... 1
Sodium (mg)... 233
%Cal-Fat...... 20%

In large pot, boil potatoes in water until soft. Drain. Transfer potatoes to large mixing bowl.

In large mixing bowl, combine potatoes, 1/2 cup warmed milk, milk powder, margarine, butter flavoring, seasoned salt and pepper. Whip with electric mixer until smooth. Add remainder of milk, if needed for proper consistency. Add green onions, parsley and Parmesan cheese. Stir until well blended.

Serve immediately, or place in covered casserole and heat up just before serving.

Yield: 8 servings

It is important to heat the milk before adding to potatoes. If cold milk is added, mashed potatoes will have a rubbery texture.

Preparation time: 15-20 minutes

Cooking time: 20-25 minutes

RED POTATOES WITH CREAMY DILL SAUCE

Per serving:
Calories...... 161
Protein (g)... 7
Fat (g)....... 0.3
Sat. Fat (g).. 0.1
Choles. (mg).. 1
Fiber (g)..... 6
Sodium (mg)... 231
%Cal-Fat...... 2%

2 pounds small red potatoes
1/4 cup flour
1 1/2 cups skim milk
2 tablespoons dry white wine
1 tablespoon finely chopped chives
1 tablespoon chopped fresh dill (or 1 teaspoon dried)
1/2 teaspoon salt, or to taste
1/4 teaspoon pepper

Scrub potatoes. Cook in boiling water until tender, about 20 to 25 minutes.

Meanwhile, in small bowl, mix flour and skim milk with wire whisk until smooth. Pour into medium saucepan and heat on stove. Add remaining ingredients. Cook until sauce comes to a boil and thickens.

After potatoes have been cooked, drain water. Cut into quarters. Add to white sauce and mix, covering potatoes with sauce.

Yield: 6 servings

Preparation time: 20 minutes

Cooking time: 20-30 minutes

HERBED RED POTATOES

4 medium red potatoes
1 tablespoon Butter Buds*
Fresh parsley or basil, finely chopped

Scrub potatoes. Cook, unpeeled, in boiling water until soft, about 30 minutes. Drain water.

Cut potatoes into quarters. Sprinkle with Butter Buds* and fresh parsley or basil. Serve immediately.

Yield: 4 servings.

Small red potatoes may be used instead. Before cooking, remove a 3/4-inch strip of peeling from around center of potato. Boil in water until tender, about 20 minutes. Drain, and sprinkle immediately with Butter Buds and parsley.*

*Contains the natural flavor of butter without the fat.

Preparation time: 10-15 minutes

Cooking time: 20-30 minutes

Per serving:
Calories...... 107
Protein (g)... 4
Fat (g)....... 0.1
Sat. Fat (g).. 0
Choles. (mg).. 0
Fiber (g)..... 5.3
Sodium (mg)... 20
%Cal-Fat...... 1%

VEGETABLE STIR-FRY

1 tablespoon lite soy sauce
1 teaspoon brown sugar
2 teaspoons olive oil
1/2 pound fresh or frozen Chinese snow peas
1/2 cup sliced fresh mushrooms
1/2 cup fresh or canned bean sprouts (drained)
1/2 red pepper, cut into narrow 2-inch strips
1 8-ounce can sliced water chestnuts, drained

Prepare vegetables. Set aside.
In small bowl, combine soy sauce and sugar, stirring well.

Per serving:
Calories...... 87
Protein (g)... 3
Fat (g)....... 2.5
Sat. Fat (g).. 0.3
Choles. (mg).. 0
Fiber (g)..... 3.5
Sodium (mg)... 166
%Cal-Fat...... 24%

Heat oil in saute pan. Add snow peas, mushrooms, bean sprouts, red pepper and water chestnuts. Stir-fry for 3 minutes. Add soy sauce mixture. Stir well and saute an additional 1 to 2 minutes, or until crisp-tender.

Yield: 4 servings.

Preparation time: 25-30 minutes

SWEET POTATO CASSEROLE

2 medium sweet potatoes
1/4 cup reserved cooking liquid
2 tablespoons packed brown sugar
1 egg substitute (1/4 cup)
2 tablespoons chopped pecans

Peel potatoes and cut into sections. Place in medium saucepan and cover with water. Bring to a boil over high heat. Reduce heat and simmer until soft, about 15 to 20 minutes.

Drain potatoes, reserving 1/4 cup liquid. In mixing bowl, combine potatoes, cooking liquid and brown sugar. Beat at high speed with electric mixer until smooth. Add egg substitute and mix well. Stir in nuts. Add more water if too thick.

Spoon into small casserole dish. Sprinkle with brown sugar. Bake, uncovered, at 350 degrees for 30 minutes.

Yield: 4 servings.

Preparation time: 15 minutes

Cooking time: 45-50 minutes

Per serving:
Calories...... 140
Protein (g)... 3
Fat (g)....... 3
Sat. Fat (g).. 0.3
Choles. (mg).. 0
Fiber (g)..... 2.5
Sodium (mg)... 39
%Cal-Fat...... 19%

GREEN BEANS AMANDINE

1 pound fresh string beans
14 ounces clear chicken broth, defatted
2 teaspoons margarine
2 tablespoons sliced almonds

Wash beans and cut off ends.

Place vegetable steamer rack in large saucepan. Pour in clear chicken broth. Add water if desired, but be sure to keep water level below steamer rack. Add beans. Bring water/broth mixture to a boil. Steam beans 15 to 20 minutes or until desired tenderness.

Lift rack out of sauce pan. Pour beans into serving dish. Top with margarine and toss until all beans are coated and margarine is melted. Sprinkle with sliced almonds. Serve immediately.

Yield: 6 servings

Preparation time: 10-15 minutes

Cooking time: 15-20 minutes

Per serving:
Calories...... 60
Protein (g)... 3
Fat (g)....... 2.9
Sat. Fat (g).. 0.5
Choles. (mg).. 0
Fiber (g)..... 2
Sodium (mg)... 238
%Cal-Fat...... 41%

SCRUMPTIOUS ASPARAGUS

2 pounds fresh asparagus spears or 2 10-ounce packages
    frozen
6 anchovy fillets
1 clove garlic, minced
3 sprigs fresh parsley, finely chopped
1 tablespoon tub margarine
1/8 teaspoon white pepper
Juice of 1 lemon

Remove tough ends from fresh asparagus spears. Steam asparagus in vegetable steamer until tender, about 10 to 15 minutes.

Meanwhile, finely chop anchovy fillets, garlic, and parsley.

Per serving:
Calories...... 51
Protein (g)... 5
Fat (g)....... 1.9
Sat. Fat (g).. 0.5
Choles. (mg).. 3
Fiber (g)..... 2
Sodium (mg)... 149
%Cal-Fat...... 28%

Melt margarine in a small saucepan. Add chopped mixture and pepper. Cook and stir occasionally over low heat for 5 minutes. Add lemon juice.

Drain asparagus thoroughly and transfer to a serving dish. Pour sauce over. Serve immediately.

Yield: 6 to 8 servings.

Sauce may be made ahead and heated just before serving.

Preparation time: 20-25 minutes

PEAS PARISIENNE

1 16-ounce package frozen peas
2 cups Boston lettuce, shredded
1 teaspoon tub margarine
2 tablespoons water
1/4 teaspoon marjoram
1/4 teaspoon salt
1/2 teaspoon sugar

Combine all ingredients in medium saucepan. Simmer for 8 to 10 minutes over medium heat until peas are cooked through. Stir occasionally and add more water if peas stick to bottom.

Yield: 4 to 6 servings.

Spinach or other greens may be substituted for the Boston lettuce.

Preparation time: 10 minutes

Cooking time: 10 minutes

Per serving:
Calories...... 85
Protein (g)... 5
Fat (g)....... 1
Sat. Fat (g).. 0.2
Choles. (mg).. 0
Fiber (g)..... 4.6
Sodium (mg)... 20
%Cal-Fat...... 10%

BEANS AND MUSHROOMS

2 10-ounce packages frozen French-style green beans
1/2 cup sliced mushrooms, preferably fresh
1/4 cup sliced green onions, including tops
2 teaspoons olive oil
1 1/2 teaspoons chopped fresh basil
2 tablespoons no-oil Italian salad dressing

Cook beans according to package directions.

Meanwhile, in a non-stick skillet, saute mushrooms and green onions in olive oil, stirring frequently. Saute for about 5 minutes, or until mushrooms turn dark in color.

Add cooked beans (drained), basil and salad dressing to mushroom mixture and heat through. Serve immediately.

Yield: 6 servings.

Preparation time: 20 minutes

Per serving:
Calories...... 35
Protein (g)... 2
Fat (g)....... 1
Sat. Fat (g).. 0.2
Choles. (mg).. 0
Fiber (g)..... 3.2
Sodium (mg)... 52
%Cal-Fat...... 21%

STEAMED CARROTS WITH ONIONS

6 large carrots, peeled and sliced
1 medium onion, sliced thin
2 teaspoons tub margarine

Slice carrots crosswise about 1/8-inch thick. Steam in vegetable steamer, or steaming basket placed in saucepan with small amount of water, for 10 minutes or until carrots are soft.

Meanwhile, melt margarine in small saute pan or skillet. Separate sliced onion into rings and saute in margarine until onion is soft and translucent, but not brown.

Mix carrots with sauteed onion and serve immediately.

Yield: 4 to 5 servings

Preparation time: 15 minutes

Per serving:
Calories...... 61
Protein (g)... 1
Fat (g)....... 1.8
Sat. Fat (g).. 0.3
Choles. (mg).. 0
Fiber (g)..... 3.4
Sodium (mg)... 56
%Cal-Fat...... 26%

SNOW CAPPED BROCCOLI

Per serving:
Calories...... 37
Protein (g)... 4
Fat (g)....... 0.7
Sat. Fat (g).. 0.3
Choles. (mg).. 2
Fiber (g)..... 2.4
Sodium (mg)... 72
%Cal-Fat...... 17%

**1 large bunch fresh broccoli, or 2 10-ounce packages
    frozen broccoli
2 egg whites
1 tablespoon low-calorie Ranch dressing
2 tablespoons grated Parmesan cheese
1/4 cup chopped green onions, including tops**

Preheat oven to 350 degrees.

Cut broccoli into spears. Steam broccoli for 10 minutes or until done.

Meanwhile, beat egg whites with an electric mixer until stiff peaks form. Gently fold in Ranch dressing, Parmesan cheese and green onions. Set aside.

Arrange cooked broccoli in a circular pattern on a 9-inch oven-proof dish or pie plate, with stem ends toward center and flowerets toward the outside.

Spoon the egg white mixture onto the center of the platter over the broccoli stems, leaving the flowerets exposed. Sprinkle lightly with additional Parmesan cheese. Bake in 350 degree oven for 12 to 15 minutes, until topping is golden.

Yield: Makes 6 to 8 servings.

Preparation time: 20-25 minutes

Cooking time: 12-15 minutes

SESAME BROCCOLI

1 bunch broccoli (or 2 10-ounce packages, frozen)
1 tablespoon tub margarine
1 tablespoon sesame seeds
Salt to taste, if desired

Wash broccoli and separate into spears. Place in vegetable steamer and steam until broccoli is crisp-tender, about 10 to 15 minutes.

Meanwhile melt margarine in small saucepan. Add sesame seeds and saute until lightly browned. Just before serving, sprinkle sesame seeds evenly over broccoli.

Yield: 6 to 8 servings.

Preparation time: 10 minutes

Cooking time: 10-15 minutes

Per serving:
Calories...... 41
Protein (g)... 3
Fat (g)....... 2
Sat. Fat (g).. 0.4
Choles. (mg).. 0
Fiber (g)..... 2.5
Sodium (mg)... 40
%Cal-Fat...... 37%

STIR-FRIED BROCCOLI

1 large stalk broccoli (3-4 cups chopped)
1 1/2 teaspoons olive oil
2 tablespoons water
1 tablespoon light soy sauce, or to taste

Peel broccoli stem. Slice stem and flowerets into bite-size pieces. (Stem slices should be no more than 1/4-inch thick.)

Pour olive oil into skillet or saute pan. Add broccoli pieces and water. Saute, covering pan when not stirring, until crisp tender, about 5 to 10 minutes. Sprinkle soy sauce over broccoli while sauteing. (Add additional water if necessary to keep broccoli from sticking or scorching.)

Yield: 4 servings

Preparation time: 10-15 minutes

Per serving:
Calories...... 33
Protein (g)... 0
Fat (g)....... 1.7
Sat. Fat (g).. 0
Choles. (mg).. 0
Fiber (g)..... 2
Sodium (mg)... 168
%Cal-Fat...... 46%

RATATOUILLE

Per serving:
Calories...... 73
Protein (g)... 3.6
Fat (g)....... 0.4
Sat. Fat (g).. 0.1
Choles. (mg).. 0
Fiber (g)..... 6.4
Sodium (mg)... 146
%Cal-Fat...... 5%

1 eggplant, 1 to 1 1/2 pounds, unpeeled
1 green pepper, sliced into 1/4 x 2-inch strips
1 large onion, thinly sliced, rings separated
1 zucchini, unpeeled and sliced thin
16-ounces canned or fresh tomatoes, chopped coarsely
1 8-ounce can "no salt added" tomato sauce
2 cloves garlic, minced
2 teaspoons olive oil (optional)
Black pepper to taste

Preheat oven to 375 degrees.

Cut eggplant into half-inch slices. Cut again into half-inch cubes. Cut up green pepper, onion and zucchini as indicated above.

In a large baking dish or casserole, place eggplant cubes. Lightly sprinkle with salt. Add separate layers of green pepper, onion and zucchini. Press down lightly with palms of hands to make more compact.

In medium-size mixing bowl, stir together chopped tomatoes, tomato sauce, and minced garlic. Pour over vegetables. Drizzle olive oil over top, if desired.

Bake, uncovered, in 375-degree oven for 1 1/4 to 1 1/2 hours. Remove from oven and wait 5 minutes before serving. Stir ratatouille well before serving.

Yield: 6 servings

Preparation time: 25-30 minutes

Cooking time: 1 1/4 hours

ZUCCHINI-MUSHROOM CASSEROLE

Vegetable cooking spray
2 medium onions, chopped
2 cloves garlic, minced
8 ounces mushrooms, sliced
3 pounds zucchini (4 large zucchini), cut in half
  lengthwise and sliced
1 28-ounce can crushed tomatoes
2 teaspoons oregano
1 teaspoon onion powder
1 teaspoon garlic powder
2 teaspoons olive oil
1/4 cup Parmesan cheese
4 egg whites
2 tablespoons Parmesan cheese

Per serving:
Calories...... 115
Protein (g)... 7.7
Fat (g)....... 3.3
Sat. Fat (g).. 1.2
Choles. (mg).. 4
Fiber (g)..... 4
Sodium (mg)... 282
%Cal-Fat...... 23%

Spray large non-stick skillet with vegetable cooking spray. With lid on, saute onions, garlic and mushrooms until tender. Add sliced zucchini to skillet and simmer, covered, over medium heat 30 minutes.

Meanwhile, in medium-size mixing bowl, combine crushed tomatoes, oregano, onion powder, garlic powder and olive oil. Add to zucchini mixture. Bring to a boil and simmer, covered, 15 minutes. Add 1/4 cup Parmesan cheese.

In small mixing bowl, combine egg whites and 2 tablespoons Parmesan cheese. Beat with wire whisk until eggs are slightly frothy. Add to skillet and cook 5 to 10 minutes or until egg whites solidify. Serve immediately.

Yield: 8 servings

Preparation time: 30 minutes

Cooking time: 1 hour

ARTICHOKE WEDGES WITH TOMATOES

Per serving:
Calories...... 71
Protein (g)... 3
Fat (g)....... 2.5
Sat. Fat (g).. 0.4
Choles. (mg).. 0
Fiber (g)..... 5.7
Sodium (mg)... 215
%Cal-Fat...... 28%

1 14-ounce can artichoke hearts, packed in water
Juice of 1 lemon
1/2 cup chopped onion
1 tablespoon olive oil
2 cloves garlic, minced
1 28-ounce can tomatoes
Pepper, to taste
2 tablespoons chopped parsley

Drain can of artichoke hearts. Cut each artichoke into 8 equal wedges. Put into medium-size bowl along with 1 cup water and juice of lemon. Set aside.

In a 10 or 12-inch frypan, saute chopped onion in olive oil over low heat until onion becomes translucent. Add garlic and saute 30 seconds longer.

Break up tomato pieces with a spoon. Add to frypan, and simmer for 3-4 minutes.

Drain artichoke mixture and add to tomato mixture. Add pepper to taste.

Simmer, partially covered, 45 minutes, stirring occasionally. If mixture becomes too thick, add water. If it is too thin, boil rapidly with cover removed. Immediately before serving, add parsley and mix well.

Yield: 6 to 8 servings.

This is a very tasty vegetable dish. The artichokes provide an excellent source of fiber.

Preparation time: 20-25 minutes

Cooking time: 45 minutes

excellnt

SPINACH-ARTICHOKE CASSEROLE

2 10-ounce packages frozen chopped spinach
1 tablespoon tub margarine
1/2 cup finely chopped onion
1 14-ounce can artichoke hearts, packed in water
3/4 cup nonfat sour cream
6 tablespoons Parmesan cheese, divided
Pepper to taste

Per serving:
Calories...... 79
Protein (g)... 6
Fat (g)....... 2.6
Sat. Fat (g).. 1.1
Choles. (mg).. 4
Fiber (g)..... 5.1
Sodium (mg)... 185
%Cal-Fat...... 27%

Preheat oven to 350 degrees.

Cook spinach according to package directions. Drain well, lightly squeezing out excess water.

Saute onion in margarine until onion becomes translucent. Drain artichoke hearts and cut into quarters.

Combine spinach, sauteed onion, artichokes, sour cream, and 1/4 cup Parmesan cheese. Place in casserole dish. Sprinkle the remaining 2 tablespoons Parmesan cheese over top.

Bake at 350 degrees for 30 minutes. Serve hot.

Yield: 8 to 10 servings

Preparation time: 20 minutes

Cooking time: 30 minutes

SPICED FRUIT COMPOTE

Per serving:
Calories...... 199
Protein (g)... 1.4
Fat (g)....... 0.3
Sat. Fat (g).. 0.1
Choles. (mg).. 0
Fiber (g)..... 4.9
Sodium (mg)... 9
%Cal-Fat...... 1%

1 16-ounce can apricot halves, in light syrup
1 16-ounce can peach halves, in light syrup
1 16-ounce can pear halves, in light syrup
1 8-ounce can pineapple tidbits, in its own juice
1/3 cup orange juice
2 tablespoons brown sugar
1 teaspoon grated orange rind
1 teaspoon grated lemon rind
4 ounces chopped dates

Drain fruit, reserving liquid from each can. Cut apricots, peaches, and pears into bite-size pieces. Combine fruits and set aside.

Combine reserved juices, orange juice, brown sugar and grated rinds in saucepan. Bring to a boil and simmer, uncovered, until liquid is reduced by half (about 10 to 15 minutes). If it's too sweet, add lemon juice to taste.

Add fruits to juice just before serving and heat through.

Yield: 8 servings

If making ahead, store fruit and juices separately. Combine just before heating and serving. This makes an excellent meat accompaniment.

Preparation time: 20 minutes

Cooking time: 20 minutes

BAKED APPLE-DATE DELIGHT

8 baking apples (with skins)
1 cup chopped dates
1/2 cup firmly packed brown sugar
1/4 cup walnuts or pecans
1 teaspoon cinnamon
1/2 teaspoon nutmeg

Preheat oven to 350 degrees.

Core apples and cut into bite-size pieces. (Do not peel.) Place in large bowl. Add remaining ingredients and mix well. Spoon into oven proof casserole.

Bake, covered, for one hour. Check after 30 to 40 minutes and uncover if too juicy.

Yield: 10 servings

Preparation time: 20-25 minutes

Cooking time: 1 hour

Per serving:
Calories...... 209
Protein (g)... 1
Fat (g)....... 2.6
Sat. Fat (g).. 0.3
Choles. (mg).. 0
Fiber (g)..... 5.4
Sodium (mg)... 4
%Cal-Fat...... 10%

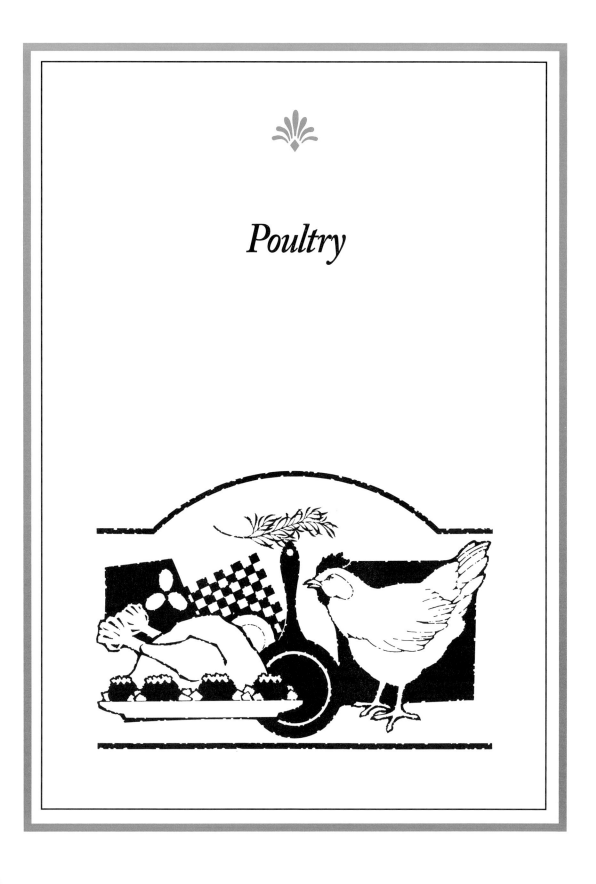

Poultry

HERBED CHICKEN-RICE CASSEROLE

Per serving:
Calories...... 369
Protein (g)... 43
Fat (g)....... 10
Sat. Fat (g).. 2.1
Choles. (mg).. 130
Fiber (g)..... 0.8
Sodium (mg)... 416
%Cal-Fat...... 25%

1 tablespoon canola oil
1/4 cup flour
2 1/2-pound fryer chicken, cut up, or 6 chicken breast
   pieces
3/4 cup uncooked white rice
1/4 teaspoon pepper
1/4 teaspoon garlic powder
1 3-ounce can sliced mushrooms, undrained
1/4 cup finely chopped onion
1 14 1/2-ounce can clear chicken broth, defatted
1 tablespoon margarine

Preheat oven to 350 degrees.

Remove skin from chicken pieces. Heat canola oil in non-stick saute pan. Dip chicken pieces in flour and brown in pan.

While it browns, put rice, pepper and garlic in a casserole dish. Stir in chopped onion. Put in mushrooms, including juice. Arrange browned chicken pieces on top. Dot with margarine. Pour chicken broth over top.

Cover and bake at 350 degrees for 1 hour.

Yield: 6 servings

If you wish to eliminate the 1 tablespoon canola oil, you can brown the chicken on a cookie sheet. Just dip in flour and broil for a few minutes in the oven.

Preparation time: 20-25 minutes

Cooking time: 1 hour

CHICKEN WITH WINE AND MUSHROOMS

6 to 8 boneless chicken breasts (about 1 1/2 pounds)
1/2 cup bread crumbs
1/4 cup Parmesan cheese
3/4 cup egg substitutes, slightly beaten
1 tablespoon olive oil
1 cup dry white wine
1 pint fresh mushrooms, sliced

Per serving:
Calories...... 316
Protein (g)... 38
Fat (g)....... 9
Sat. Fat (g).. 2.6
Choles. (mg).. 100
Fiber (g)..... 0.6
Sodium (mg)... 280
%Cal-Fat...... 26%

Preheat oven to 350 degrees.

Remove all visible fat from chicken breasts and pound to flatten slightly.

In large skillet, heat olive oil.

Meanwhile, roll chicken breasts first in Parmesan cheese, then dip in egg and bread crumbs. Place in skillet and brown both sides. Remove from skillet and place in baking dish.

Pour 1 cup wine into same skillet. Bring to a boil and simmer for 3 minutes. Next add fresh mushrooms and cook 5 to 10 additional minutes. Pour wine and mushroom sauce over chicken.

Cover and bake at 350 degrees for one hour.

Yield: 6 servings.

This recipe is very tasty and goes well with the Bulgur with Steamed Vegetables. (Recipe, page 340)

Preparation time: 25 minutes

Cooking time: 1 hour

CHICKEN A LA KING

Per serving:
Calories...... 494
Protein (g)... 41
Fat (g)....... 8
Sat. Fat (g).. 2.3
Choles. (mg).. 89
Fiber (g)..... 8
Sodium (mg)... 862
%Cal-Fat...... 16%

1 pound chicken meat, skinless and visible fat removed
8 ounces fresh mushrooms, sliced (or 4 ounces canned
**   mushrooms)**
1 cup frozen peas
2 ounces chopped pimiento, drained
1/2 cup flour
1 14 1/2-ounce can clear chicken broth, defatted
3/4 cup evaporated skim milk
1/4 cup sherry
Salt and pepper to taste
8 slices whole wheat bread, toasted

Boil chicken in water for 25 minutes. Drain and cool slightly. Cut up chicken into bite-size pieces.

Meanwhile steam mushrooms and peas until tender.

Pour defatted chicken broth into medium-size bowl. Add flour and mix with wire whisk until lumps disappear.

Pour broth and flour mixture into large saucepan placed over medium heat. Add milk and sherry. Bring to a boil, stirring occasionally with wire whisk. Continue stirring until sauce thickens and has a smooth consistency. Add chicken, vegetables and drained pimiento. Heat through. Add salt and pepper to taste.

Serve over toasted bread.

Yield: 4 servings

This recipe is also a great way to use up leftover turkey breast — just substitute the turkey breast for the chicken.

Preparation time: 35 minutes

CHICKEN AND DUMPLINGS

1 pound boneless chicken breast
1 cup frozen peas
1 cup sliced carrots
1 large onion, cut into eighths
1/2 cup flour
1 14 1/2-ounce can clear chicken broth, defatted
1 1/4 cups skim milk
Salt and pepper to taste

Dumplings:
1 cup flour
2 teaspoons baking powder
1/2 teaspoon salt
1/2 cup milk
2 tablespoons canola oil

Per serving:
Calories...... 417
Protein (g)... 39
Fat (g)....... 10
Sat. Fat (g).. 1.6
Choles. (mg).. 78
Fiber (g)..... 3.7
Sodium (mg)... 745
%Cal-Fat...... 22%

Cut all visible fat from chicken breasts. Boil chicken in water for 25 minutes. Drain and cut into bite-size pieces. Set aside.

Meanwhile, place peas, sliced carrots and onion into vegetable steamer. Steam until vegetables are tender.

Skim fat from top of chicken broth. Pour into medium-size bowl. Add flour and mix with wire whisk until smooth.

Pour broth mixture into large saucepan placed over medium heat. Add milk. Bring to a boil, stirring occasionally. Continue stirring until sauce thickens and has a smooth consistency. Add chicken and vegetables and heat through. Season to taste. Pour into shallow casserole dish.

Preheat oven to 400 degrees.

To make dumplings:

In a medium-size bowl, combine flour, baking powder and salt. Mix well. Add milk and oil and mix just until moistened. Place heaping tablespoons of dough over top of chicken casserole.

Bake at 400 degrees, covered, for 15 minutes. Remove lid. Bake an additional 5 minutes.

Yield: 4 to 6 servings

Preparation time: 30-40 minutes

Cooking time: 20 minutes

CHICKEN-GARBANZO STIR FRY

Per serving:
Calories...... 356
Protein (g)... 30
Fat (g)....... 7.4
Sat. Fat (g).. 1.4
Choles. (mg).. 48
Fiber (g)..... 6.2
Sodium (mg)... 220
%Cal-Fat...... 21%

1/2 to 3/4 pound boneless chicken breast, cut into
   bite-size pieces
1 19-ounce can garbanzo beans (chick peas), drained
2 teaspoons olive oil
1/4 cup chopped green onions, including tops
1 red or green pepper, cut into narrow bite-size pieces
3 tablespoons no-oil Italian dressing
1 tablespoon cornstarch
1/2 cup water
2 tablespoons chopped pimiento
1/4 cup slivered almonds (optional)
Lite soy sauce or lemon juice (optional)
Rice or pasta, cooked

Cut up green onions and red pepper as indicated above. Set aside. Cut up chicken.

Spray non-stick skillet or saute pan with vegetable cooking spray. Stir-fry chicken over medium-high heat for approximately 2 minutes, or until meat turns white. Add garbanzo beans, drained, and stir-fry for an additional minute. Add olive oil, green onions, and pepper. Stir-fry approximately 2 to 3 more minutes, until pepper is crisp-tender.

Meanwhile make sauce by combining Italian dressing, cornstarch and water in small mixing bowl.

Add chopped pimiento, almonds (if desired), and cornstarch mixture to skillet. Mix well and continue cooking until sauce thickens. Serve over rice or pasta and sprinkle with Lite soy sauce or lemon juice.

Yield: 4 servings.

A tasty, quick dish that is ideal when time is limited. Protein is supplied by both the beans and chicken, thus less meat is required to get adequate protein.

Preparation time: 25-30 minutes

STIR-FRIED CHICKEN AND VEGETABLES

3/4 pound boneless chicken breast
1/4 cup dry sherry
1/4 cup dark corn syrup
1/4 cup water
2 tablespoons cornstarch
3 tablespoons Lite soy sauce
2 tablespoons apple cider vinegar
3 tablespoons water
1/2 pound fresh snow peas
1/2 head cauliflower
2 large stalks of broccoli
1 clove garlic, minced
Brown or white rice
Soy sauce to taste

Per serving:
Calories...... 365
Protein (g)... 38
Fat (g)....... 4.8
Sat. Fat (g).. 1.2
Choles. (mg).. 64
Fiber (g)..... 7
Sodium (mg)... 536
%Cal-Fat...... 12%

Cut chicken breast into bite-size pieces. Set aside. Prepare vegetables by cutting cauliflower and broccoli into bite-size pieces and cutting off ends of snow peas. Set aside.

Prepare seasoning sauce: Combine sherry, corn syrup, water, cornstarch, soy sauce and vinegar. Blend thoroughly. Set aside.

Saute chicken pieces in non-stick saute pan until brown (no oil necessary). Next, add three tablespoons water to saute pan. Add snow peas, cauliflower, broccoli and minced garlic. Steam 4 to 5 minutes. Vegetables should be bright in color and slightly crispy. Add seasoning sauce and heat until sauce comes to a boil and thickens. Mix all ingredients well.

Serve over cooked rice. Sprinkle with soy sauce, if desired.

Yield: 4 to 5 servings.

You may substitute turkey breast for the chicken if desired.

Preparation time: 30 -35 minutes

CRUNCHY CHICKEN CASSEROLE

Per serving:
Calories...... 338
Protein (g)... 28
Fat (g)....... 7.8
Sat. Fat (g).. 1.6
Choles. (mg).. 65
Fiber (g)..... 2.9
Sodium (mg)... 583
%Cal-Fat...... 21%

3/4 to 1 pound boneless chicken breast
1 cup brown or white rice, uncooked
1 cup celery, diced
1/4 cup onion, diced
1 8-ounce can sliced water chestnuts, drained
1 4-ounce can sliced mushrooms, including liquid
2 tablespoons lemon juice
1/2 teaspoon salt
2 tablespoons light mayonnaise
1 1/2 cups water, divided
1 chicken bouillon cube
2 1/2 tablespoons flour
1 tablespoon tub margarine
1 3/4 cups corn flakes cereal

Cook chicken breasts by boiling in water for 30 minutes. Cut into bite-size pieces. Cook rice according to package directions. Cut up celery and onion.

In large mixing bowl, combine chicken, cooked rice, celery, onion, water chestnuts, mushrooms, including liquid, lemon juice, salt and mayonnaise. Set aside.

Dissolve chicken bouillon in medium skillet with 1 1/4 cups water. Heat on stove. Meanwhile, combine remaining 1/4 cup cold water and flour in small bowl, mixing until it becomes a smooth paste. Add flour paste to liquid in skillet, heating until it thickens and comes to a full boil.

Add gravy to other ingredients and carefully stir together until well blended. Spoon into 9 x 13-inch pan and spread evenly.

Melt margarine in medium skillet. Toss corn flakes in margarine until flakes are evenly coated. Sprinkle over top of casserole.

Bake in preheated oven at 350 degrees for 35 minutes, or until heated through.

Yield: 6 servings

Rice and chicken may be cooked the night before or early in the day. Remaining preparation time is then much shorter. This casserole is very moist as well as is low in fat.

Preparation time: 30-35 minutes

Cooking time: 1 hour, divided

SPICY CHICKEN AND PASTA

2 teaspoons canola oil
6 chicken breasts, boneless or with bones, skin removed
8 ounces rotini pasta (corkscrew-shaped)
1 clove garlic, minced
1 green pepper, chopped
1 bunch broccoli, cut into bite-size pieces
2 16-ounce cans tomatoes (no salt added), coarsely
   chopped
1/2 teaspoon salt, or to taste
2 tablespoons chopped parsley
1/4 teaspoon black pepper
1 teaspoon dried oregano
2 tablespoons Parmesan cheese

Per serving:
Calories...... 435
Protein (g)... 46
Fat (g)....... 7.7
Sat. Fat (g).. 2.2
Choles. (mg).. 98
Fiber (g)..... 5.1
Sodium (mg)... 371
%Cal-Fat...... 18%

Bring 2 quarts of water to a boil in large saucepan. Cook pasta according to package directions. Drain and set aside.

Meanwhile, heat canola oil in deep 12-inch skillet over medium heat. Add chicken breasts and brown on both sides. Cook an additional 5 minutes. Remove from skillet and cover.

Add garlic, green pepper and broccoli to skillet. Stir-fry for two minutes. Stir in chopped tomatoes, salt, parsley, pepper and oregano. Add chicken. Bring to a boil, reduce heat, and simmer, covered, for 10 to 15 minutes, stirring occasionally. Add cooked and drained pasta, mixing well.

Transfer to a serving dish. Sprinkle with Parmesan cheese.

Yield: 6 servings.

Preparation time: 30-40 minutes

CHICKEN CORDON BLEU

Per serving:
Calories...... 312
Protein (g)... 38
Fat (g)....... 10.9
Sat. Fat (g).. 4.4
Choles. (mg).. 98
Fiber (g)..... 1.3
Sodium (mg)... 594
%Cal-Fat...... 33%

4 boneless chicken breasts
4 thin slices ham
4 slices Swiss cheese (1/2 oz. each)
1/4 cup flour
1/4 teaspoon seasoned salt
1/4 teaspoon pepper
2 teaspoons margarine, melted
1/2 pound fresh mushrooms, sliced
2 tablespoons lemon juice
2 tablespoons sherry
1 tablespoon Worcestershire sauce
1 tablespoon chopped fresh parsley
3 tablespoons cold water
1 1/2 tablespoons flour

Preheat oven to 350 degrees.

Pound chicken breasts to 1/4-inch thickness. On each flattened piece of chicken, place one slice of ham and one slice of Swiss cheese. Roll and secure with a toothpick.

Combine flour, salt and pepper. Roll the breasts in the flour mixture. Brown the rolled chicken breasts in margarine in a medium-size skillet. After browned on all sides (about 10 minutes), place in an 8 or 9-inch square baking dish.

Meanwhile, saute sliced mushrooms in lemon juice, sherry and Worcestershire sauce until tender. Add chopped parsley. Mix 1 1/2 tablespoons of flour with cold water until a smooth paste. Add to the mushroom mixture. Stir over medium heat until sauce thickens. Pour sauce over chicken breasts.

Bake at 350 degrees for 25 to 30 minutes until hot and bubbly. Serve with seasoned rice.

Yield: 4 servings.

Preparation time: 25-30 minutes

Cooking time: 25-30 minutes

BREAST OF CHICKEN BEAUFORT

6 boneless chicken breasts
2 ounces lean ham, finely chopped
1/4 cup finely chopped onion
1/4 cup egg substitute
1 cup soft bread crumbs
1 tablespoon chopped fresh parsley
1 tablespoon dry sherry
1/2 teaspoon salt
Dash cayenne pepper
1 clove garlic, minced
7 ounces back fin crabmeat

Sauce:
1 14 1/2-ounce can clear chicken broth, defatted
1/4 cup flour
1 teaspoon lemon juice
1/2 cup dry sherry
3 tablespoons tomato paste

Per serving:
Calories...... 280
Protein (g)... 40
Fat (g)....... 6.3
Sat. Fat (g).. 1.4
Choles. (mg).. 111
Fiber (g)..... 0.6
Sodium (mg)... 785
%Cal-Fat...... 17%

Preheat oven to 350 degrees.

Pound chicken breasts to 1/4-inch thickness. Combine next 10 ingredients to make stuffing. Place 1/6 of stuffing on each flattened chicken breast. Roll and secure with toothpicks. Place in 9-inch square baking dish. Bake, covered, in 350 degree oven for 30 minutes. Drain juices from baking dish.

To make sauce, combine flour and chicken broth in small saucepan. Mix with wire whisk until all lumps disappear. Heat until sauce comes to a boil and thickens. Add remaining ingredients and mix well until smooth. Pour over chicken breasts and bake an additional 30 minutes, uncovered.

To serve, transfer chicken breasts to serving platter. Pour sauce over.

Yield: 6 servings.

Preparation time: 30 minutes

Cooking time: 1 hour

CHICKEN SEAFOOD ARTICHOKE CASSEROLE

1 14-ounce can artichokes, <u>drained</u>
1 pound boneless chicken breast, cooked
1 pound shrimp, cooked and cleaned
3/4 pound fresh mushrooms, sliced

Sauce:
1 1/2 cups milk
1/4 cup flour
1/4 cup sherry
1 1/2 teaspoons Worcestershire sauce
1/2 teaspoon salt
1/4 teaspoon pepper
3 tablespoons Parmesan cheese
Paprika
2 tablespoons chopped fresh parsley
6 to 8 cups cooked rice

(handwritten note: Can add ~1/4 tsp paprika to sauce)

Cut artichokes lengthwise into quarters and arrange in bottom of 9-inch square baking dish. Cut up cooked chicken into bite-size pieces. Arrange shrimp and chicken evenly in baking dish.

In large skillet, saute sliced mushrooms until tender. (No oil needed, but keep lid on to prevent sticking.) Drain. Spread mushrooms evenly over top of casserole. *(handwritten note: make sure to cook moisture out & drain)*

Meanwhile, make sauce: Pour milk and flour into a medium-size skillet. Stir briskly with a wire whisk until all lumps disappear. Bring to a boil over medium heat, stirring frequently, until sauce thickens. Add sherry, Worcestershire sauce, salt and pepper.

Pour sauce over casserole. Sprinkle with Parmesan cheese, paprika and parsley.

Bake, uncovered, at 350 degrees for 40 minutes.

Serve over rice.

Yield: 8 servings.

Back fin crabmeat may be substituted for the shrimp, if desired.

Preparation time: 35-40 minutes (if shrimp are already cleaned)

Cooking time: 40 minutes

CHICKEN CACCIATORE

1 pound boneless chicken breast, cut into bite-size pieces
Vegetable cooking spray
2 tablespoons water
2 green peppers, cut into 1/2 x 1-inch pieces
2 medium onions, sliced
2 cloves garlic, minced
1/2 pound fresh mushrooms, sliced, or 4 oz. canned
1 16-ounce can tomatoes, chopped
1 8-ounce can tomato sauce
1/4 teaspoon pepper
1 teaspoon dried oregano or basil
1/2 teaspoon celery seed
1/4 cup dry white wine
1 pound pasta, preferable flat noodles
Parmesan cheese (optional)

Per serving:
Calories...... 647
Protein (g)... 45
Fat (g)....... 6.5
Sat. Fat (g).. 1.9
Choles. (mg).. 72
Fiber (g)..... 5.6
Sodium (mg)... 309
%Cal-Fat...... 9%

Spray large, non-stick skillet with vegetable cooking spray. In skillet, over medium heat, brown chicken breast pieces. Remove chicken.

Add two tablespoons water to skillet. Add cut up vegetables -green peppers, onions, garlic and mushrooms. Steam until tender but not brown. Check frequently to make sure water doesn't boil away. Add more if necessary. Return chicken to skillet.

Meanwhile, roughly chop canned tomatoes in food processor. Pour into medium-size bowl. Add tomato sauce, pepper, oregano and celery seed. Mix well. Pour over chicken and vegetables in skillet. Cover and simmer 30 minutes.

Stir in 1/4 cup dry white wine. Cook chicken, uncovered, 15 minutes longer, or until desired consistency. Stir occasionally.

Meanwhile, cook pasta according to package directions. Drain. Mix small amount of tomato sauce into pasta to keep from sticking.

To serve, spoon chicken cacciatore over pasta. Sprinkle with Parmesan cheese, if desired.

Yield: 4 servings.

Preparation time: 30 minutes

Cooking time: 45 minutes

BEIJING CHICKEN STIR-FRY

Per serving:
Calories...... 388
Protein (g)... 34
Fat (g)....... 9
Sat. Fat (g).. 1.6
Choles. (mg).. 72
Fiber (g)..... 4.7
Sodium (mg)... 548
%Cal-Fat...... 22%

3/4 pound boneless chicken breast
2 tablespoons cornstarch, divided
3 tablespoons Lite soy sauce, divided
2 tablespoons dry sherry
1 clove garlic, minced
1 tablespoon sesame seeds, toasted
1 cup water
3 teaspoons vegetable oil, divided
1 16-ounce can bean sprouts or 1/2 pound fresh bean
** sprouts**
1 bunch green onions and tops, cut into 2-inch lengths
1 8-ounce can water chestnuts, drained
12 ounces pasta, cooked, preferably dumpling pasta

Cut chicken breast into narrow strips. Combine 1 tablespoon cornstarch, 1 tablespoon soy sauce, sherry and minced garlic in medium bowl. Stir in chicken and let stand for 10 minutes.

Meanwhile, spray small non-stick skillet with vegetable cooking spray. Place over medium heat. Add sesame seeds and heat, stirring occasionally, until seeds turn light brown. Remove from heat and set aside.

Combine water, remaining 1 tablespoon cornstarch and 2 tablespoons soy sauce in small bowl. Set aside.

Heat 2 teaspoons oil in wok or non-stick saute pan until hot. Add chicken and stir-fry 3 minutes, or until chicken strips are fully cooked. Remove.

Add remaining 1 teaspoon oil to pan and stir-fry bean sprouts, green onions and water chestnuts for 3 minutes. Add about 2 tablespoons water if vegetables stick to pan.

Stir in chicken, soy sauce/water mixture and toasted sesame seeds. Cook and continue stirring until mixture comes to a boil and thickens. Serve immediately over hot pasta.

Yield: 4 servings.

Preparation time: 30-35 minutes

CHICKEN L'ORANGE

4 boneless chicken breasts
Lemon-pepper seasoning, to taste
Vegetable cooking spray

Mandarin Orange Sauce:
1/3 cup brown sugar
1/3 cup granulated sugar
1/4 teaspoon salt
1 tablespoon cornstarch
1 cup orange juice
1 teaspoon Dijon mustard
11-ounce can mandarin oranges in light syrup, drained
1 to 2 tablespoons orange liqueur (optional)

Per serving:
Calories...... 344
Protein (g)... 28
Fat (g)....... 4
Sat. Fat (g).. 1.1
Choles. (mg).. 73
Fiber (g)..... 1.6
Sodium (mg)... 223
%Cal-Fat...... 10%

Preheat gas or charcoal grill on medium heat.

Lightly sprinkle lemon pepper on both sides of chicken breasts. Place aluminum foil on grill, spray with cooking spray, and place chicken breasts on foil. Grill 8 to 10 minutes on each side, or just until meat is no longer pink in middle. Do not overcook. (Chicken breasts may also be prepared in a non-stick skillet, sprayed with cooking spray.)

Meanwhile, make sauce. In small saucepan, combine sugars, salt and cornstarch. Slowly stir in juice until smooth. Stir in mustard with a wire whisk. Place over medium heat and bring to a boil. Simmer until transparent and thickened, about 3 minutes. Stir in drained mandarin oranges, and, if desired, orange liqueur. Heat slightly, but do not boil.

To serve, place chicken breasts on serving platter and spoon sauce over top.

Yield: 4 servings.

Mandarin Orange Sauce is also delicious served over fish, especially Orange Roughy or Red Snapper.

Preparation time: 25 minutes

COQ AU VIN

Per serving:
Calories...... 367
Protein (g)... 30
Fat (g)....... 6.5
Sat. Fat (g).. 1.4
Choles. (mg).. 65
Fiber (g)..... 4
Sodium (mg)...539
%Cal-Fat...... 16%

4 boneless chicken breast halves
2 teaspoons olive oil
12 whole mushrooms, scrubbed
12 small white onions, peeled
2/3 cup sliced green onion, including tops
1 clove garlic, crushed
2 cups Burgundy wine
1 cup canned condensed chicken broth, undiluted
1/4 cup flour
1/2 teaspoon seasoned salt
1/2 teaspoon dried thyme
1/8 teaspoon black pepper
8 small red potatoes, scrubbed (1 1/4-inch diameter)
Fresh parsley for garnish

Remove skin from chicken and pound to 1/4-inch thickness.
Heat olive oil in Dutch oven. Add chicken and brown on both sides. Remove and set aside.

Add mushrooms and white onions to Dutch oven. Cook until slightly browned. (You may need to add one to two tablespoons water if they begin to stick. If so, cover pan while browning.) Remove and set aside.

Add green onions and crushed garlic to Dutch oven. Saute 2 minutes. (Add additional water, if necessary.) Immediately add Burgundy and begin to heat.

Meanwhile, with wire whisk, mix flour into condensed chicken broth until lumps disappear. Add broth mixture, salt, thyme and pepper to Dutch oven. Bring to a boil. Stir until sauce thickens.

Remove from heat. Return chicken, mushrooms and onions to Dutch oven. Cover and refrigerate for 2 hours or overnight.

Preheat oven to 375 degrees. Just before baking, add potatoes to chicken mixture. Bake, covered, about 1 hour and 50 minutes, or until chicken and potatoes are tender. Garnish with parsley.

Yield: 4 servings

Preparation time: 30-35 minutes

Cooking time: 1 hour, 50 minutes

GRILLED BREAST OF CHICKEN SANDWICH

4 boneless chicken breast halves
1/2 cup no-oil Italian dressing
Honey mustard (to taste)
Lettuce
Tomato, sliced
4 large hamburger buns

Per serving:
Calories...... 281
Protein (g)... 31
Fat (g)....... 5.6
Sat. Fat (g).. 1.5
Choles. (mg).. 73
Fiber (g)..... 1.8
Sodium (mg)... NA
%Cal-Fat...... 19%

Remove all visible fat from chicken breasts. Pound to 1/4-inch thickness. Place chicken breasts in mixing bowl and pour salad dressing over, evenly covering meat. Marinate at least 2 hours or overnight.

Preheat outdoor grill. Place aluminum foil on grill, spray with vegetable cooking spray, and cook chicken breasts over medium heat approximately 8 minutes per side. Do not overcook. Transfer to platter.

To assemble sandwich, place chicken breast on bun, top with honey mustard (or catsup), tomato and lettuce.

Yield: 4 servings

This provides a tasty alternative to hamburgers or hotdogs cooked on a grill. The big bonus is that it is much lower in fat and just as easy to prepare.

Preparation time: 10-15 minutes

Cooking time: 15-20 minutes

Marinating time: 2 hours

BARBECUED SHREDDED TURKEY BREAST

Per serving:
Calories...... 290
Protein (g)... 28
Fat (g)....... 5.3
Sat. Fat (g).. 1.3
Choles. (mg).. 68
Fiber (g)..... 1.6
Sodium (mg)... 898
%Cal-Fat...... 17%

1 6 to 7-pound whole turkey breast (2 1/2 – 3 pounds turkey meat)
1 3/4 cups brewed strong coffee
1 1/2 cups Worcestershire sauce
1/4 cup water
1 1/2 cups catsup
5 tablespoons lite margarine
1/4 cup packed brown sugar
3 teaspoons garlic powder
2 teaspoons onion powder
2 teaspoons black pepper
16 to 18 sandwich rolls

Cook turkey breast in a covered pot of boiling water for 3 hours. Remove from water and allow to cool slightly. Remove meat from bone and shred. Set aside.

Combine remaining ingredients (except sandwich rolls) in 4-quart saucepan. Add shredded turkey breast and let simmer for 30 minutes or longer over low heat, stirring occasionally.

Serve on sliced hard rolls or hamburger buns.

Yield: 16 to 18 servings.

The liquid left over from cooking the turkey breast makes an excellent stock for chicken or turkey soup, or it can be used for cooking rice. To defat it, let it cool in the refrigerator, then remove the fat from the top. It can be refrigerated for several days or frozen until ready to use.

Preparation time: 30 minutes

Cooking time: 3 hours, 30 minutes

TURKEY PARMIGIANA

1 pound turkey breast slices, about 1/4-inch thick
2 teaspoons olive oil
1/2 cup crushed cornflake crumbs
1/4 cup grated Parmesan cheese
1 egg substitute
1 8-ounce can no-salt added tomato sauce
1/2 teaspoon dried oregano, crushed
1/2 teaspoon sugar
Dash garlic powder
2 thin slices mozzarella cheese, halved (2 ounces)

Per serving:
Calories...... 324
Protein (g)... 44
Fat (g)....... 8.6
Sat. Fat (g).. 3.6
Choles. (mg).. 110
Fiber (g)..... 1.1
Sodium (mg)... 411
%Cal-Fat...... 24%

Pound turkey breast slices with meat pounder to tenderize. Set aside.

In a medium-size bowl, combine crushed cornflake crumbs, Parmesan cheese, and a dash of pepper. Pour egg substitute into a small bowl.

Heat olive oil in large skillet or saute pan.

Dip turkey breast slices first in egg, then in crumb mixture. Place in saute pan and brown on both sides. Cook for 20 minutes longer.

Meanwhile, in small saucepan, combine tomato sauce, oregano, sugar and garlic powder. Heat to boiling, stirring occasionally. Pour sauce over meat. Top with cheese.

Turn on oven broiler. Transfer meat to an oven-proof serving dish. Broil close to heat until cheese bubbles and turns golden, about 3 to 4 minutes. Serve immediately.

Yield: 4 servings.

If time is short, cheese can be melted on top of chicken in saute pan, by putting the lid on for about 4 - 5 minutes, rather than transferring to another dish and broiling. Chicken breasts, pounded to 1/4-inch thickness, may be substituted for turkey breast.

Preparation time: 30 minutes

Cooking time: 30 minutes

STUFFED TURKEY CUTLETS

Per serving:
Calories...... 256
Protein (g)... 27
Fat (g)....... 9.3
Sat. Fat (g).. 0.9
Choles. (mg).. 66
Fiber (g)..... 1
Sodium (mg)... 372
%Cal-Fat...... 24%

4 turkey breast cutlets (1 pound total)
1 cup herb-seasoned stuffing mix
1 medium carrot, shredded
1 egg substitute
2 tablespoons canola oil

Sauce:
1 cup water
1 chicken bouillon cube
1/4 cup flour
1/2 cup cold water
1 teaspoon lemon juice
1/2 cup Chablis wine
2 teaspoons minced parsley

Preheat oven to 350 degrees.

Pound turkey breast cutlets slightly to tenderize. Combine stuffing mix, carrot, egg substitute and cooking oil in a small mixing bowl.

To assemble, lay turkey cutlets flat and spoon 1/4 of stuffing on one end of each cutlet. Fold other end over and secure with a toothpick. Place in a 9-inch square baking dish. Bake, covered, in 350 degree oven for 30 minutes.

Meanwhile, make sauce. Place chicken bouillon cube and 1 cup water in medium-size skillet. Heat until bouillon cube is dissolved. In a small bowl, mix flour and 1/2 cup cold water with a wire whisk until all lumps disappear. Add to skillet and stir until sauce thickens. Add lemon juice, wine and parsley and mix well.

Pour 1/2 of sauce (one cup) over turkey cutlets and bake, uncovered, for an additional 30 minutes. Transfer cutlets to a platter and spoon remaining sauce (warmed) over top.

Yield: Serves 4

Preparation time: 25-30 minutes

Cooking time: 1 hour

NONFAT TURKEY GRAVY

Meat juices from roasted whole turkey or turkey breast (defatted)*
1/4 cup flour
1/2 cup cold water
1/4 teaspoon salt (or to taste)
Pepper to taste

Per serving:
Calories...... 27
Protein (g)... 2
Fat (g)....... 0.4
Sat. Fat (g).. 0.1
Choles. (mg).. 0
Fiber (g)..... 0
Sodium (mg)... NA
%Cal-Fat...... 5%

Add enough water to meat juices to make 1 1/2 cups liquid. Pour into medium-size frypan and heat.

Meanwhile, in a small bowl, using a wire whisk, stir flour into cold water until all lumps disappear.

Gradually add flour mixture to meat juices, stirring constantly with a wire whisk. Bring to a boil. Reduce heat and simmer 5 to 10 minutes. Season to taste.

To defat the turkey juices, pour all the drippings into a bowl. Add ice cubes and place in freezer. After 10 - 15 minutes the fat will layer at the top and solidify. Separate the top fat layer and use the dark juices on the bottom for the gravy. Chicken, turkey or beef broth may be substituted for defatted meat juices plus water.

An alternate method is especially good if you cook whole turkey or turkey breast often. You simply save the meat juices from one turkey meal for the next turkey's gravy. For example, the first time you prepare a turkey or turkey breast, you will save the meat juices for your next turkey meal.

Prepare the drippings as follows: Pour the meat juices into an airtight plastic container. Refrigerate overnight. The next morning, remove the congealed fat from the top. Freeze the defatted meat juices and use in making gravy the next time you serve turkey.

Yield: 2 cups gravy, or 6 servings

Preparation time: 10-15 minutes

Beef, Pork, & Veal

ROUND STEAK CHILE

Per serving:
Calories...... 365
Protein (g)... 31
Fat (g)....... 6
Sat. Fat (g).. 1.9
Choles. (mg).. 47
Fiber (g)..... 11.2
Sodium (mg)... 881
%Cal-Fat...... 14%

1/2 pound round steak, ground (all visible fat removed)
1 cup chopped onion
1 green pepper, chopped
1 16-ounce can tomatoes, broken up
2 16-ounce cans dark red kidney beans, drained and
   rinsed
1 8-ounce can tomato sauce, no salt added
1/4 teaspoon salt, optional
2 teaspoons chili powder, or to taste
2 bay leaves

Have butcher grind round steak or grind it yourself in food processor.

In heavy skillet, combine meat, onion and green pepper. Cook until meat is lightly browned and vegetables are tender. Stir in remaining ingredients. Simmer, covered, for 30 minutes to 1 hour.

Remove bay leaves and serve immediately.

Yield: 4 servings

The amount of fat in this recipe is greatly reduced over traditional chile recipes by using round steak rather than ground beef, and by using less beef and more kidney beans.

Preparation time: 20 minutes

Cooking time: 30 minutes to 1 hour

BEEF STEW

1 1/2 pounds round steak, all visible fat removed, cut into
    1-inch cubes
Vegetable cooking spray
1 15 1/2-ounce can Northern beans, drained and rinsed
1 16-ounce can tomatoes, chopped
4 small onions, quartered
4 carrots, cut into 1/2-inch slices
4 small potatoes, cut into bite-size pieces
1 cup celery, chopped
1/2 pound fresh mushrooms, sliced
1 cup clear beef broth, defatted
1 cup dry white wine
2 tablespoons Worcestershire sauce
1/4 teaspoon ground pepper
1/4 cup flour

Per serving:
Calories...... 423
Protein (g)... 43
Fat (g)....... 7.4
Sat. Fat (g).. 2.5
Choles. (mg).. 78
Fiber (g)..... 9
Sodium (mg)... 508
%Cal-Fat...... 17%

Preheat oven to 350 degrees.

Spray large skillet with vegetable cooking spray. Brown meat cubes on stove over medium heat. Transfer meat and juice to large oven-proof casserole. Add next seven ingredients to casserole dish.

In medium-size bowl, combine beef broth, wine, Worcestershire sauce and pepper. Add flour, mixing with a wire whisk until all lumps are gone. Pour over meat and vegetables. Stir to mix.

Cover and bake in 350 degree oven 2 1/2 to 3 hours. Stir occasionally.

Yield: 6 servings

Preparation time: 35-40 minutes

Cooking time: 2 1/2 to 3 hours

BEEF BOURGUIGNON

**2 pounds round steak, all visible fat removed, cut into
    1-inch cubes**
Vegetable cooking spray
2 cups chopped onion
4 medium carrots, cut into bite-size chunks
2 celery stalks, chopped
1 clove garlic, minced
2 cups Burgundy wine
1 14 1/2-ounce can clear beef broth, defatted
1 tablespoon catsup
2 tablespoons Worcestershire sauce
1/2 teaspoon salt, or to taste
1/4 teaspoon pepper, or to taste
1/2 teaspoon thyme
1/4 cup flour
1/2 cup water
1 8-ounce can sliced mushrooms, drained
1 pint pearl onions, parboiled and peeled
1/4 cup chopped fresh parsley
1 pound Dumpling pasta or egg noodles

Preheat oven to 350 degrees.

Spray large skillet with vegetable cooking spray. Saute beef cubes until thoroughly browned. With slotted spoon, transfer beef cubes to large oven-proof casserole. In same skillet, saute chopped onion, carrots, celery and garlic until onion becomes translucent. Add to meat in casserole.

In same skillet, combine wine, beef broth, catsup, Worcestershire sauce, salt, pepper and thyme. In small bowl, mix flour and water with wire whisk until smooth. Add to wine mixture, stirring constantly, until it comes to a boil. Pour over casserole. Add mushrooms and whole onions to casserole.

Cover and bake at 350 degrees for 3 hours, or until meat and vegetables are tender.

Just before serving, sprinkle chopped parsley over casserole.

Meanwhile prepare pasta according to package directions. Serve the beef bourguignon over pasta.

Yield: 6 to 8 servings

Preparation time: 45-50 minutes

Cooking time: 3 hours

MARINATED BEEF STIR-FRY

3/4 pound round steak, all visible fat removed
1/2 cup diagonally sliced green onions (1-inch slices)
4 cups sliced bok choy (about 5 stalks)*
2 carrots, shredded
1 8-ounce can bamboo shoots, drained
2 teaspoons olive oil
Hot cooked rice (3 to 4 cups)

Marinade:
2 tablespoons reduced-sodium soy sauce
2 tablespoons dry sherry
1 tablespoon hoisin sauce (hot bean sauce)
2 teaspoons grated gingerroot
1 clove garlic minced

Per serving:
Calories...... 354
Protein (g)... 24
Fat (g)....... 7.5
Sat. Fat (g).. 2.2
Choles. (mg).. 55
Fiber (g)..... 4.3
Sodium (mg)... 352
%Cal-Fat...... 20%

Cut beef on the bias into bite-size pieces 1/8-inch thick. (To make slicing easier, partially freeze beef in freezer about 45 minutes prior to cutting.)

Prepare marinade by combining all ingredients in small mixing bowl. Add beef and marinate at room temperature 30 minutes or in refrigerator for 2 hours. Stir occasionally.

Meanwhile, cut up green onions, bok choy, and carrots as directed.

Preheat a wok or large skillet over medium-high heat. Add olive oil. Add onions and bok choy; stir-fry for 2 minutes. Add carrots and bamboo shoots; stir-fry about 3 minutes or until vegetables are crisp-tender. Remove vegetables from pan.

Add beef and marinade to skillet and stir-fry for 3 to 4 minutes or until meat is cooked. Add vegetables and heat through. Serve immediately over rice.

Yield: 6 servings

To slice bok choy, first cut each celery-like stalk in half lengthwise, including dark green top. Next, cut stalk as you would chop celery, about 1/4-inch thick. Coarsely chop leafy greens at top of stalk.

Preparation time: 30-40 minutes

Marinating time: 30 minutes to 2 hours

SWISS STEAK

Per serving:
Calories...... 263
Protein (g)... 35
Fat (g)....... 8
Sat. Fat (g).. 2.5
Choles. (mg).. 78
Fiber (g)..... 1.8
Sodium (mg)... 263
%Cal-Fat...... 29%

1 1/2 pounds round or flank steak, cut 1-inch thick
1/4 cup flour
1/2 teaspoon salt
1/8 teaspoon black pepper
2 teaspoons canola oil
1 cup chopped onion
3 fresh tomatoes, or 1 16-ounce can tomatoes, chopped finely
2 carrots, peeled and chopped finely
1 tablespoon chopped fresh thyme or 1 teaspoon dried

Trim meat of all visible fat.

Combine flour, salt and pepper. Pound flour into meat using a meat mallet or the dull edge of a large knife.

In large skillet or Dutch oven, brown meat on both sides in hot oil.

In a medium-size mixing bowl, combine chopped onion, tomatoes and carrots. Pour over meat. Cover, bring to a boil, and reduce heat. Simmer over low heat for 1 1/2 hours or until tender. Turn meat once or twice during cooking time.

Remove meat to a warm platter and slice, diagonally, into 1/4-inch thick slices. Pour the vegetable sauce over the slices of meat. Some sauce may be reserved for passing at the table. Serve immediately.

Yield: 6 servings

If desired, you can puree the sauce in a food processor. There is enough sauce not only for the meat, but for whatever side dish of rice, potatoes or polenta, you choose to serve with it.

Preparation time: 20-25 minutes

Cooking time: 1 1/2 hours

PEPPER STEAK

1 pound round or flank steak, trimmed of all visible fat
2 green peppers (or 1 red and 1 green pepper), cut into
1/2 x 1-inch strips
2 large tomatoes, cut into small wedges*
Vegetable cooking spray
1 clove garlic, minced
1 cup beef broth, fat skimmed from top
2 tablespoons lite soy sauce
1 tablespoon sherry
2 tablespoons water
1 tablespoon cornstarch
3 to 4 cups prepared rice

Per serving:
Calories...... 520
Protein (g)... 42
Fat (g)....... 11.6
Sat. Fat (g).. 3.8
Choles. (mg).. 108
Fiber (g)..... 2.6
Sodium (mg)... 564
%Cal-Fat...... 20%

Cut steak across the grain into 1/8-inch strips (or have this done by butcher). Cut up peppers and tomatoes as indicated above; cover, and set aside.

Spray large nonstick skillet with vegetable cooking spray. Brown meat strips over medium-high heat, until browned on all sides. Add minced garlic and stir-fry 1/2 minute longer. Add beef broth. Bring to a boil, reduce heat and simmer, covered, 30 to 40 minutes, or until meat is tender.

Add green or red peppers and simmer, covered, about 8 minutes. Add tomatoes and simmer an additional 5 minutes.

Meanwhile, in small mixing bowl, combine soy sauce, sherry, water, and cornstarch. Add to center of skillet and bring to a boil without stirring. Cook one minute longer, stirring until mixture thickens and thoroughly coats meat and vegetables.

Serve immediately over hot rice. Sprinkle with additional soy sauce, if desired.

Yield: 4 servings

If you prefer, tomatoes may be peeled.

Preparation time: 30-35 minutes

Cooking time: 45-50 minutes

MARINATED BEEF TENDERLOIN

Per serving:
Calories...... 245
Protein (g)... 32
Fat (g)....... 11.5
Sat. Fat (g).. 4.1
Choles. (mg).. 96
Fiber (g)..... 0
Sodium (mg)... NA
%Cal-Fat...... 39%

With pork tenderloin:
Fat..........5.3
%Cal-Fat.....24%

1 beef tenderloin (about 4 to 6 pounds), trimmed
1/2 cup lite soy sauce
1/4 cup dry sherry
1 tablespoon Worcestershire sauce
1 clove garlic, minced
1 tablespoon sugar
1/2 teaspoon ground ginger
1/4 teaspoon black pepper

Remove all visible fat and connective tissue from tenderloin.

Prepare marinade by mixing together soy sauce, sherry, Worcestershire sauce, garlic, sugar, ginger and pepper.

Pour marinade over tenderloin. Cover and refrigerate 2 to 8 hours, or overnight (the longer the better).

Preheat oven to 425 degrees.

Remove tenderloin from marinade. Place on rack in open pan. Tuck under small end so meat will cook evenly. Roast in 425 degree oven 45 minutes to 1 hour, or until internal temperature of beef is 140 degrees (rare). Cook longer if you prefer tenderloin to be cooked to medium. Wait 5 minutes before slicing.

Yield: Approximately 16 4-ounce servings (cooked)

If a whole tenderloin is too much meat, ask your butcher to cut a half tenderloin for you. Prepare as indicated above and roast at 425 degrees for 45 to 50 minutes.

*This marinade is also excellent for pork tenderloin. Prepare as above and bake at 375 degrees for 30 to 40 minutes, or until internal temperature reaches 155–160 degrees. It may also be baked in a shallow pan **with** the marinade, if the marinating time is short, or if a stronger flavor is desired.*

Preparation time: 10-15 minutes

Cooking time: 45-60 minutes

Marinating time: 2 to 24 hours

BEEF-BEAN BURGER

1/2 pound extra-lean ground round
1 small onion, chopped
1 15-ounce can black-eyed peas, drained and rinsed
2 tablespoons catsup
1/2 cup dry bread crumbs
1 egg substitute (1/4 cup)
1/2 teaspoon cumin
1/4 teaspoon salt (optional)

Per serving:
Calories...... 250
Protein (g)... 25
Fat (g)....... 5.2
Sat. Fat (g).. 1.7
Choles. (mg).. 40
Fiber (g)..... 5.2
Sodium (mg)... 374
%Cal-Fat...... 19%

In medium-size bowl, combine ground round and chopped onion.

Place drained black-eyed peas and catsup into food processor. Process until pureed. Add to mixing bowl along with remaining ingredients. Mix well. (Burgers are easier to form if the meat-bean mixture is refrigerated at least 30 minutes.)

Spray large skillet with vegetable cooking spray. Form meat mixture into 5 or 6 patties, depending on preferred size. Fry over medium heat approximately 8 minutes per side. Serve on hamburger buns or hard rolls.

Yield: 5 to 6 patties

These burgers taste like a cross between a soy burger and a beef burger. You still get the taste of beef, but the texture is different from standard beef burgers. The big benefit of these burgers is the much lower fat quantity and the addition of fiber (from the beans.)

Preparation time: 15-20 minutes

Cooking time: 15 minutes

APPLE-DATE STUFFED TENDERLOIN

Per serving:
Calories...... 276
Protein (g)... 33
Fat (g)....... 5.5
Sat. Fat (g).. 2
Choles. (mg).. 106
Fiber (g)..... 1.6
Sodium (mg)... 280
%Cal-Fat...... 18%

1 1/4 to 1 1/2 pounds pork tenderloin, trimmed of all visible fat
1/4 cup dry white wine
2 tablespoons Worcestershire sauce
3/4 cup chunky applesauce
1/3 cup chopped dates
3 tablespoons brown sugar
1/4 teaspoon salt
1/2 teaspoon cinnamon
Sprigs of parsley for garnish

Form a "pocket" in the pork tenderloin(s) by cutting a slit lengthwise down the center, about 3/4 of the way through to the other side. Be careful not to slit the other side. Open up slit tenderloin(s) and lay flat in a shallow baking dish.

Combine wine and Worcestershire sauce. Pour over pork tenderloin(s) and marinate, covered, for 1 to 3 hours in refrigerator, or 30 minutes at room temperature.

Preheat oven to 375 degrees. Spray a 7 1/2 x 11 x 2-inch baking dish with vegetable cooking spray.

In a small bowl, combine applesauce, dates, brown sugar, salt, and cinnamon. Spoon mixture into pocket(s) of tenderloin(s). Close pockets loosely with wooden toothpicks. Place in prepared baking dish.

Bake at 375 degrees for approximately 30 to 40 minutes or until meat thermometer reads 157 to 160 degrees. (Do not overcook.) Let meat stand five minutes before slicing. Garnish with sprigs of fresh parsley.

Quick Preparation Method: Do not marinate tenderloin, but instead lightly salt "pocket." Prepare applesauce mixture, stuff pocket, and bake as instructed above.

Yield: 5 servings

Preparation time: 20-25 minutes

Cooking time: 30-40 minutes

Marinating time: 30 minutes to 3 hours

PORK MEDALLIONS WITH MUSHROOM SAUCE

1 1/2 pounds pork tenderloin(s), trimmed of all visible fat
Vegetable cooking spray
8 ounces sliced fresh mushrooms
2 tablespoons water
1/4 cup finely chopped onion
1 teaspoon chopped fresh rosemary, or 1/2 teaspoon
   dried rosemary
1/4 teaspoon pepper
1/4 teaspoon garlic powder
6 tablespoons dry sherry
3 tablespoons lite soy sauce
1 1/2 tablespoons lime juice
1 1/2 teaspoons sugar
Fresh rosemary sprigs (for garnish)

Per serving:
Calories...... 230
Protein (g)... 34
Fat (g)....... 5.7
Sat. Fat (g).. 2
Choles. (mg).. 106
Fiber (g)..... 0.7
Sodium (mg)... 482
%Cal-Fat...... 22%

Cut tenderloin(s) into six equal pieces. Pound or press each tenderloin slice to 3/4-inch thickness.

Spray large skillet with vegetable cooking spray. Place over medium-high heat and brown tenderloin slices for about two minutes on each side. Transfer tenderloin to platter and keep warm.

Add mushrooms, water, onion, rosemary, pepper and garlic to skillet. Cover and saute for 5 minutes or until mushrooms turn dark brown.

In a separate bowl, combine sherry, soy sauce, lime juice and sugar. Add to mushroom mixture in skillet.

Return tenderloin slices to skillet. Spoon mushroom sauce over slices. Cover and simmer for 15 to 20 minutes, turning meat over after 8 to 10 minutes. (Meat should have *no* pink inside.) Place pork tenderloin slices on serving plate. Cover with mushroom mixture. Garnish with sprigs of fresh rosemary, if desired.

Yield: 6 4-ounce servings

Preparation time: 30-35 minutes

Cooking time: 15-20 minutes

STIR-FRY GINGERED PORK

Per serving:
Calories...... 446
Protein (g)... 34
Fat (g)....... 7.1
Sat. Fat (g).. 1.9
Choles. (mg).. 85
Fiber (g)..... 4.3
Sodium (mg)... 510
%Cal-Fat...... 14%

1 pound pork tenderloin, trimmed of visible fat, cut into thin, bite-size strips
1/4 cup dry sherry
2 tablespoons lite soy sauce
2 tablespoons water
1 teaspoon sugar
1 cup clear beef broth, defatted
4 teaspoons cornstarch
2 teaspoons canola oil
2 teaspoons grated gingerroot
4 green onions including tops, finely diced
2 medium carrots, cut into julienne strips
1/2 pound fresh spinach, washed and coarsely chopped
1 8-ounce can bamboo shoots, drained
4 cups hot cooked rice
Soy sauce to taste

Cut pork tenderloin on the bias into thin bite-size strips. In small mixing bowl, combine sherry, soy sauce, water and sugar. Add pork, stirring to coat well. Cover and marinate at room temperature 30 minutes or 2 hours in the refrigerator, stirring occasionally.

Drain pork, reserving marinade. Add beef broth and cornstarch to marinade. Stir until well blended. Set aside.

Heat oil in wok or heavy skillet over medium-high heat. Stir-fry gingerroot for 20 seconds. Add pork and stir-fry 3 to 4 minutes or until pork is no longer pink. Remove pork, keeping warm. Add green onions and carrots; stir-fry 2 minutes. Add chopped spinach and stir-fry an additional 3 minutes, or until vegetables are crisp tender and spinach has wilted. Add bamboo shoots and heat through.

Return pork to skillet. Add marinade mixture. Cook and stir until it comes to a boil and thickens. Mix to evenly coat meat and vegetables. Serve immediately over rice.

Yield: 4 to 6 servings

Preparation time: 35-45 minutes

Marinating time: 30 minutes to 2 hours

PORK TENDERLOIN WITH MUSTARD SAUCE

1 1/2 pounds pork tenderloin(s), trimmed of visible fat
Salt and pepper to taste (optional)
1/4 cup prepared honey mustard
1 tablespoon water

Per serving:
Calories...... 216
Protein (g)... 33
Fat (g)....... 5.7
Sat. Fat (g).. 2
Choles. (mg).. 71
Fiber (g)..... 0
Sodium (mg)... 140
%Cal-Fat...... 24%

Preheat oven to 375 degrees.

In small bowl, combine honey mustard and water. Microwave on low for 15 seconds. Mix well until it becomes a smooth paste.

Spray roasting rack or broiler pan with non-stick cooking spray. Place trimmed tenderloin on prepared rack. Sprinkle lightly with salt and pepper, if desired. Spread half the honey mustard over top. Roast at 375 degrees for 20 minutes. Spread remaining honey mustard on tenderloin and cook an additional 10 to 20 minutes or until meat thermometer registers 157 to 160 degrees. (Avoid overcooking.) Let meat stand 5 minutes before serving.

To serve, cut into serving pieces and place on a platter. Garnish with fresh sprigs of parsley. Additional honey mustard sauce may be passed at the table, if desired.

Yield: 6 4-ounce servings

This is a very simple meat dish to prepare, perfect when time is limited. It can also be cooked on a preheated outdoor grill over medium heat. Place aluminum foil on the cooking rack, spray with vegetable cooking spray to avoid sticking, and cook approximately the same length of time as indicated above. Use a meat thermometer to be sure meat has been thoroughly cooked on the inside.

A good accompaniment for this dish is Rice-Mushroom Casserole (Recipe, page 338), a steamed vegetable of choice and a fresh green salad.

Preparation time: 10 minutes

Cooking time: 30-40 minutes

PORK TENDERLOIN FLORENTINE

1 1/2 pounds pork tenderloin
**2 10-ounce packages frozen chopped spinach, thawed
    and drained (squeeze lightly to remove excess water)**
2 cups soft bread crumbs (about 3 slices)
1/4 cup finely chopped fresh parsley
1/2 cup grated Parmesan cheese
1 teaspoon minced garlic
2 egg substitutes (1/2 cup)
1 teaspoon lemon pepper
1/4 teaspoon salt

Preheat oven to 375 degrees.

Slit the pork tenderloin lengthwise down the center, cutting about 3/4 of the way through to the other side. (If you have 2 tenderloins, do the same with both.) Open up slit tenderloin(s) and lay flat.

In large mixing bowl, combine thawed and drained spinach with remaining ingredients to make spinach pesto stuffing. Spoon mixture evenly over pork tenderloin(s), mounding slightly. Place on shallow baking pan, sprayed with vegetable cooking spray.

Bake at 375 degrees for approximately 30 to 40 minutes or until meat thermometer reads 157 to 160 degrees. Cut into six equal portions. Serve immediately.

Yield: 6 servings

Preparation time: 25-30 minutes

Cooking time: 30-40 minutes

PORK MARENGO

2 3/4 pounds pork tenderloin, trimmed of visible fat, cut
  into 3/4- inch cubes
Vegetable cooking spray
1 cup chopped onion
1 cup chopped celery
1 clove garlic, minced
1 cup dry white wine, divided
2 8-ounce cans tomato sauce
2 bay leaves
1 teaspoon dried oregano
1/2 teaspoon rosemary
1 teaspoon salt
1/2 teaspoon pepper
2 sprigs parsley, chopped finely
1 pound mushrooms, sliced
2 tablespoons lemon juice
2 tablespoons light margarine, divided
1 tablespoon flour
2 tablespoons cold water
2 tablespoons fresh parsley, finely chopped
20 ounces dumpling pasta, or egg noodles

Per serving:
Calories...... 533
Protein (g)... 48
Fat (g)....... 9.2
Sat. Fat (g).. 2.8
Choles. (mg).. 130
Fiber (g).... 5
Sodium (mg).. 646
%Cal-Fat..... 16%

Trim all visible fat from tenderloin and cut into 3/4-inch cubes. Spray large non-stick skillet with vegetable cooking spray. Add meat cubes and saute until light gray. Remove from skillet with slotted spoon.

Add onion, celery and garlic to meat juices in skillet. Saute until onion becomes translucent, about 5 minutes.

Stir in 1/2 cup wine, tomato sauce, bay leaves, oregano, rosemary, salt, pepper, parsley and sauteed pork. Bring to a boil. Reduce heat and simmer 1 1/2 hours. Remove bay leaves.

Meanwhile, slice mushrooms. Toss with lemon juice. In medium-size skillet, melt 1 tablespoon margarine. Add mushrooms and saute until tender, about 5 to 10 minutes. Add remaining 1/2 cup wine and sauteed mushrooms to pork mixture.

Mix flour and cold water to make a paste. Add to skillet. Simmer, covered, 15 minutes longer. Meanwhile, prepare pasta according to package directions. Drain and toss with 1 tablespoon margarine to prevent pasta from sticking together.

Transfer pork mixture to a serving dish. Sprinkle with parsley. Serve over pasta.

Yield: 8 to 10 generous servings.

Recipe can be made ahead and refrigerated. Reheat in 350 degree oven for 30 to 40 minutes.

Preparation time: 1 hour

Cooking time: 1 3/4 hours

VEAL SALTIMBOCCA

Per serving:
Calories...... 225
Protein (g)... 31
Fat (g)....... 8.4
Sat. Fat (g).. 4.2
Choles. (mg).. 85
Fiber (g)..... 0.6
Sodium (mg)... 451
%Cal-Fat...... 33%

6 veal cutlets pounded 1/8-inch thick
3 slices lean ham, halved (about 3 ounces total)
1 medium tomato, peeled and chopped
2 tablespoons finely chopped green onion
3 ounces grated mozzarella cheese (part-skim)
1/2 teaspoon ground sage
1/3 cup dry bread crumbs
1/4 cup grated Parmesan cheese
2 tablespoons fresh chopped parsley
1 egg substitute (1/4 cup)

Preheat oven to 350 degrees.

Pound veal until it reaches desired thickness. Place the 6 veal cutlets on a flat surface. Top each with slice of ham (cut to size of cutlet), chopped tomato, and green onion. Sprinkle mozzarella cheese and ground sage over top.

Fold in sides and roll up like a jelly role. Secure with toothpicks.

Combine bread crumbs, Parmesan cheese and parsley. Dip veal rolls first in egg substitute, then bread crumb mixture. Place in shallow, oblong casserole dish. Bake, covered, at 350 degrees for 1 hour. Remove lid for last 10 minutes of baking.

Place on serving dish and remove toothpicks. Garnish with fresh sprigs of parsley.

Yield: 6 servings

Preparation time: 30 minutes

Cooking time: 1 hour

VEAL PICCATA WITH MUSHROOMS

8 ounces fresh mushrooms, sliced
1/2 cup dry white wine
Juice of 1/2 lemon
3/4 pound veal cutlets, sliced 1/4-inch thick*
1/4 teaspoon salt
1/8 teaspoon pepper
1/4 cup flour
2 teaspoons olive oil
1 cup clear chicken broth
2 tablespoons chopped fresh parsley

Per serving:
Calories...... 231
Protein (g)... 28
Fat (g)....... 6.8
Sat. Fat (g).. 0.5
Choles. (mg).. 75
Fiber (g)..... 1.1
Sodium (mg)... 374
%Cal-Fat...... 15%

Combine mushrooms, wine and lemon juice in saucepan. Bring to a boil, reduce heat, and simmer, uncovered, about 10 minutes, until mushrooms are tender. Set aside.

Meanwhile, pound veal cutlets until 1/2 original thickness. (Use a rolling pin or smooth side of meat mallet.) Sprinkle lightly with salt and pepper. Dredge with flour.

Heat olive oil in large nonstick saucepan. Place floured veal cutlets in pan and brown on both sides. Add chicken broth and simmer 3 minutes. Add mushroom mixture and cook, uncovered, 5 to 10 minutes, or until sauce begins to thicken and is reduced by approximately one-half.

Sprinkle with chopped parsley during last minute of cooking time. Transfer to a serving platter. Garnish with lemon wedges. Serve immediately.

Yield: 4 servings

You may also use veal cutlets, cut 1/8-inch thick by the butcher. In this case there is no need to pound them thinner. However, they are usually more tender, if pounded.

Preparation time: 35-40 minutes

VEAL ROLLS DIVAN

Per serving:
Calories...... 309
Protein (g)... 35
Fat (g)....... 8
Sat. Fat (g).. 3.2
Choles. (mg).. 83
Fiber (g)..... 3.7
Sodium (mg)... 566
%Cal-Fat...... 23%

6 veal cutlets (about 3 ounces each), pounded 1/8-inch thick
1 tablespoon margarine
1/2 cup chopped onion
1 1/2 cups packaged cornbread stuffing mix
1/4 cup plus 2 tablespoons hot water
1/4 cup egg substitute
Vegetable cooking spray
2 10-ounce packages frozen broccoli spears, thawed
1/3 cup all-purpose flour
1/2 cup skim milk
1 14-ounce can clear chicken broth (or from own stock)
3 tablespoons dry white wine
1/4 cup grated Parmesan cheese
Garnish with cherry tomatoes or radish roses (optional)

Preheat oven to 350 degrees.

Pound veal cutlets to desired thickness.

Saute onion in margarine, until soft but not brown.

Make stuffing: In large mixing bowl, combine stuffing mix, hot water, egg substitute, and sauteed onion. Mix until will blended. Place about 1/3 cup stuffing on each cutlet. Roll veal loosely, starting at narrow end. (Since cutlets generally overlap sufficiently, there is seldom a need to fasten with toothpicks. However, if veal tends to unfold, use toothpicks to fasten.)

Spray large skillet with vegetable cooking spray. Brown veal rolls on all sides. Simmer an additional 10 minutes, covered. Remove veal from skillet and set aside.

Meanwhile, thaw broccoli spears in microwave. Set aside.

Using a wire whisk, blend flour into skim milk until all lumps disappear. Pour into same skillet used for cooking veal. Immediately add chicken broth. Stir constantly and bring to a boil over medium heat. After mixture thickens, stir in wine.

Assemble dish: Place thawed broccoli spears crosswise in 11 x 7 1/2 x 2 1/2-inch baking dish. Top with veal rolls. Pour half the sauce over broccoli and veal. Cover and bake at 350 degrees for 30 minutes. Remove from oven.

Add Parmesan cheese to remaining sauce. Pour cheese sauce over veal dish. Broil 3 to 5 minutes or until sauce is lightly browned.Serve immediately. Garnish plates with cherry tomatoes or radish roses.

Yield: 6 servings

Preparation time: 40 minutes

Cooking time: 35 minutes

Safe Grilling Tips

* Select the leanest cuts of meat.

* Trim all visible fat from meat before grilling. This will help prevent flare-ups from dripping fat.

* Choose fish or chicken over beef and pork, since they are generally lower in fat. (Lean beef and pork are still appropriate on occasion.)

* Avoid eating charred parts of meat.

* If you grill frequently (several times a week), consider precooking (microwaving or parboiling) the meat so it is not on the grill as long. Grill immediately after precooking.

* To keep fat from dripping onto the coals and producing smoke, place aluminum foil on top of grate and place food directly on the foil, turning up the sides slightly to contain the meat juices; or put a metal drip pan beneath the food to be grilled.

* Baste with barbecue sauce or marinate in low-fat salad dressings, or other marinades low in fat.

* Serve food from the grill on a clean platter, not one that has raw, possibly contaminated, meat juices on it.

* Grill vegetables with little or no added fat.

* Mesquite produces more PAHs than hardwood because it is a softwood and burns at a higher temperature. Therefore, you may want to limit its use.

* Clean the grill after each use.

Fish & Seafood

ORANGE ROUGHY WITH MUSHROOM SAUCE

Per serving:
Calories...... 289
Protein (g)... 35
Fat (g)....... 5.8
Sat. Fat (g).. 1
Choles. (mg).. 82
Fiber (g)..... 1.4
Sodium (mg)... 704
%Cal-Fat...... 18%

1 1/2 pounds orange roughy fish fillets
8 ounces fresh mushrooms, sliced
1/2 cup water
1/2 cup dry sherry
1/4 cup low-sodium soy sauce
1/4 cup lime juice, divided
2 teaspoons sugar
1/4 cup flour
1 tablespoon olive oil
1/2 bunch green onions, chopped
2 cloves garlic, minced
1/2 teaspoon black pepper

Slice mushrooms in food processor. Place in medium-size covered skillet (no oil necessary) and cook on low until mushrooms darken. Drain mushrooms, reserving liquid. Set aside.

In a medium-size mixing bowl, combine juice from mushrooms, 1/2 cup water, sherry, soy sauce, 2 tablespoons lime juice and sugar. Set aside.

Rinse fish and pat dry. Rub fish with remaining 2 tablespoons lime juice. Next, rub flour evenly over both sides of fish.

Heat olive oil in large, heavy skillet, preferably non-stick. When oil is hot, place fish in skillet and sear each side for 2 to 3 minutes. Carefully transfer fish to a platter.

Add mushrooms, chopped green onions, minced garlic and pepper to hot skillet. Cook for 1 1/2 minutes. Reduce heat. Add sherry mixture and fish fillets, and bring to a boil. Cover and simmer an additional 5 to 10 minutes, until fish is opaque and flakes easily with a fork.

Transfer fish to a serving platter and pour mushroom sauce over. Serve immediately.

Yield: Makes 4 large servings.

This recipe is also excellent with red snapper.

Preparation time: 35-40 minutes

KIWI ORANGE ROUGHY

4 orange roughy fillets (1 1/2 pounds)
1/4 teaspoon garlic powder
1/4 teaspoon pepper
1/4 teaspoon dried oregano flakes
1 tablespoon Butter Buds*
1/4 cup lime juice
1 tablespoon canola oil
2 kiwifruit, peeled and sliced
1/4 cup slivered almonds (optional)

Per serving:
Calories...... 213
Protein (g)... 33
Fat (g)....... 5.6
Sat. Fat (g).. 0.7
Choles. (mg).. 82
Fiber (g)..... 1.4
Sodium (mg)... 140
%Cal-Fat...... 24%

Preheat oven to 350 degrees. Wash fish fillets and pat dry.

Combine garlic powder, pepper and oregano. Sprinkle over fillets. Place fillets in a 12 x 8 x 2-inch non-stick baking dish.

Combine Butter Buds and lime juice. Drizzle fillets first with canola oil, then lime juice mixture.

Cover and bake at 350 degrees for 20 minutes or until fish flakes easily with a fork.

Transfer fillets to serving platter. Carefully arrange 3 or 4 kiwifruit slices on top of each fillet. Sprinkle with slivered almonds, if desired.

Yield: 4 servings

The kiwifruit adds interesting color and flavor to the fish.

*Contains natural butter flavor without the oil or cholesterol. Available at most food stores.

Preparation time: 15 minutes

Cooking time: 20 minutes

GRILLED SWORDFISH WITH ANCHOVY SAUCE

Per serving:
Calories...... 306
Protein (g)... 43
Fat (g)....... 9.7
Sat. Fat (g).. 2.9
Choles. (mg).. 82
Fiber (g)..... 0.3
Sodium (mg)... 636
%Cal-Fat...... 30%

1 1/2 to 2 pounds swordfish steaks (sliced 3/4 to 1-inch thick)

Anchovy Sauce:
2 teaspoons tub margarine
1 2-ounce can anchovy fillets in olive oil, drained and chopped finely
2 cloves garlic, minced
3 sprigs fresh parsley, finely chopped
1/4 teaspoon white pepper
Juice of 1 lemon
1/4 cup flour
1 1/2 cups skim milk
2 tablespoons whole capers

Preheat gas grill or set oven control to broil.

Make anchovy sauce: Melt margarine in small saucepan. Add chopped anchovy fillets, garlic, parsley, and pepper. Cook and stir occasionally over low heat for 5 minutes. Add lemon juice. Set aside.

In a medium-size saucepan, whisk together flour and milk until all lumps disappear. Place over medium heat. Bring to a boil, stirring frequently, and continue cooking until sauce thickens. Add anchovy mixture and heat almost to a boil. Stir in capers. Keep warm until ready to serve.

Meanwhile, wash swordfish steaks and pat dry. Grill or broil approximately 5 minutes per side, or until fish flakes easily with a fork. (Grill over hot coals, or broil on lightly greased broiler rack, placed 4 inches from heat.)

To serve, place swordfish steaks on serving platter, and spoon anchovy sauce over each steak.

Yield: 4 or 5 6-ounce servings

To remove excess oil from anchovy fillets, pat dry with a paper towel. This sauce is also excellent over other firm flesh fish, including salmon, shark and red snapper.

Preparation time: 30-35 minutes

STUFFED FLOUNDER

2 teaspoons tub margarine
1/4 cup finely chopped onion
2 tablespoons finely chopped green pepper
1 cup fresh or canned crabmeat, drained and shell
   fragments removed
1/2 cup dry bread crumbs
3 tablespoons egg substitute
1 tablespoon finely chopped fresh parsley
1/2 teaspoon seasoned salt
1/4 teaspoon pepper
4 fresh flounder fillets (about 1 1/2 pounds total weight)

Sauce:
1/4 cup flour
1 1/2 cups skim milk
1/2 teaspoon seasoned salt
1/3 cup dry white wine
2 tablespoons Parmesan cheese
1/2 teaspoon paprika
1 tablespoon Parmesan cheese

Per serving:
Calories...... 360
Protein (g)... 48
Fat (g)....... 6.5
Sat. Fat (g).. 2.1
Choles. (mg).. 117
Fiber (g)..... 1.1
Sodium (mg)... 741
%Cal-Fat...... 18%

Preheat oven to 400 degrees.

In saucepan, saute onion and green pepper in margarine until tender. Add crabmeat, breadcrumbs, egg substitute, parsley, salt and pepper. Mix well.

Spread mixture over flounder fillets. Roll fillets and place seam side down in 12 x 7 1/2 x 2-inch baking dish.

Make sauce: Using a wire whisk, mix together flour and skim milk in mixing bowl until all lumps disappear. Pour into skillet placed over medium heat. Add salt, wine and 2 tablespoons Parmesan cheese. Bring to a boil, continually stirring until mixture thickens.

Pour sauce over fish. Sprinkle with paprika and 1 tablespoon Parmesan cheese. Bake in 400 degree oven for 35 minutes, or until fish flakes easily with fork. Transfer fish to serving dish. Spoon excess sauce from pan over fish. Serve immediately.

Yield: 4 servings

Preparation time: 30 minutes

Cooking time: 35 minutes

POACHED SALMON

Per serving:
Calories...... 163
Protein (g)... 22
Fat (g)....... 7.2
Sat. Fat (g).. 1.1
Choles. (mg).. 62
Fiber (g)..... 0
Sodium (mg)... 292
%Cal-Fat...... 38%

1 pound salmon, steaks or fillet
4 cups water
2 tablespoons lemon juice
1 teaspoon salt
1 bay leaf

In a large skillet or saucepan, combine water, lemon juice, salt and bay leaf. Bring to a boil. Carefully place salmon in pan and bring to a second boil. Simmer for 10 minutes. Remove from pan with a spatula. Chill.

(If pan is not large enough to cook salmon in one layer, cook half at a time. Same water mixture can be used again.)

Yield: 4 servings

Preparation time: 10 minutes

Cooking time: 10 minutes

MARINATED SALMON

Per serving:
Calories...... 216
Protein (g)... 36
Fat (g)....... 9.1
Sat. Fat (g).. 1.0
Choles. (mg).. 94
Fiber (g)..... 0
Sodium (mg)... NA
%Cal-Fat...... 38%

1 1/2 to 2 pounds salmon fillets
1/2 cup no-oil Italian dressing

Wash salmon fillets and pat dry. Place in shallow baking dish. Pour Italian dressing over top and marinate for 4 to 6 hours.

Remove fillets from marinade. Broil 4 inches from heat on lightly greased broiler rack or grill over hot coals until fish flakes easily with a fork. (Generally, allow about 5 minutes per side for fish 1-inch thick. Adjust the time, based on intensity of heat and thickness of fish.)

Yield: 4 or 5 6-ounce servings

Preparation time: 5-10 minutes

Cooking time: 10 minutes

SALMON STIR-FRY

1 can (16 ozs.) salmon
1/2 pound fresh or frozen Chinese snow peas
1 cup sliced fresh mushrooms
1 red or green pepper, cut into narrow strips
1 8-ounce can sliced water chestnuts, drained
1 clove garlic, minced
2 teaspoons olive oil
2 teaspoons cornstarch
1/4 teaspoon cayenne pepper
Brown rice (4 cups cooked)
Lite soy sauce or lemon juice

Per serving:
Calories...... 444
Protein (g)... 30
Fat (g)....... 11.8
Sat. Fat (g).. 2.7
Choles. (mg).. 50
Fiber (g)..... 5
Sodium (mg)... 621
%Cal-Fat...... 25%

Prepare vegetables: Cut off tops of snow peas; slice mushrooms and red pepper; and drain water chestnuts. Set aside.

Drain salmon, reserving liquid. Break salmon into chunks. Set aside.

Heat olive oil in large skillet or saute pan. Stir-fry vegetables and minced garlic for 5 minutes.

Add water to reserved salmon liquid to make 1/2 cup liquid. Mix in cornstarch and cayenne. Pour liquid over vegetables and cook until it begins to boil. Add chunks of salmon and toss until well coated.

Serve over brown rice. Sprinkle with Lite soy sauce or lemon juice.

Yield: 4 servings

Preparation time: 25-30 minutes

Cooking time: 50 minutes (for brown rice)

SALMON TERIYAKI

Per serving:
Calories...... 255
Protein (g)... 30
Fat (g)....... 9
Sat. Fat (g).. 1.2
Choles. (mg).. 88
Fiber (g)..... 0
Sodium (mg)... NA
%Cal-Fat...... 36%

1 to 1 1/2 pounds salmon fillets
2 tablespoons Lite soy sauce
1/4 cup Chablis wine
1/4 teaspoon paprika
1 1/2 teaspoons sugar

Wash salmon fillets and pat dry.

Prepare marinade by combining soy sauce, wine, paprika, and sugar. Place fillets in shallow container and pour marinade over. Marinate for 30 minutes at room temperature, or 1 to 2 hours in refrigerator.

Meanwhile, set oven control to broil.

Spray broiler rack with vegetable cooking spray. Remove salmon from marinade and place on rack. Spoon 2 tablespoons of marinade over top of fish. Broil approximately 4 to 6 inches from heat, skin side down, for 8 to 10 minutes, or until fish flakes easily with a fork.

Place on platter and serve immediately. Garnish with lemon wedges.

Yield: 4 servings

Preparation time: 10-15 minutes

Cooking time: 10 minutes

Marinating time: 30 minutes to 2 hours

LIGHT FRIED FISH FILLETS

**1 to 1 1/2 pounds fish fillets: flounder, sole, orange
   roughy, red snapper, or catfish
2 egg substitutes (1/2 cup)
1 tablespoon sherry
1/2 cup Italian style bread crumbs
2 teaspoons olive oil
Lemon slices and fresh sprigs of parsley for garnish**

Per serving:
Calories...... 270
Protein (g)... 40
Fat (g)....... 7.6
Sat. Fat (g).. 2.3
Choles. (mg).. 87
Fiber (g)..... 0.4
Sodium (mg)... 379
%Cal-Fat...... 27%

In a small bowl, combine egg substitutes and sherry.
On a platter or paper plate, place bread crumbs.

Heat olive oil in a large nonstick fry pan. Dip fish first in egg mixture, then in bread crumbs. Place in preheated frypan. Fry 4 to 6 minutes per side, or until fish flakes easily with a fork. Avoid overcooking, which dries out the fish.

Transfer fish to serving platter. Garnish with fresh sprigs of parsley and lemon slices. Squeeze fresh lemon over fish, or serve with nonfat tartar sauce (Recipe, page 196), or seafood cocktail sauce.

Yield: 4 servings

Preparation time: 15 minutes

Cooking time: 10 minutes

DIJON/ONION-TOPPED FISH

**6 small fish steaks, 1-inch thick (1 1/2 to 2 pounds)
Dash pepper
2 egg whites
2 tablespoons grated Parmesan cheese
2 tablespoons Dijon-style mustard
2 tablespoons chopped green onions (including tops)**

Per serving (using flounder/sole):
Calories...... 135
Protein (g)... 24
Fat (g)....... 3.3
Sat. Fat (g).. 0.7
Choles. (mg).. 56
Fiber (g)..... 0
Sodium (mg)... 214
%Cal-Fat...... 22%

Set oven control to broil and/or 550 degrees. Sprinkle fish steaks with pepper. Place fish on lightly greased broiler rack placed about 4 inches from heat. Broil until light brown, about

5 minutes. Turn, and broil for an additional 5 minutes, or until fish flakes easily with a fork.

Meanwhile, beat egg whites until stiff but not dry. Fold in Parmesan cheese, mustard and onions. Spread mixture over fish. Broil until topping is golden brown, about 1 1/2 minutes. Serve immediately.

Yield: 6 servings

This sauce is excellent with salmon or halibut steaks, but is also good on a variety of other fish. Garnish with fanned green onion tops.

Preparation time: 15-20 minutes

CRAB CAKES

Per serving:
Calories...... 152
Protein (g)... 16
Fat (g)....... 2.5
Sat. Fat (g).. 0.5
Choles. (mg).. 52
Fiber (g)..... 0.6
Sodium (mg)... 498
%Cal-Fat...... 17%

1 pound lump crabmeat
1 egg substitute (1/4 cup)
3/4 cup evaporated skim milk
1 1/4 cups dry bread crumbs
1/4 teaspoon cayenne pepper
3/4 teaspoon dry mustard
1 teaspoon seasoned salt
2 teaspoons Worcestershire sauce
1 tablespoon tub margarine, melted

Preheat oven on broil setting.

Carefully look over crabmeat and remove shells. Combine all ingredients, except margarine, mixing thoroughly.

Spray cookie sheet with vegetable cooking spray. Press crab mixture into 8 patties, about 3/4-inch thick. Place on cookie sheet. Brush tops of cakes with melted margarine. Broil, with oven door open, 5 inches from heat source, about 4 minutes on each side, or until lightly browned.

Yield: 8 crab cakes

Preparation time: 20-25 minutes

Cooking time: 8 minutes

SCALLOPS FLORENTINE

1 1/2 pounds fresh bay or sea scallops
1 10-ounce package frozen chopped spinach
1/4 cup all-purpose flour
1/2 teaspoon salt
1/4 teaspoon pepper
1 1/2 tablespoons olive oil
4-6 cloves garlic, minced

Per serving:
Calories...... 200
Protein (g)... 25
Fat (g)....... 5.3
Sat. Fat (g).. 0.7
Choles. (mg).. 45
Fiber (g)..... 1.7
Sodium (mg)... 481
%Cal-Fat...... 24%

Wash scallops in cold water. Drain and pat dry. Set aside.
Microwave spinach to thaw completely. Lightly squeeze excess moisture from spinach. (Do not squeeze completely dry.)
Combine flour, salt and pepper in medium-size mixing bowl. Toss scallops in flour mixture to coat completely.
Heat olive oil in large nonstick skillet. Add minced garlic. When garlic oil becomes hot, add scallops and saute about 5 minutes, or until scallops become firm and opaque. (Do not overcook scallops or they will become rubbery.) Add spinach and toss until heated through, about 4 to 5 additional minutes. Serve immediately.

Yield: 4 to 6 servings

This dish is delicious with a rice casserole, crusty French bread and a crisp green salad.

Preparation time: 25 minutes

ARTICHOKE-SCALLOP LINGUINE

Per serving:
Calories...... 453
Protein (g)... 31
Fat (g)....... 6.8
Sat. Fat (g).. 0.8
Choles. (mg).. 37
Fiber (g)..... 6.4
Sodium (mg)... 770
%Cal-Fat...... 14%

2 teaspoons olive oil
4 green onions, chopped (including tops)
2 cloves garlic, minced
2 tablespoons fresh basil, minced, or 2 teaspoons dried
1/2 teaspoon salt
Dash red pepper
1 16-ounce can tomatoes
1/2 cup dry white wine
2 tablespoons tomato paste
1 pound bay scallops, rinsed and drained
1 14-ounce can artichoke hearts, cut lengthwise into
   quarters
8 ounces linguine
2 tablespoons slivered almonds, toasted
Parmesan cheese (optional)

In heavy skillet, heat olive oil over medium heat. Add green onions and minced garlic. Saute 2 minutes. Add basil, salt, pepper, tomatoes, wine and tomato paste. Bring to a boil, breaking tomatoes up into small chunks with a spoon. Cover. Simmer for 20 minutes.

Add scallops and quartered artichoke hearts to tomato mixture. Cook until scallops are cooked, about 5 minutes.

Meanwhile, cook linguine according to package directions and drain. Toss with scallop mixture, mixing well. Transfer to shallow bowl or platter. Sprinkle with slivered almonds and Parmesan cheese, if desired.

Yield: 4 servings

Preparation time: 25 minutes

Cooking time: 25 minutes

PASTA WITH SCALLOPS AND WINE

12 ounces fresh sea scallops, drained and rinsed
2 teaspoons olive oil
1 cup chopped onion
1 cup dry white wine
1 chicken bouillon cube
1 tablespoon fresh basil, finely chopped, or 1 teaspoon dried
1/8 teaspoon freshly ground pepper
1 1/2 cups chopped tomato (fresh or canned)
12 ounces dumpling pasta or "eggless" egg noodles, cooked
1/4 cup grated Parmesan cheese
1/2 cup fresh minced parsley

Per serving:
Calories...... 332
Protein (g)... 22
Fat (g)....... 6.9
Sat. Fat (g).. 1.9
Choles. (mg).. 33
Fiber (g)..... 3
Sodium (mg)... 455
%Cal-Fat...... 19%

Cut large scallops in half and set aside. (Do not cut small scallops.)

In large saucepan cook onion in olive oil until tender but not brown. Stir in wine, bouillon cube, basil and pepper. Bring to a boil over medium heat. Simmer, uncovered, for 12 to 15 minutes, or until liquid is reduced to about 1/2 the original amount. Add scallops and chopped tomatoes. Cover and simmer about 5 minutes or just until scallops are cooked. (They will be white and more firm when cooked.)

Meanwhile, cook pasta according to package directions. Toss pasta with scallop mixture, Parmesan cheese, and parsley until ingredients are well blended. Serve immediately.

Yield: 4 servings

12 ounces of medium-size fresh or frozen shrimp may be substituted for the scallops. This is a delicious meal to serve on a special occasion. Scallop mixture may be made a day ahead of time, and heated up at last minute, before tossing with pasta, cheese and parsley.

Preparation time: 30-35 minutes

SCALLOPS TERIYAKI

Per serving:
Calories...... 241
Protein (g)... 22
Fat (g)....... 4.5
Sat. Fat (g).. 0.4
Choles. (mg).. 38
Fiber (g)..... 2.2
Sodium (mg)... NA
%Cal-Fat...... 18%

1 pound sea scallops
1 medium onion, sliced and quartered
1 green or red pepper, chopped in 1/4 x 1-inch pieces
1 8-ounce can sliced water chestnuts, drained
2 tablespoons sherry

Seafood Teriyaki Marinade:
1/2 cup lite soy sauce
2 teaspoons lemon juice
2 tablespoons brown sugar
2 cloves garlic, minced
1 teaspoon ground ginger
1 tablespoon vegetable oil
1 tablespoon sherry

Rinse scallops. Prepare marinade by mixing together soy sauce, lemon juice, brown sugar, garlic, ginger, vegetable oil and sherry. Pour marinade over scallops and refrigerate 1 to 3 hours.

Meanwhile, chop onion and pepper as specified above. Drain water chestnuts and set aside.

Spray nonstick frypan or saute pan with vegetable cooking spray. Add onions and peppers and saute over medium heat 3 minutes. (Add 2 tablespoons water if vegetables stick.)

Remove scallops from marinade. Add to frypan. Cook over medium heat, stirring frequently until scallops are firm and opaque (about 5 minutes). Add water chestnuts and sherry and heat through. Serve immediately over rice.

Yield: 4 servings

Preparation time: 30-35 minutes

Marinating time: 1-3 hours

SCALLOPS EN BROCHETTE

1 pound fresh sea scallops
2 tablespoons honey mustard
1 egg substitute (1/4 cup)
1/2 cup Italian bread crumbs
1 pint cherry tomatoes
2 green peppers, cut into 1-inch squares
1 large onion, cut into bite-size pieces
Salt and pepper to taste

Per serving:
Calories...... 202
Protein (g)... 24
Fat (g)....... 2.6
Sat. Fat (g).. 0.4
Choles. (mg).. 38
Fiber (g)..... 2.4
Sodium (mg)... 407
%Cal-Fat...... 12%

Preheat gas or charcoal grill.

Wash scallops in cold water. Drain and pat dry. Prepare vegetables (cherry tomatoes, green peppers and onion). Set aside.

Combine honey mustard and egg substitute in small bowl.

Dip scallops first in egg mixture, next in bread crumbs.

Thread scallops and vegetables on 8 skewers, starting with green pepper square, followed by cherry tomato, onion and scallop. Repeat until skewers are full. End with green pepper square.

Grill over medium heat for 10 to 15 minutes, until scallops are lightly browned.

Serve with plain or seasoned rice.

Yield: 4 servings

Preparation time: 40-45 minutes

Cooking time: 10-15 minutes

SHRIMP SUKIYAKI

Per serving:
Calories...... 384
Protein (g)... 27
Fat (g)....... 6.3
Sat. Fat (g).. 1.1
Choles. (mg).. 165
Fiber (g)..... 6.5
Sodium (mg)... 850
%Cal-Fat...... 14%

12 ounces medium-size raw shrimp, peeled and deveined
1 medium yellow onion, thinly sliced
1 pound fresh spinach, trimmed, washed and drained
1 bunch green onions and tops, cut into 2-inch lengths
1/4 pound fresh mushrooms, sliced
5 tablespoons lite soy sauce, divided
2 tablespoons cornstarch, divided
1/2 cup water
2 tablespoons brown sugar, firmly packed
1 tablespoon olive oil
2 tablespoons water
1 cup uncooked brown or white rice

Cook rice according to package directions.

Meanwhile, clean shrimp (thaw, if frozen). Prepare yellow onion, spinach, green onions and mushrooms as indicated above. Set aside.

In small mixing bowl, combine 1/4 cup lite soy sauce, 1 tablespoon cornstarch, 1/2 cup water and brown sugar. Set aside.

Blend remaining 1 tablespoon soy sauce and 1 tablespoon cornstarch in a small bowl. Stir in shrimp until well coated.

Heat olive oil in large skillet. Add shrimp and stir-fry for 3 minutes. Remove.

Add 2 tablespoons water and yellow onion to skillet; cook 1 minute. Add spinach, green onions, mushrooms and soy sauce mixture. Cover and cook until spinach wilts, stirring occasionally. Return shrimp to skillet. Cook 5 to 7 minutes or until vegetables are tender and shrimp is pink.

Serve immediately over rice. Sprinkle with lemon juice or additional soy sauce if desired.

Yield: 4 servings.

Preparation time: 50-60 minutes

SHRIMP JAMBALAYA

1 tablespoon olive oil
1 clove garlic, minced
1 green pepper, chopped
1 medium onion, chopped fine
1 16-ounce can whole tomatoes, chopped
1 tablespoon Worcestershire sauce
1 pound fresh or frozen shrimp, cleaned
2 cups water
1/2 teaspoon salt or to taste
1/4 teaspoon thyme
1/8 teaspoon pepper
1/4-1/2 teaspoon cayenne pepper, or to taste
1 cup uncooked long grain rice

Per serving:
Calories...... 237
Protein (g)... 19
Fat (g)....... 4
Sat. Fat (g).. 0.6
Choles. (mg).. 172
Fiber (g)..... 2.1
Sodium (mg)... 449
%Cal-Fat...... 15%

Cut up green pepper and onion as indicated above.

Heat olive oil in heavy 10-inch skillet. Add minced garlic, green pepper and onion. Saute 5 minutes. Add chopped tomatoes and Worcestershire sauce to skillet.

Thaw shrimp, if frozen, and drain. Add shrimp to skillet along with water and seasonings. Bring to a boil. Stir in rice. As soon as mixture returns to a boil, reduce heat. Simmer, covered, about 30 minutes, or until all liquid is absorbed.

Yield: 6 1-cup servings

For a variation, substitute 2 to 3 cups cooked chicken or turkey meat. Another delicious variation is to use 1/2 pound shrimp and 1/2 pound scallops. Cornbread provides a nice complement to this meal.

Preparation time: 25 minutes

Cooking time: 30 minutes

SHRIMP CACCIATORE

Per serving:
Calories...... 514
Protein (g)... 36
Fat (g)....... 5.5
Sat. Fat (g).. 1
Choles. (mg).. 172
Fiber (g)..... 6.8
Sodium (mg)... 618
%Cal-Fat...... 10%

1/4 pound fresh mushrooms, sliced
1 medium onion, chopped
1 green pepper, coarsely chopped
1 15-ounce can no-salt-added tomatoes, chopped
2 cups prepared spaghetti sauce
1/2 teaspoon dried oregano
1 tablespoon fresh basil or 1 teaspoon dried
1/2 teaspoon garlic powder
1/4 teaspoon black pepper
1/4 cup dry white wine
1 1/2 pounds fresh shrimp, shelled and deveined
1 pound spaghetti, uncooked
Parmesan cheese to taste

Place sliced mushrooms and chopped onion and pepper in large frypan. Cover and saute until vegetables are tender. (No cooking oil necessary.)

Chop tomatoes coarsely in food processor. Add to vegetables in frypan. Also add prepared spaghetti sauce, oregano, basil, garlic powder, pepper and white wine. Bring to a boil and simmer, uncovered, 20 minutes or until sauce thickens slightly. Stir in cleaned shrimp and bring to a boil. Simmer 5 minutes.

Meanwhile, cook spaghetti according to package directions. Drain.

To serve, place desired portion of spaghetti on individual plates. Top with tomato-shrimp sauce. Sprinkle Parmesan cheese to taste.

Yield: 6 servings

To prevent spaghetti from sticking together, add 1/4 cup tomato sauce to spaghetti immediately after it is drained.

Preparation time: 25-30 minutes
(if shrimp are already cleaned)

Cooking time: 25 minutes

SHRIMP CREOLE

1 large onion, chopped
1/2 cup finely chopped celery
1 green pepper, chopped finely
2 cloves garlic, minced
2 teaspoons olive oil
1 28-ounce can tomatoes, chopped*
1 teaspoon sugar
1/2 teaspoon chili powder
1/4 teaspoon black pepper
1 tablespoon Worcestershire sauce
1/4 teaspoon basil
1/4 teaspoon thyme
Tabasco sauce to taste
1 pound fresh medium-size shrimp, peeled and deveined
2 tablespoons fresh parsley, chopped
1 teaspoon cornstarch
2 teaspoons water
Rice (3 to 4 cups cooked)

Per serving:
Calories...... 444
Protein (g)... 31
Fat (g)....... 5.4
Sat. Fat (g).. 0.9
Choles. (mg).. 172
Fiber (g)..... 4.2
Sodium (mg)... 572
%Cal-Fat...... 11%

In large saucepan, cook onion, celery, green pepper, and garlic in olive oil until tender, but not brown. Add chopped tomatoes, sugar, chili powder, pepper, Worcestershire sauce, basil, thyme and Tabasco sauce. Simmer, covered, 30 to 45 minutes.

Add shrimp and parsley to saucepan. Bring to a boil, and simmer an additional 20 minutes.

Mix cornstarch with water in small bowl. Stir into sauce and continue stirring until mixture thickens. Serve over rice.

Yield: 4 servings

To reduce sodium, use no-salt-added canned tomatoes.

Preparation time: 35 minutes (if shrimp already cleaned)

Cooking time: 50-60 minutes

Meatless Main Dishes

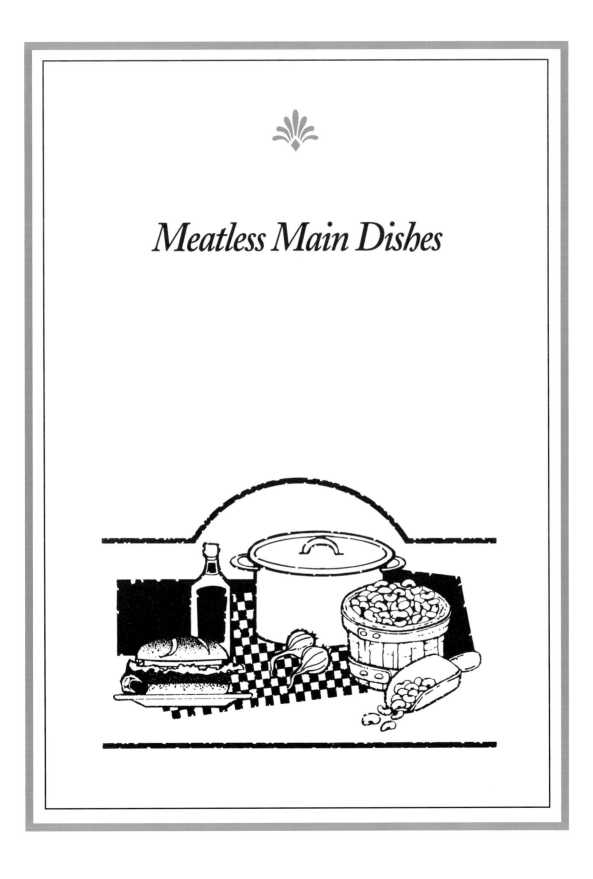

VEGETARIAN CHILI

Per serving:
Calories...... 309
Protein (g)... 14
Fat (g)....... 3.4
Sat. Fat (g).. 0.7
Choles. (mg).. 0
Fiber (g)..... 12.6
Sodium (mg)... 764
%Cal-Fat...... 9%

3 cans (15 ounces) kidney beans, drained and rinsed
1 cup water
1 vegetable bouillon cube
1 cup raw bulgur
1/2 teaspoon minced garlic
1 1/2 cups chopped onion
1 cup chopped carrots
1 cup chopped green peppers
1 tablespoon olive oil
3 large fresh tomatoes, or 1 15-ounce can tomatoes, chopped
2 8-ounce cans tomato sauce
2 tablespoons dry red wine
Juice of 1/2 lemon
2 teaspoons chili powder (or more, to taste)
Water as needed, at least one cup
Salt to taste

Drain and rinse kidney beans in a colander. Set aside.

Bring water to a boil. Add bouillon cube and stir until dissolved. Pour over raw bulgur. Cover and let stand at least 15 minutes.

In large skillet, sauté garlic, onions, carrots and green peppers in olive oil until tender. (About 10 minutes)

Add kidney beans, bulgur and remaining ingredients to skillet and simmer 45 minutes or longer. Add water as needed for desired consistency.

Yield: 6 to 8 servings.

A hearty chili which tastes great with cornbread. It is also very good served over pasta, with or without the bulgur.

Preparation time: 25-30 minutes

Cooking time: 45 minutes

BEAN STROGANOFF

1 large onion, minced
16 ounces fresh mushrooms, sliced
2 teaspoons olive oil
5 tablespoons flour
1 14 1/2-ounce can clear beef broth, defatted*
2 tablespoons tomato paste
2 teaspoons prepared mustard
1 teaspoon Worcestershire sauce
1/4 teaspoon pepper
1/2 teaspoon sugar
1/4 teaspoon garlic powder
3/4 cup sherry
3 16-ounce cans pinto beans, drained and rinsed
3/4 cup plain nonfat yogurt
16 ounces dumpling pasta, or "eggless" egg noodles

Per serving:
Calories...... 460
Protein (g)... 20
Fat (g)....... 3.2
Sat. Fat (g).. 0.5
Choles. (mg).. 0
Fiber (g)..... 13.7
Sodium (mg)... 634
%Cal-Fat...... 7%

In large skillet, saute mushrooms and onions in olive oil.

In medium-size mixing bowl, mix flour and beef broth with a wire whisk until smooth. Add to skillet. Add remaining ingredients except yogurt and pasta. Bring to a boil and simmer 30 minutes to blend flavors.

Remove from heat and stir in yogurt. Serve over Dumpling pasta or eggless egg noodles.

Yield: 8 servings

Vegetable bouillon dissolved in 2 cups boiling water may be substituted for the beef broth.

Preparation time: 35-40 minutes

Cooking time: 30 minutes

LENTIL BURRITOS

1 1/2 cups dried lentils
3 1/2 to 4 cups water
1 bay leaf
1 clove garlic, minced
1/2 teaspoon salt
1/4 teaspoon dried thyme
1 small onion chopped (1/4 to 1/2 cup)
1/2 cup chili salsa
6 10-inch flour tortillas
1 medium tomato chopped
2 ounces reduced-calorie cheddar cheese, shredded

Wash lentils. Combine lentils, 3 1/2 cups water, and next four ingredients in saucepan. Bring to a boil, reduce heat, and simmer 1 1/2 hours. Stir occasionally and add additional water if necessary. Remove bay leaf.

Add chopped onion and chili salsa to saucepan. Cook bean mixture, uncovered, over medium heat 5 minutes, stirring frequently.

Meanwhile, wrap tortillas tightly in aluminum foil; heat in a 350 degree oven 10 minutes, or until warmed. (If not wrapped tightly, they will dry out and become hard.)

To assemble burrito, spoon 1/6 of the bean mixture (about 1/3 cup) on each tortilla near one edge. Top with chopped tomato and shredded cheese. Fold the edge nearest the filling over the top of the filling, just covering it. Fold in the two sides, like an envelope, then roll up. Serve immediately.

Yield: 6 10-inch burritos

Preparation time: 20-25 minutes

Cooking time: 1 1/2 hours

PUERTO RICAN BLACK BEANS AND RICE

1 pound dried black beans
1 cup chopped onion
1 green pepper, chopped
2 cloves garlic, minced
1 tablespoon olive oil
3 cups water
1 16-ounce can tomatoes, chopped
1 tablespoon wine vinegar
1/2 teaspoon sugar
1 teaspoon salt
1/8 teaspoon Tabasco sauce
5 - 6 cups cooked rice (1 1/2 cups uncooked)
1/4 cup chopped green onions
Salsa (optional)

Per serving:
Calories...... 486
Protein (g)... 20
Fat (g)....... 3.5
Sat. Fat (g).. 0.7
Choles. (mg).. 0
Fiber (g)..... 14.1
Sodium (mg)... 368
%Cal-Fat...... 7%

Wash beans and soak 8 hours or overnight. Drain.

Saute onion, green pepper and garlic in olive oil until vegetables are tender.

In a large kettle, combine beans, sauteed vegetables, water, tomatoes, vinegar, sugar, salt and Tabasco sauce. Bring to a boil. Cover and simmer about 2 hours or until beans are tender.

Meanwhile, prepare rice according to package directions (without added salt or margarine).

To serve, spoon black beans over rice. Sprinkle with green onions. Top with salsa, if desired.

Yield: 6 to 8 servings

Preparation time: 25-30 minutes

Cooking time: 2 hours

HEARTY BEAN STEW OVER PASTA

Per serving:
Calories...... 599
Protein (g)... 27
Fat (g)....... 7.4
Sat. Fat (g).. 1
Choles. (mg).. 0
Fiber (g)..... 14.5
Sodium (mg)... 814
%Cal-Fat...... 11%

2 16-ounce cans red kidney beans, rinsed and drained
1 19-ounce can garbanzo beans, rinsed and drained
3 large carrots, peeled and cut into 1/4-inch slices
1/2 cup chopped onion
1 16-ounce can tomatoes, chopped
1 8-ounce can (no salt added) tomato sauce
1/2 cup dry white wine
1 tablespoon olive oil
2 teaspoons chili powder
2 tablespoons fresh parsley, finely chopped
1/2 teaspoon garlic powder
1/4 teaspoon pepper
8 ounces dumpling pasta
Parmesan cheese (optional)

In a Dutch oven or large saucepan, combine all ingredients except pasta and Parmesan cheese. Bring to a boil, reduce heat, and simmer, covered, 1 hour or until vegetables are tender.

Meanwhile, cook pasta according to package directions. Drain. Serve bean stew over pasta. Sprinkle with Parmesan cheese, if desired.

Yield: 4 to 6 servings

Preparation time: 20-25 minutes

Cooking time: 1 hour

BLACK-EYED PEAS, ARTICHOKE HEARTS AND LINGUINE

2 teaspoons olive oil
1 carrot, peeled and chopped
1/2 cup chopped onions
2 cloves garlic, minced
2 16-ounce cans black-eyed peas, rinsed and drained
1 14-ounce can artichoke hearts, drained and quartered
1/4 cup black olives, sliced
1 8-ounce can tomato sauce
1/2 cup water
1/4 cup chopped parsley
12 ounces linguine, broken in half
1/4 cup grated Parmesan cheese

Per serving:
Calories...... 612
Protein (g)... 28
Fat (g)....... 8
Sat. Fat (g).. 2.2
Choles. (mg).. 5
Fiber (g)..... 14.2
Sodium (mg)... 806
%Cal-Fat...... 12%

Heat olive oil in large saucepan. Add chopped carrot, onions and garlic. Saute 5 minutes. Add remaining ingredients, except linguine and Parmesan cheese. Bring to a boil, reduce heat, and simmer 30 minutes.

Meanwhile, cook linguine according to package directions. Drain and put into serving dish. Spoon 1/2 of the bean mixture over the linguine. Mix well. Spoon remaining sauce over top of linguine and sprinkle with Parmesan cheese.

Yield: 4 servings

Preparation time: 20-25 minutes

Cooking time: 30 minutes

VEGETARIAN CHOW MEIN

Per serving:
Calories...... 398
Protein (g)... 13
Fat (g)....... 3
Sat. Fat (g).. 0.5
Choles. (mg).. 0
Fiber (g)..... 7
Sodium (mg)... 866
%Cal-Fat...... 7%

1/4 cup dry white wine
3 tablespoons lite soy sauce
2 tablespoons cornstarch
1 teaspoon instant chicken bouillon granules
1 cup cold water
2 teaspoons olive oil
1 teaspoon grated gingerroot
2 medium carrots, cut julienne style
1/2 cup sliced onions, rings separated
2 medium zucchini, halved lengthwise and sliced
   1/4-inch thick
1 4-ounce can mushrooms, drained
8 ounces fresh bean sprouts (or 16-ounce can, drained)
1 16-ounce can pinto beans, rinsed and drained
1 8-ounce can sliced water chestnuts, drained
Hot cooked rice (about 4 cups)
Soy sauce to taste

Combine wine, soy sauce, cornstarch, bouillon granules and water. Set sauce aside.

Cut up vegetables (carrots, onion, and zucchini) as indicated above. Set aside.

In a wok or large skillet, preheat olive oil over medium-high heat. Stir-fry gingerroot for 15 seconds. Add carrots, onions, zucchini and mushrooms; stir-fry about 4 to 6 minutes or until vegetables are crisp-tender. Stir in bean sprouts; stir-fry 1 minute.

Stir sauce. Add to center of wok or skillet. Cook and stir until thickened. Add pinto beans, and water chestnuts. Stir until vegetables and beans are evenly coated with sauce. Cover and cook 1 minute longer. Serve immediately over hot cooked rice. Sprinkle with soy sauce, if desired.

Yield: 4 to 6 servings

For a variation, 8 ounces fresh tofu (bean curd), cut into 1/2-inch cubes, may be substituted for the pinto beans. Add tofu at the same time as the pinto beans.

Preparation time: 35-40 minutes

EGYPTIAN POCKET SANDWICH

3 large slices pita bread
1 16-ounce can fava beans, drained
1/2 teaspoon garlic powder
1/2 teaspoon cumin
1/4 cup water
2 small cucumbers, chopped
1 tomato, chopped
1 tablespoon fresh parsley, minced
1 tablespoon olive oil
1 tablespoon lemon juice
Tahini-Lemon Sauce (recipe below)

Per serving:
Calories..... 272
Protein (g).. 13
Fat (g)...... 7
Sat.Fat (g).. 0.9
Choles. (mg).. 0
Fiber (g)..... 6.1
Sodium (mg)... 414
%Cal-Fat...... 23%

Cut large pita bread slices in half and open up to make a pocket. Cover and set aside.

In medium saucepan, combine drained fava beans, garlic powder, cumin and water. Bring bean mixture to a boil over medium heat. Reduce heat and simmer, partially covered, for 30 minutes. Mixture should not be watery, but about the consistency of a light paste. Add more water if too thick.

Make salad mixture by combining chopped cucumbers, chopped tomato, parsley, olive oil, and lemon juice. Set aside.

Make Tahini-Lemon Sauce, following recipe below.

Assemble pocket sandwich: First put approximately 1/4 cup fava bean mixture into pocket, followed by 1/4 cup salad mixture. Top with 1 tablespoon Tahini-Lemon Sauce. Serve immediately. (Pita bread may be warmed in microwave before filling, if desired.)

TAHINI-LEMON SAUCE
1/3 cup sesame tahini
1/4 cup lemon juice
2-3 cloves garlic, minced
1/4 cup cold water
1/4 teaspoon salt
1/4 teaspoon pepper

Combine all ingredients in food processor. Blend until smooth. Sauce may be served immediately. If stored in refrigerator, it will stay fresh for several weeks. It will thicken slightly after chilling overnight in refrigerator.

Yield: Makes 6 large 1/2 pocket sandwiches.

Preparation time: 35-45 minutes

BEANBURGERS

Per serving:
Calories...... 337
Protein (g)... 16
Fat (g)....... 7.2
Sat. Fat (g).. 1.3
Choles. (mg).. 0
Fiber (g)..... 5.9
Sodium (mg)... 634
%Cal-Fat...... 19%

3/4 cup dry lentils
3 cups water
1 medium onion, chopped finely
1/2 cup dry bread crumbs
1 egg substitute (1/4 cup)
2 tablespoons chopped walnuts
1/4 cup chili sauce
1/2 teaspoon prepared mustard
1/2 teaspoon salt
Dash cayenne
1 tablespoon tub margarine
5 large buns

Rinse lentils. Place lentils and water in saucepan. Bring to a boil and simmer, covered, 45 to 50 minutes, or until tender. Drain. Transfer to mixing bowl and mash with a fork.

Add onion, bread crumbs, egg substitute, walnuts, chili sauce, mustard, salt and cayenne to mixing bowl. Mix well. Shape into five patties, about 1/2 to 3/4-inch thick.

Melt margarine in skillet. Cook beanburgers in margarine over medium heat about 4 minutes per side, or until lightly browned.

Serve on a bun with condiments and garnishes of choice: mayonnaise (fat-free or light), catsup, mustard, pickles, green onions and/or sliced tomatoes.

Yield: 5 burgers

The beanburger mix can be made ahead and stored in the refrigerator for up to 4 days. If a longer storage time is desired, make into patties and freeze.

Preparation time: 20 minutes

Cooking time: 55 minutes

CAROLYN'S BARBECUED BEANS

1/2 cup black beans, dry
1/2 cup lima beans, dry
1/2 cup red kidney beans, dry
1/2 cup black-eyed peas,dry
1 cup navy beans, dry
2 teaspoons salt
1/2 cup chopped onion
1 carrot, chopped
1 apple with peel, cored and diced
2 tablespoons molasses
1/2 cup catsup
1/2 cup spicy barbecue sauce
2 tablespoons firmly packed brown sugar
1 teaspoon prepared mustard

Per serving:
Calories...... 242
Protein (g)... 12
Fat (g)....... 1.2
Sat. Fat (g).. 0.2
Choles. (mg).. 0
Fiber (g)..... 10.6
Sodium (mg)... 757
%Cal-Fat...... 4%

Wash and sort beans. Soak overnight or at least 6 hours.* Drain.

In large kettle, place presoaked beans. Pour in enough water to make water level 2 inches above beans. Add salt and onion. Cook 1 to 1 1/2 hours or until tender. Drain, reserving 1 1/2 cups of bean broth. Add remaining ingredients, including reserved broth. Bring to a boil and simmer for 30 minutes.

Yield: 8 servings

Instead of soaking beans overnight, an alternate method may be used: Place beans in large kettle and cover with water, 2 inches above level of beans. Heat until boiling. Boil 2 minutes and remove from heat. Let beans sit, covered, for at least 1 hour before draining. (Beans may soak this way all day long.)

Add fresh water (2 inches above level of beans), onion and salt. Cook beans 45 to 60 minutes, or until they are tender. Drain, reserving 1 1/2 cups of bean broth. Add remaining ingredients, including reserved broth, and simmer 30 minutes.

Preparation time: 20-30 minutes

Cooking time: 1 1/2 to 2 hours

STUFFED BAKED POTATOES

Per serving:
Calories...... 339
Protein (g)... 11
Fat (g)....... 3.1
Sat. Fat (g).. 1.2
Choles. (mg).. 6
Fiber (g)..... 8.1
Sodium (mg)... 398
%Cal-Fat...... 3%

4 large baking potatoes
1 16-ounce can vegetarian baked beans
1/2 cup chopped scallions or chives
2 ounces reduced-calorie cheddar cheese, shredded
Nonfat sour cream (optional)

Bake potatoes in oven or microwave until soft. (Bake for about 1 hour at 350 degrees in oven, or 15 to 18 minutes in microwave on high setting.)

Heat baked beans on stove.

To serve, slash potatoes across top, spread open, and fill with baked beans. Sprinkle scallions, and cheddar cheese on top, and if desired, nonfat sour cream.

Yield: 4 servings

This is a quick, nutritious, low-fat meal. It is popular with children because they can assemble it themselves. Serve with your favorite bread and a crisp fruit salad, such as Slim Waldorf Salad. (Recipe, page 216)

Preparation time: 10 minutes

Cooking time: 1 hour (18 minutes microwave)

SPINACH FRITTATA

2 teaspoons canola oil
1 10-ounce package frozen chopped spinach, thawed
   and drained
1 medium-size zucchini, coarsely chopped
1 small onion, finely chopped
1 teaspoon minced garlic
6 egg substitutes (1 1/2 cups)
1/4 cup skim milk
1/4 teaspoon pepper
1/4 teaspoon dried oregano
1/4 teaspoon dried basil
1/4 teaspoon salt
1/2 cup grated Parmesan cheese

Per serving:
Calories...... 105
Protein (g)... 11
Fat (g)....... 4.8
Sat. Fat (g).. 1.6
Choles. (mg).. 6
Fiber (g)..... 1.8
Sodium (mg)... 302
%Cal-Fat...... 39%

Thaw spinach and squeeze lightly to remove excess water.

Heat oil in large skillet. Add spinach, zucchini, onion and garlic to skillet and saute until vegetables are tender, about 5 to 10 minutes. Remove from heat and let cool slightly.

In large mixing bowl, beat egg substitutes and milk with a wire whisk. Add pepper, oregano, basil and salt. Stir in Parmesan cheese and vegetables.

Spray 9-inch pie pan with vegetable cooking spray. Pour egg mixture into pie pan. Bake in 350 degree oven for 25 to 30 minutes or until puffed and slightly browned. Serve hot.

Yield: 8 servings

This frittata may be baked a day in advance and stored in the refrigerator. Heat just before serving, either in the oven, covered, or in the microwave. This is an excellent choice for a brunch.

Preparation time: 25-30 minutes

Cooking time: 25-30 minutes

EGG FOO YONG

Per serving:
Calories...... 60
Protein (g)... 6
Fat (g)....... 1.4
Sat. Fat (g).. 0.3
Choles. (mg).. 0
Fiber (g)..... 1
Sodium (mg)... 163
%Cal-Fat...... 21%

4 egg substitutes (1 cup)
1/4 cup all-purpose flour
1 16-ounce can mixed Oriental vegetables, drained
1/4 cup minced green onions
1/2 teaspoon seasoned salt
1/8 teaspoon black pepper
Vegetable cooking spray

In a medium-size mixing bowl, combine egg substitutes and flour. Mix with a wire whisk until all lumps disappear. Add Oriental vegetables, green onions, seasoned salt, and pepper. Mix until well blended.

Spray a 10-inch non-stick skillet or saute pan with a vegetable cooking spray. Place over medium-high heat. Add 1/4 cup egg mixture; press down with spatula until about 4 inches in diameter. (Cook 2 or 3 at a time in skillet.)

Cook the egg foo yong 1 to 2 minutes, or until it starts to lightly brown on bottom; turn with spatula and cook other side, about 1 to 2 minutes. Transfer to warmed serving platter. Repeat with remaining mixture.

Serve immediately with Duck Sauce or Hot Sweet Mustard Sauce.

Yield: 6 small servings

For a variation, 6 ounces of crabmeat or 3/4 cup diced shrimp, chicken or turkey may be added.

Preparation time: 20-25 minutes

VEGETABLE-PASTA STIR-FRY

1 pound linguine
1 tablespoon canola oil
2 cloves garlic, minced
1 medium eggplant, cut into 1/2-inch cubes
1 red pepper, cut into 1-inch strips
1 medium onion, chopped
1/4 cup Burgundy wine
1/2 teaspoon salt
1 16-ounce can garbanzo beans, drained and rinsed
4 medium tomatoes, chopped
1/4 cup pitted ripe olives, sliced
1/2 cup fresh parsley, chopped
2 teaspoons tub margarine
1/4 cup grated Parmesan cheese
Additional Parmesan cheese (optional)

Per serving:
Calories...... 338
Protein (g)... 14
Fat (g)....... 7.8
Sat. Fat (g).. 1.5
Choles. (mg).. 3
Fiber (g)..... 8.4
Sodium (mg)... 425
%Cal-Fat...... 21%

Prepare vegetables (eggplant, red pepper, onion, tomatoes, olives and parsley) by cutting/chopping as indicated above. Set aside.

Cook linguine in boiling water according to package directions.

Meanwhile, preheat oil in wok or large skillet over medium-high heat; add garlic and stir-fry for 15 seconds. Add eggplant, pepper and onion; stir-fry 3 minutes. Add wine and salt, and mix well. Steam for 5 minutes.

Add beans, tomatoes, olives and parsley. Cover and cook 5 additional minutes.

After pasta is cooked, drain, and place in large bowl. Add vegetables, margarine and Parmesan cheese. Toss gently until well mixed. Serve immediately. Sprinkle additional Parmesan cheese over top, if desired.

Yield: 6 servings

Preparation time: 35-45 minutes

SPINACH-NOODLE CASSEROLE

Per serving:
Calories...... 257
Protein (g)... 23
Fat (g)....... 4.8
Sat. Fat (g).. 2.3
Choles. (mg).. 10
Fiber (g)..... 3
Sodium (mg)... 690
%Cal-Fat...... 17%

8 ounces "eggless" egg noodles, uncooked
Vegetable cooking spray
1/2 pound fresh mushrooms, sliced
1 medium onion, chopped
1 10-ounce package frozen chopped spinach, thawed
    and pressed dry
1/4 cup dry white wine
3 egg substitutes (3/4 cup)
3 cups low-fat cottage cheese
1/2 cup Parmesan cheese
1 teaspoon seasoned salt
2 tablespoons wheat germ
2 tablespoons Parmesan cheese

Preheat oven to 375 degrees.

Cook noodles according to package directions. Drain. Set aside.*

Meanwhile, spray skillet or saute pan with vegetable cooking spray. Saute mushrooms and onions until vegetables are tender. Stir in spinach. Pour in wine. Steam until wine evaporates (about 2 minutes).

In large mixing bowl, stir together egg substitutes, cottage cheese, 1/2 cup Parmesan cheese, and seasoned salt. Add mushroom-spinach mixture. Add cooked noodles and wheat germ. Spread in 9 x 13-inch pan. Sprinkle remaining Parmesan cheese over top.

Bake at 375 degrees for 30 minutes, covered; and an additional 15 minutes, uncovered.

Yield: 8 servings

If cooked noodles need to be held awhile before mixing them with other ingredients, they should be placed over steaming hot water in a colander. Steam will keep them hot without further cooking, and stickiness will be minimized.

Preparation time: 30-35 minutes

Cooking time: 45 minutes

VEGETARIAN LASAGNA

1 cup chopped onion
2 teaspoons olive oil
1 10-ounce package frozen chopped spinach, thawed
    and squeezed dry
1 cup all-purpose flour
3 cups skim milk
1/2 cup Parmesan cheese
3/4 teaspoon seasoned salt
1/4 teaspoon pepper
1 teaspoon dried oregano, crushed
8 ounces lasagna noodles, cooked and drained
1/4 cup Parmesan cheese
2 ounces part-skim mozzarella cheese, shredded

Per serving:
Calories...... 455
Protein (g)... 25
Fat (g)....... 9.6
Sat. Fat (g).. 4.6
Choles. (mg).. 21
Fiber (g)..... 4.2
Sodium (mg)... 643
%Cal-Fat...... 19%

In a large, covered skillet, cook chopped onion in olive oil until onion is tender but not brown. Add chopped spinach and mix together.

In large mixing bowl, combine flour with milk using a wire whisk until all lumps disappear. Pour into skillet. Add 1/2 cup Parmesan cheese, seasoned salt, pepper, and oregano. Cook over medium heat, stirring occasionally, until mixture comes to a boil and thickens. Simmer, covered, over low heat until ready to assemble lasagna.

Meanwhile cook lasagna noodles according to package directions.
Drain and pat dry with paper towels.

Arrange a single layer of lasagna noodles in the bottom of a lightly greased 12 x 7 1/2 x 2-inch baking dish. Top with 1/3 of the spinach mixture. Repeat the layers 2 more times. Sprinkle 1/4 cup Parmesan cheese over top, followed by mozzarella cheese.

Bake, uncovered, at 350 degrees 30 to 35 minutes, or until cheese is lightly browned on top. Let stand 10 minutes before serving.

Yield: 4 to 6 servings

Preparation time: 30-35 minutes

Cooking time: 35 minutes

EGGPLANT PARMESAN

Per serving:
Calories...... 177
Protein (g)... 11
Fat (g)....... 5.6
Sat. Fat (g).. 2.5
Choles. (mg).. 10
Fiber (g)..... 3
Sodium (mg)... 485
%Cal-Fat...... 29%

1 large eggplant
2 egg substitutes (1/2 cup)
3/4 cup Italian bread crumbs
1 cup prepared spaghetti sauce
1 cup tomato sauce (no salt added)
1/4 cup Parmesan cheese
2 1/2 ounces part-skim mozzarella cheese

Preheat oven to 425 degrees.

Spray large cookie sheet with vegetable cooking spray. Cut eggplant (unpeeled) into 1/4-inch-thick slices. Dip each slice first in egg substitutes and then bread crumbs. Place in single layer on cookie sheet. Bake at 425 degrees 10 minutes. Turn over and bake an additional 10 minutes.

Meanwhile, make tomato sauce by combining prepared spaghetti sauce and tomato sauce (no salt added) in small bowl. Season to taste.

Reduce oven heat to 350 degrees.

Assemble eggplant Parmesan in a 2 to 3-quart casserole dish. Place 2 or 3 tablespoons tomato sauce on bottom of baking dish. Next arrange layer of eggplant slices on top of sauce. Top with 1/3 of sauce and 1/3 of Parmesan cheese. Repeat layers 3 times or until all ingredients are used up, ending with sauce and Parmesan cheese on top. Cover with thin layer of mozzarella cheese.

Bake, covered, at 350 degrees 20 minutes. Broil, uncovered, an additional 3 to 5 minutes or until cheese is lightly browned.

Yield: 6 large servings

Preparation time: 30 minutes

Cooking time: 30 minutes

DEEP-DISH SICILIAN PIZZA

1 pound frozen bread dough, white or whole wheat
1 1/4 cups spaghetti sauce, or seasoned tomato sauce
1 14-ounce can artichoke hearts in water, drained and chopped
1 medium onion, sliced thin, rings separated
1/2 green pepper, sliced in 2-inch narrow strips
1/4 cup Parmesan cheese
2 ounces (1/2 cup) shredded mozzarella cheese (optional)

Per slice:
Calories...... 231
Protein (g)... 8
Fat (g)....... 4.2
Sat. Fat (g).. 1.1
Choles. (mg).. 2.5
Fiber (g)..... 4
Sodium (mg)... 597
%Cal-Fat...... 16%

With mozzarella:
Fat (g)........5.4
%Cal-Fat.....20%

Thaw dough overnight in refrigerator or at room temperature for 2 hours.

Place dough in greased bowl, cover, and let rise in warm place until it has doubled in size (about 45 to 60 minutes).

Spray 14-inch deep-dish pizza pan with vegetable cooking spray. Punch dough down. On floured surface, roll out into large circle. Place in pizza pan. Spread with fingers to make dough fit to edges of pan. Cover dough and let rise in warm place 45 to 60 minutes.

Preheat oven to 400 degrees.

Pour spaghetti sauce over dough. Arrange vegetables on top. (Other toppings may be substituted, depending on individual preferences.) Sprinkle Parmesan cheese, and if desired, mozzarella cheese over top.

Bake at 400 degrees 20 to 25 minutes, or until cheese melts and crust turns light brown.

Yield: 1 14-inch pizza, or 8 slices

Preparation time: 15-20 minutes

Cooking time: 20-25 minutes
(Plus 1 1/2 to 2 hours for dough to rise)

Pasta, Rice & Grains

FETTUCINE WITH ARTICHOKES IN WHITE SAUCE

Per serving:
Calories...... 267
Protein (g)... 11
Fat (g)....... 6.2
Sat. Fat (g).. 1.5
Choles. (mg).. 3
Fiber (g)..... 5.3
Sodium (mg)... 289
%Cal-Fat...... 21%

2 tablespoons olive oil
2 tablespoons flour
1 1/2 cups chicken stock, or one 14 1/2-ounce can clear
    chicken broth, defatted
3 cloves of garlic, crushed, or 1 teaspoon minced garlic
2 tablespoons fresh lemon juice
Freshly ground pepper, to taste
1 14-ounce can artichoke hearts, drained and cut into
    bite-size pieces
12 ounces fettucini or linguine, uncooked
1/4 cup fresh parsley, minced
1/4 cup Parmesan cheese
2 tablespoons tub margarine, optional

In a large heavy skillet, heat olive oil and flour over moderately low heat, for 3 minutes. Stir in chicken stock, and cook over medium heat until mixture comes to a boil.

Add garlic, lemon juice, and pepper to skillet. Cook for 5 minutes over low heat, stirring occasionally. Add artichoke hearts and cook, uncovered, for an additional 8 minutes.

Meanwhile, cook fettucini according to package directions, and drain.

Pour fettucini into large serving dish. Immediately add parsley, Parmesan cheese, artichoke sauce, and margarine, if desired. Toss until well mixed. Serve immediately.

Pass additional Parmesan cheese to sprinkle over top.

Yield: 6 to 8 servings

A delicious lower-fat alternative to Fettucini Alfredo, which contains large amounts of butter and cream.

Preparation time: 20-30 minutes

PASTA WITH RED CLAM SAUCE

3 6 1/2-ounce cans minced clams, drained
1 medium onion, chopped fine
2 teaspoons olive oil
1/2 cup dry white wine
1 15-ounce can tomatoes (no salt added)
2 cups prepared spaghetti sauce
16 ounces pasta
Parmesan cheese

Per serving:
Calories...... 555
Protein (g)... 38
Fat (g)....... 8
Sat. Fat (g).. 1.3
Choles. (mg).. 70
Fiber (g)..... 4.8
Sodium (mg)... 625
%Cal-Fat...... 13%

Drain clams. Set aside.

Saute chopped onion in olive oil in medium-size skillet until onions are soft. Add wine and clams. Cook until liquid is reduced by one-half.

Chop tomatoes in food processor. Add to skillet along with prepared spaghetti sauce. Simmer, uncovered, for 15 to 30 minutes.

Meanwhile, prepare pasta as directed on package. Drain. Place in large serving bowl. Spoon clam sauce over top. Sprinkle with Parmesan cheese.

Yield: 4 to 6 servings

Preparation time: 15-20 minutes

Cooking time: 20-30 minutes

PASTA WITH WHITE CLAM SAUCE

3 6 1/2-ounce cans chopped clams, including juice
2 teaspoons olive oil
1/2 cup chopped onion
1 - 2 cloves garlic, minced
1/2 cup dry white wine
1 teaspoon dried basil
4 teaspoons cornstarch
1/4 cup Parmesan cheese
2 tablespoons fresh chopped parsley
1 pound linguine or angel hair pasta

Heat olive oil in medium-size skillet over low heat. Add onions and saute until they become translucent. Add garlic and saute an additional 1/2 minute.

Meanwhile, drain juice from 2 cans of clams, reserving liquid.

Add drained clams and 1 can of clams with liquid to skillet. Add wine and basil. Bring to a boil and simmer about 10 to 15 minutes.

Add cornstarch to reserved liquid from clams. Mix well with wire whisk. Add to skillet and continue to cook over low heat until mixture returns to a boil and thickens.

Meanwhile, cook pasta according to package directions. Drain well.

In large bowl, combine drained pasta, clam sauce, Parmesan cheese and parsley. Toss until well mixed. Serve immediately. Sprinkle with additional Parmesan cheese, if desired.

Yield: 4 to 6 servings

Garnish with open clam shells on top for a nice effect.

Preparation time: 20-25 minutes

BAKED ZITI

Vegetable cooking spray
1 medium onion, chopped
2 cloves garlic, minced
1 28-ounce can crushed tomatoes
1 16-ounce can tomatoes, finely chopped
1 8-ounce can tomato sauce
1/4 cup minced parsley
2 teaspoons dried basil
2 teaspoons fennel
1/4 cup dry white wine
1 tablespoon Parmesan cheese
1/4 teaspoon pepper
1 1/2 teaspoons sugar
Salt to taste
1 pound pasta, penne rigate or cut ziti
1/2 pound ricotta low-fat cheese
4 ounces part-skim mozzarella cheese, shredded
1/4 cup Parmesan cheese, grated

Per serving:
Calories...... 407
Protein (g)... 21
Fat (g)....... 7.1
Sat. Fat (g).. 3.9
Choles. (mg).. 22
Fiber (g)..... 4.6
Sodium (mg)... 557
%Cal-Fat...... 16%

Spray large skillet with vegetable cooking spray. Add chopped onion and garlic and saute until onion becomes translucent. Add 2 tablespoons water, if necessary, to keep onion from sticking.

Add crushed tomatoes, chopped tomatoes, tomato sauce, parsley, basil, fennel, wine, 1 tablespoon Parmesan cheese, pepper and sugar to skillet. Bring to a boil. Cover and simmer on low 1 to 1 1/2 hours. Add water if sauce is too thick. Salt to taste, if desired.

Meanwhile, cook pasta according to package directions. Drain. Rinse with cold water immediately to prevent pasta from sticking together.

Assemble in 9 x 13-inch pan: Spread about 1 1/4 cups sauce on bottom of pan. Top with 1/3 of the cooked ziti. Crumble 1/4 pound ricotta cheese and sprinkle 2 ounces mozzarella cheese over ziti. Repeat layers of sauce, ziti, ricotta and mozzarella. Pour about 1 1/2 cups sauce over top. Add remaining 1/3 of the ziti and the remaining sauce (about 1 1/2 cups). Sprinkle Parmesan cheese over top.

Bake, uncovered, in 350 degree oven 30 minutes, or until heated through. Remove from oven and let sit for 5 minutes before serving.

Yield: 6 to 8 servings

Baked ziti can be assembled a day in advance, covered and refrigerated until ready to bake. To bake, cover with aluminum foil and bake at 350 degrees 45 minutes, removing foil for last 20 minutes of baking.

Preparation time: 30-35 minutes

Cooking time: 1 1/2 to 2 hours

TUNA FETTUCCINE

12 ounces spinach fettuccine
1/2 cup sliced green onion, including tops
2 teaspoons tub margarine
1/4 cup all-purpose flour
2 cups skim milk
1/2 teaspoon seasoned salt
1/4 cup Parmesan cheese
1 6 1/2 ounce can tuna in spring water, drained
1/4 cup sliced, pitted ripe olives

Cook fettuccine according to package directions. Drain. To keep warm, place in colander over pot of hot water and cover.

Meanwhile, in medium skillet, saute green onion in margarine.

With a wire whisk, combine flour and milk in mixing bowl. Add to onions in skillet. Slowly heat until mixture comes to a boil and thickens. Add seasoned salt, Parmesan cheese, tuna (broken into chunks) and olives. Heat through.

To serve, spoon tuna mixture over fettuccine.

Yield: 4 servings

Preparation time: 20-25 minutes

Per serving:
Calories...... 497
Protein (g)... 32
Fat (g)....... 6
Sat. Fat (g).. 2
Choles. (mg).. 15
Fiber (g)..... 4.8
Sodium (mg)... 589
%Cal-Fat...... 11%

SPAGHETTI AND MEATBALLS

1 pound ground turkey breast*
2 egg substitutes (1/2 cup)
1 cup seasoned breadcrumbs
1/2 cup finely chopped onion
1 tablespoon Parmesan cheese
1 tablespoon olive oil
Marinara sauce (Recipe, page 331)
1 pound spaghetti pasta
Parmesan cheese

In large bowl, mix together first five ingredients until well blended.

Heat olive oil in 10-inch skillet. Form ground turkey mixture into 1 1/4-inch balls and brown in skillet.

Meanwhile, mix together in medium-size bowl the marinara sauce ingredients.

After meatballs have browned, pour sauce over. Simmer for 20 to 60 minutes.

While sauce and meatballs are simmering, cook pasta according to package directions.

To serve, drain pasta and place on large tray or in large spaghetti bowl. Stir in 1/2 cup sauce to prevent pasta from sticking together. Arrange several meatballs on top. Sprinkle with Parmesan cheese. Have additional sauce and meatballs to pass at table.

Yield: 6 servings

The ground turkey commercially available at grocery stores contains both light and dark turkey meat, plus some fat and skin, which amounts to about 2 1/2 teaspoons of fat (12 grams) per 3-ounce serving. Skinless turkey breast, with the fat removed, that you can grind yourself or have your butcher grind, contains only 1/2 teaspoon fat (2.5 grams) per 3-ounce serving. However, even the commercially available ground turkey, in most cases, contains 25% less fat than "lean" ground beef.

Preparation time: 30 minutes

Cooking time: 30–60 minutes

QUICK MARINARA SAUCE WITH PASTA

Per serving:
Calories...... 457
Protein (g)... 15
Fat (g)....... 4.3
Sat. Fat (g).. 0.9
Choles. (mg).. 0
Fiber (g)..... 4.8
Sodium (mg)... 521
%Cal-Fat...... 8%

1 16-ounce can tomatoes (no salt added), chopped finely in food processor
2 cups prepared spaghetti sauce
2 tablespoons dry white wine
1/4 cup bean paste* (optional)
Dash freshly ground black pepper
1/4 teaspoon garlic powder
1 teaspoon dried basil
Parmesan cheese, to taste
16 ounces pasta

To make marinara sauce, combine all ingredients except cheese and pasta in a medium-size skillet. Bring to a boil and simmer, uncovered, for at least 20 minutes.

Meanwhile, cook pasta according to package directions. Drain. Place in a large bowl. Stir in 1/4 cup marinara sauce to keep pasta from sticking together.

To serve, spoon marinara sauce over pasta and sprinkle with Parmesan cheese.

*To make bean paste, use a 16-ounce can of beans, either black eyed peas, northern beans, garbanzo beans or kidney beans. Drain beans, reserving 2 tablespoons liquid. Puree beans and reserved liquid in food processor until smooth. Refrigerate until ready to use. Keeps in refrigerator for up to 2 weeks.

Yield: 4 cups sauce, enough for 4 to 6 servings

Sodium in prepared spaghetti sauces is very high. By adding "no salt added" tomatoes or tomato sauce to a prepared sauce as this recipe specifies, the sodium content is approximately cut in half. Bean paste adds additional protein and makes the sauce slightly thicker.

Tip: Add hot taco sauce (to taste) to leftover bean paste for a delicious and nutritious dip—perfect for cold vegetables or melba rounds.

Preparation time: 15-20 minutes

Cooking time: 20-40 minutes

ZITI WITH CREAMY MUSHROOM SAUCE

1 pound ziti pasta
2 teaspoons olive oil
8 ounces fresh mushrooms, sliced
1 cup clear chicken broth, defatted
1 cup skim milk
1/3 cup flour
1/2 teaspoon seasoned salt
1/8 teaspoon white pepper
1/4 cup Parmesan cheese
Salt to taste
Parmesan cheese to taste

Per serving:
Calories...... 368
Protein (g)... 15
Fat (g)....... 4.5
Sat. Fat (g).. 1.3
Choles. (mg).. 4
Fiber (g)..... 4.4
Sodium (mg)... 412
%Cal-Fat...... 11%

Cook pasta according to package directions. Drain.

Meanwhile, heat olive oil in a medium-size skillet. Add sliced mushrooms and cook until mushrooms become soft and turn dark in color.

Place a large skillet over medium heat. Pour in chicken broth.

In a small mixing bowl or measuring cup, add flour to skim milk. Stir briskly with a wire whisk until all lumps disappear. Add to chicken broth along with seasoned salt and pepper. Heat until mixture comes to a boil and thickens. Add cooked mushrooms, including juice, and heat through.

To serve, place cooked ziti in a large bowl. Pour mushroom sauce over and toss to coat. Add Parmesan cheese and mix well. Serve immediately. Add salt or additional Parmesan cheese to taste, if desired.

Yield: 6 side-dish servings

Preparation time: 20-25 minutes

FRESH HERBED TOMATO SAUCE (WITH PASTA)

Per serving:
Calories...... 427
Protein (g)... 16
Fat (g)....... 5.1
Sat. Fat (g).. 1.5
Choles. (mg).. 4
Fiber (g)..... 4.6
Sodium (mg)... 332
%Cal-Fat...... 11%

2 teaspoons olive oil
3 - 4 cloves garlic, minced
**6 medium vine-ripened tomatoes, chopped finely in food
  processor***
**1 1/2 tablespoons fresh minced basil, or 1 1/2 teaspoons
  dried**
1/2 teaspoon salt, or to taste
1 pound pasta
1/4 cup grated Parmesan cheese

Heat olive oil in two-quart saucepan over medium heat. Add garlic and cook until tender.

Stir in tomatoes, basil and salt. Bring to a boil and simmer, stirring occasionally, 45 minutes or until sauce is desired thickness.

Meanwhile, cook your favorite pasta according to package directions. Drain. (Do not rinse.) Add small amount of sauce to pasta to keep from sticking together.

Serve immediately. Top with sauce and sprinkle with Parmesan cheese.

Yield: 4 to 6 servings.

Fresh, vine-ripened tomatoes produce a much sweeter tomato sauce than hot house tomatoes or canned tomatoes. This recipe does not call for peeling the tomatoes, but you may prefer to do so.

Preparation time: 15-20 minutes

Cooking time: 45 minutes

FETTUCINE WITH SHRIMP AND MUSSELS

3/4 pound large fresh shrimp
18 to 24 fresh mussels (in shells)
2 tablespoons olive oil
1 teaspoon minced garlic
3 tablespoons flour
1 3/4 cups chicken stock, or one 14 1/2-ounce can clear
    chicken broth, defatted
1/4 cup dry white wine
1 tablespoon lemon juice
Freshly ground pepper, to taste
1/4 cup fresh parsley, chopped
1/4 cup grated Parmesan cheese
12 ounces fettucine or linguine
2 tablespoons tub margarine, optional

Per serving:
Calories...... 435
Protein (g)... 25
Fat (g)....... 10.1
Sat. Fat (g).. 2.4
Choles. (mg).. 140
Fiber (g)..... 3
Sodium (mg)... 490
Cal-Fat...... 20%

Preheat oven to 325 degrees.

Clean shrimp. Set aside.

Rinse mussels and remove any debris. Place on large cookie sheet in preheated oven. Bake 5 to 10 minutes or until shells open. Remove from oven. Set aside.

Meanwhile, heat olive oil in large skillet placed over medium heat. Add minced garlic and saute for 1 minute. Stir in flour, mixing well. Add chicken broth, stirring constantly with a wire whisk until mixture comes to a boil and thickens. Stir in wine, lemon juice, and pepper.

Add shrimp and mussels to skillet. Cook 3 to 4 minutes, uncovered, until shrimp turn pink in color. Stir occasionally.

Meanwhile, cook fettucine according to package directions. Remove mussels from skillet. Set aside, keeping warm.

To assemble, place drained fettucine in large serving dish. Immediately pour shrimp mixture, parsley and Parmesan cheese over top. Add margarine, if desired. Toss until well blended. Add mussels and toss lightly. Serve immediately. Pass additional Parmesan cheese to sprinkle over top.

Yield: 4 servings

Preparation time: 30-40 minutes

PARMESAN RICE

Per serving:
Calories...... 208
Protein (g)... 8
Fat (g)....... 2.5
Sat. Fat (g).. 1
Choles. (mg).. 3
Fiber (g)..... 2
Sodium (mg)... 330
%Cal-Fat...... 11%

2 cups rice, uncooked
1 bunch green onions, chopped
1 red pepper, chopped
1/4 cup salsa (medium)
1 cup canned chick peas, drained
1/2 cup chopped parsley
1 tablespoon fresh basil, chopped
2 egg substitutes (1/2 cup)
1/2 cup skim milk
1 teaspoon salt
1/4 teaspoon pepper
1 teaspoon garlic powder
1 tablespoon white wine vinegar
1 tablespoon sugar
1/2 cup Parmesan cheese

Cook rice according to package directions.

Meanwhile, in large casserole dish (5 quart), combine chopped green onions, red pepper, salsa, chick peas, parsley, and basil.

In a medium-size mixing bowl, combine remaining ingredients, except Parmesan cheese. Beat with a wire whisk. Set aside.

Add rice to casserole dish. Mix well. Add egg mixture and Parmesan cheese. Stir until all ingredients are well mixed. Sprinkle additional Parmesan cheese lightly over top.

Bake at 350 degrees 30 minutes.

Yield: 10 1-cup servings.

Preparation time: 30-35 minutes

Cooking time: 30 minutes

WILD RICE BAKED CASSEROLE

1 cup wild rice, uncooked
2 tablespoons tub margarine
1 large onion, chopped
1 large stalk celery, chopped
1 cup long-grain white rice, uncooked
2 14-ounce cans clear chicken broth, defatted
2 tablespoons light soy sauce
1/4 cup dry white wine

Per serving:
Calories...... 200
Protein (g)... 7
Fat (g)....... 3.8
Sat. Fat (g).. 0.7
Choles. (mg).. 0
Fiber (g)..... 2
Sodium (mg)... 520
%Cal-Fat...... 14%

Preheat oven to 350 degrees.

Place wild rice in a medium saucepan and cover with about 2 inches of water. Bring to a boil and simmer 20 minutes. Drain water and set rice aside.

Meanwhile, in large skillet, melt margarine. Add chopped onion and celery. Saute until onion becomes translucent, but not brown. Add white rice and saute 2 to 3 minutes, or until rice is lightly browned. Stir in wild rice.

Transfer to a covered 2 1/2-quart casserole dish. (At this stage, casserole may be refrigerated for several hours or overnight.)

Before you are ready to bake casserole, combine chicken broth, soy sauce and wine in medium saucepan. Bring to a boil. Pour over rice in casserole dish. Bake in 350 degree oven 1 hour or until all liquid is absorbed.

Yield: 8 servings

Preparation time: 20-25 minutes

Cooking time: 1 hour

SAFFRON RICE

Per serving:
Calories...... 263
Protein (g)... 11
Fat (g)....... 4
Sat. Fat (g).. 1.8
Choles. (mg).. 5
Fiber (g)..... 1.2
Sodium (mg)... 520
%Cal-Fat...... 14%

4 cups chicken broth, homemade or canned, defatted
2 teaspoons tub margarine
1/4 cup finely chopped onion
1 cup uncooked white rice
1/4 cup dry white wine
Pinch of saffron
1/4 cup freshly grated Parmesan cheese

Bring chicken broth to a boil and keep it barely simmering over low heat.

Meanwhile, melt margarine in heavy saucepan. Add chopped onion, and saute until onion is soft but not brown. Add the rice and saute 2 minutes. Add wine and simmer until liquid is reduced by 1/2 (about 2 minutes).

Add half the broth and the saffron to the saucepan, and cook, uncovered, over medium heat, stirring frequently. As the broth is absorbed, add more, about 1/2 cup at a time. Continue cooking, adding broth as needed, until rice is tender, but not soft. The total cooking time, after the broth is added, should be about 30 minutes. Stir constantly toward the end of the cooking time to avoid sticking.

Remove from heat. Stir in the Parmesan cheese. Cover until ready to serve.

Yield: 4 servings

The saffron lends a delicate flavor and a beautiful soft yellow color to the rice.

To reduce sodium, use homemade chicken broth, or dilute the canned broth with water.

Preparation time: 15-20 minutes

Cooking time: 30 minutes

SPANISH RICE

1 cup uncooked white rice
2 teaspoons olive oil
1 medium onion, chopped finely
1 clove garlic, minced
1 8-ounce can tomato sauce
3 tablespoons salsa (medium or hot)
1 1/2 cups water

Heat olive oil in large skillet. Add rice, onion and garlic, and saute until rice turns golden brown. Add remaining ingredients and bring to a boil. Reduce heat and simmer 25 minutes or until liquid is absorbed and rice is tender.

Yield: 4 servings

Preparation time: 15 minutes

Cooking time: 25 minutes

Per serving:
Calories...... 236
Protein (g)... 5
Fat (g)....... 3
Sat. Fat (g).. 0.5
Choles. (mg).. 0
Fiber (g)..... 2.3
Sodium (mg)... 198
%Cal-Fat...... 12%

RICE-MUSHROOM CASSEROLE

1 pound fresh mushrooms, sliced
2 14-ounce cans clear chicken broth, defatted
3/4 cup water
1/2 cup wild rice, uncooked
1 1/2 cups long grain rice, uncooked
1 tablespoon tub margarine

Wash mushrooms and slice. Place in skillet (no oil necessary), cover, and simmer on low until mushrooms turn dark in color. Stir occasionally. Drain, saving juice from mushrooms. Set aside.

Meanwhile, in a large saucepan, combine chicken broth, water and wild rice. Bring to a boil, and simmer for 10 minutes.

Add long grain rice, juice from mushrooms, and margarine to saucepan. Bring to a second boil. Reduce heat and simmer, for

Per serving:
Calories...... 187
Protein (g)... 7
Fat (g)....... 2.2
Sat. Fat (g).. 0.5
Choles. (mg).. 0
Fiber (g)..... 2.2
Sodium (mg)... 337
%Cal-Fat...... 10%

approximately 30 minutes longer, or until liquid is fully absorbed.

Stir in mushrooms. Serve immediately.

Yield: 8 servings

Preparation time: 30 minutes

Cooking time: 30 minutes

GREEN RICE CASSEROLE

Per serving:
Calories...... 208
Protein (g)... 9
Fat (g)....... 4
Sat. Fat (g).. 1
Choles. (mg).. 3
Fiber (g)..... 2.2
Sodium (mg)... 400
%Cal-Fat...... 18%

3 to 4 cups cooked long grain rice
1 10-ounce package frozen chopped spinach, thawed
1/2 cup chopped green onions with tops
1/4 cup minced parsley
1/4 cup slivered almonds
2 teaspoons lemon juice
1/4 teaspoon salt
1/4 teaspoon garlic powder
2 egg substitutes (1/2 cup)
3/4 cup skim milk
1/4 cup Parmesan cheese
2 tablespoons light soy sauce

Cook rice according to package directions. Thaw spinach in microwave. Squeeze lightly to remove excess moisture.

Combine first eight ingredients in large mixing bowl.

In small mixing bowl, mix together eggs, milk, Parmesan cheese and soy sauce with a wire whisk. Add to rice mixture, stirring until uniformly mixed.

Pour into 3-quart casserole dish. Cover. Bake at 350 degrees 30 to 40 minutes.

Yield: 8 servings

Preparation time: 20-25 minutes

Cooking time: 1 to 1 1/4 hours

BAKED BULGUR WITH FRUIT

2 vegetable bouillon cubes (or 1 large cube)
2 cups boiling water
1 cup bulgur
1/2 teaspoon basil
1/2 cup dark raisins
1/2 cup chopped golden apple, with peel
1/4 cup coarsely chopped pecans

Preheat oven to 350 degrees.

Dissolve bouillon in boiling water. Pour into 2-quart casserole. Add remaining ingredients and stir to mix. Cover and bake at 350 degrees 40 minutes.

Yield: 4 to 6 servings

Preparation time: 15 minutes

Cooking time: 40 minutes

Per serving:
Calories...... 202
Protein (g)... 5
Fat (g)....... 4.4
Sat. Fat (g).. 0.5
Choles. (mg).. 0
Fiber (g)..... 7.8
Sodium (mg)... 452
%Cal-Fat...... 19%

BULGUR WITH STEAMED VEGETABLES

1/4 cup chopped carrots
1/4 cup chopped celery
1/4 cup chopped onion
3 tablespoons water, divided
1 cup bulgur
1 1/2 cups water
1 chicken bouillon cube
2 tablespoons chopped fresh parsley

In a non-stick saute pan or medium frypan, add chopped vegetables and 2 tablespoons water. Steam 2 minutes.

Add bulgur and one additional tablespoon water. Toss for 3 to 5 minutes until vegetables have softened and bulgur is golden brown.

Per serving:
Calories...... 106
Protein (g)... 4
Fat (g)....... 0.6
Sat. Fat (g).. 0.1
Choles. (mg).. 0
Fiber (g)..... 6.7
Sodium (mg)... 236
%Cal-Fat...... 5%

Add 1 1/2 cups water and bouillon cube and bring to a boil. Reduce heat to medium-low. Simmer, uncovered, about 15 minutes, or until all liquid has been absorbed. Stir in chopped parsley immediately before serving.

Yield: 4 to 6 servings.

Excellent served with boneless chicken breasts and bright, crisp green salad or fresh tomato slices.

Preparation time: 15-20 minutes

Cooking time: 15 minutes

POLENTA

3 cups water
1 cup coarse yellow cornmeal
1 cup cold water
1 teaspoon salt
2 teaspoons tub margarine (optional)

Bring 3 cups water to a boil in medium-size saucepan.

Meanwhile, combine cornmeal with 1 cup cold water and salt. Add slowly to boiling water. Reduce heat and cook, stirring constantly, until cornmeal mixture returns to a boil.

Cook, uncovered, stirring frequently, about 5 to 15 minutes, depending on the coarseness of the cornmeal. The cooking is complete when the mixture thickens and the cornmeal is soft.

Serve immediately, either plain or with a small amount of margarine.

Yield: 4 cups or 6 servings

Polenta is sometimes used as a substitute for spaghetti in Northern Italy. It is commonly served with the sauce or gravy accompanying a meat or fish dish.

Preparation time: 15-30 minutes

Per serving:
Calories...... 110
Protein (g)... 3
Fat (g)....... 1
Sat. Fat (g).. 0.1
Choles. (mg).. 0
Fiber (g)..... 3.3
Sodium (mg)... 542
%Cal-Fat...... 9%

POTATO GNOCCHI

3 cups water
1 cup skim milk
3 cups instant mashed potato flakes
2 egg substitutes (1/2 cup)
3 1/2 cups all-purpose flour, divided
1 teaspoon salt

Combine 3 cups water and 1 cup skim milk in medium saucepan. Bring to a boil. Remove from heat and stir in 3 cups instant mashed potatoes. (This makes stiff mashed potatoes.) Transfer to a large mixing bowl.

Add egg substitutes (or 3 lightly beaten egg whites), 1/2 cup flour and salt to mashed potatoes. Mix should be very sticky.

Knead in 3 cups of flour, one cup at a time. (This can be done with an electric mixer using a dough attachment.)

On a well floured surface, roll dough into 1/2-inch diameter tubes, about 10 inches long. Cut into one-inch lengths. Place on a tray lined with wax paper. Separate layers of gnocchi with additional wax paper.

Add 1 tablespoon canola oil and 1/2 teaspoon salt to large pot of water. Bring to a boil. Add gnocchi, stirring frequently. Bring to a second boil and cook 10 to 12 minutes, stirring occasionally. Drain well in a colander.

Serve topped with your favorite tomato sauce or white sauce.

Yield: 3 pounds of dough, 8 large servings

Making this dough can be a fun family project on a Sunday afternoon. Allow at least one hour to make pasta. Gnocchi is a soft chewy pasta that is a favorite with many Italian families.

Preparation time: 1 to 1 1/2 hours

Cooking time: 15 minutes

Per serving:
Calories...... 282
Protein (g)... 10
Fat (g)....... 1.2
Sat. Fat (g).. 0.2
Choles. (mg).. 0
Fiber (g)..... 2.5
Sodium (mg)... 329
%Cal-Fat...... 4%

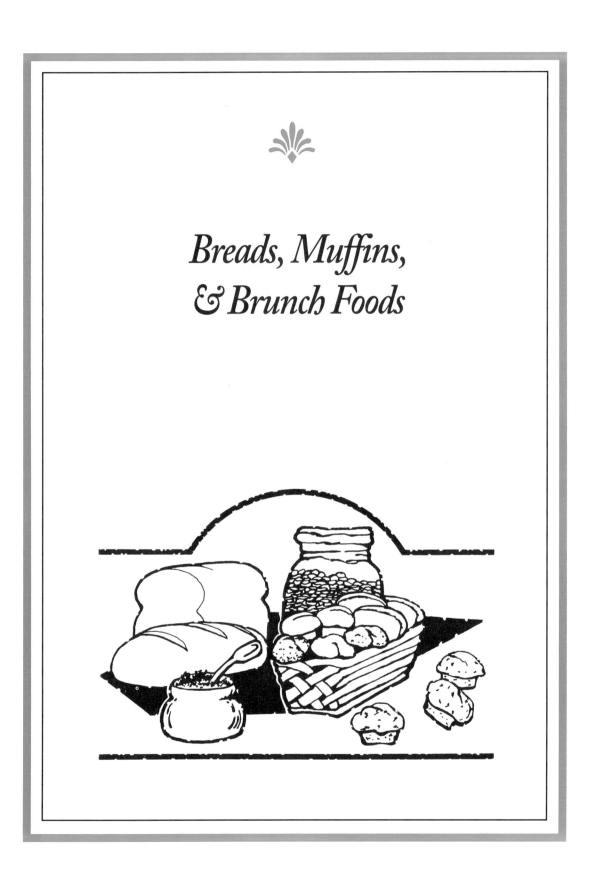

Breads, Muffins, & Brunch Foods

HONEY GRAIN BREAD

Per slice:
Calories...... 118
Protein (g)... 3
Fat (g)....... 2.5
Sat. Fat (g).. 0.3
Choles. (mg).. 0
Fiber (g)..... 2
Sodium (mg)... 37
%Cal-Fat...... 19%

3 cups whole wheat flour
2 cups all-purpose flour
1 cup quick-cooking oats
1/2 teaspoon salt
2 packages active dry yeast
1 1/2 cups water
1/4 - 1/2 cup honey
1/3 cup safflower oil
3 egg whites or 1/2 cup egg substitutes
1/2 - 1 1/2 cups all-purpose flour

Place 3 cups whole wheat flour, 2 cups all-purpose flour, oats, salt and yeast in bowl. Mix well.

Combine water, honey and safflower oil in saucepan; heat to 120 to 130 F. Slowly add warm liquids to flour mixture by hand or with an electric mixer or food processor (using dough attachment) until well mixed, about one minute.

Add egg whites. Mix well, for about one minute.

Add remaining flour, 1/2 cup at a time, until dough becomes elastic, or if using an electric appliance, until dough clings to attachment and cleans sides of bowl, about 3 minutes. Continue to knead for 7 to 10 minutes, by hand or machine, until dough is smooth and elastic.

Place in lightly greased bowl, turning to grease top. Cover, let rise in warm place, until doubled in bulk, about 40 to 60 minutes.

Punch dough down. Divide dough in half. Shape each half into a loaf. Place each loaf in a non-stick 8 1/2 x 4 1/2 x 2 1/2-inch bread pan.

Bake at 350 degrees for 30 to 40 minutes. Remove from pans and cool on wire racks for 10 minutes. Immediately put in plastic bag to maintain moistness.

Yield: 2 loaves or 34 1/2-inch slices

Preparation time: 30 minutes

Baking time: 30-40 minutes

Rising time: 40-60 minutes

OATMEAL BREAD

1 cup rolled oats
2 cups boiling water
1 teaspoon salt
1/2 cup molasses
3 tablespoons margarine, soft
2 packages active dry yeast
1/3 cup lukewarm water
6 1/2 to 7 cups all-purpose flour
1 cup raisins

Per slice:
Calories...... 126
Protein (g)... 3
Fat (g)....... 1.1
Sat. Fat (g).. 0.2
Choles. (mg).. 0
Fiber (g)..... 1.3
Sodium (mg)... 73
%Cal-Fat...... 8%

Pour oats into large mixing bowl. Pour boiling water over and soak oats for 1/2 hour. Add salt, molasses and margarine.

Soften yeast in 1/3 cup lukewarm water (100 - 110 degrees). Add to mixing bowl. Add flour and raisins and knead well (about 10 minutes), either by hand or using electric mixer with dough hook. Dough should be elastic, but not sticky.

Place in large greased bowl and let rise in warm place until double in bulk, about 1 hour. Punch down. Divide dough in half, form into two loaves, and place in greased 9 x 5 x 3-inch loaf pans. Let rise until double in bulk, about 30 to 40 minutes.

Bake in 325 degree preheated oven for 50 minutes, or until loaves are golden brown. Remove from pans after 15 minutes. Wrap to keep moist.

Yield: 2 loaves or 36 1/2-inch slices

Preparation time: 40-45 minutes

Baking time: 50 minutes

Rising time: 1 1/2 hours

QUICK FRENCH BREAD

Per slice:
Calories...... 77
Protein (g)... 2
Fat (g)....... 0.6
Sat. Fat (g).. 0.1
Choles. (mg).. 0
Fiber (g)..... 0.6
Sodium (mg)... 100
%Cal-Fat...... 8%

1 package active dry yeast
1 cup warm water (105 - 115 degrees)
1 tablespoon tub margarine
3 1/2 to 3 3/4 cups all-purpose flour, divided
1 teaspoon salt

Glaze (optional):
1 egg substitute (1/4 cup)
1 tablespoon water

Dissolve yeast in warm water. Add margarine.

With steel blade in food processor bowl, add 2 cups flour and salt. Turn machine on and off to combine. Add yeast mixture and process until combined. Gradually add remaining flour and process until dough is no longer sticky and collects into a ball. The dough should be slightly stiff.

Place dough in lightly greased bowl, cover with a towel, and let rise in warm place for 1 hour or until double in size.

Turn the dough out onto a lightly floured board, punch it down, and knead again. Divide the dough in half and form into two loaves. Place shaped loaves on lightly greased baking sheet. Let rise until double in size, about 1 hour.

Mix egg and water to make a glaze. Brush gently over top. Bake in 375 degree oven for 20 to 25 minutes, until loaves are golden brown and sound hollow when tapped.

Yield: 2 medium loaves (24 slices)

This simple dough may also be used to make 2 10-inch pizza crusts.

Preparation time: 20-25 minutes

Baking time: 20-25 minutes

Rising time: 2 hours

ITALIAN OLIVE-ONION BREAD

2 cups whole wheat flour
2 1/2 cups all-purpose flour
2 tablespoons sugar
1 teaspoon salt
2 packages active dry yeast
1 1/4 cups water
2 tablespoons cooking oil
2 egg substitutes (1/2 cup)
1/2 - 1 1/2 cups all-purpose flour
1/2 cup chopped onion
1/3 cup green pimiento olives, coarsely chopped
1/3 cup black olives, coarsely chopped

Place wheat flour, 2 1/2 cups all-purpose flour, sugar, salt, and yeast in mixing bowl. (An electric mixer, fitted with dough hook, works best.) Mix well.

Combine water and oil in small saucepan. Heat over low heat until very warm (120 - 130 degrees F.)

Gradually add warm liquid to flour mixture, mixing well. Add egg substitutes and mix until well blended.

Combine 1/2 cup flour with chopped onion and olives. Add to mixing bowl and mix until olives and onions are blended throughout.

Add remaining flour, 1/2 cup at a time, and knead until dough becomes smooth and elastic. (If using an electric mixer, dough should no longer stick to sides of bowl. Knead with dough hook for 7 to 10 minutes.)

Place in a lightly greased bowl, turning to grease top. Cover and let rise in a warm place until doubled in size, about 1 hour.

Punch dough down and divide in half. Shape each half into a loaf. Place each loaf in a non-stick 8 1/2 x 4 1/2 x 2 1/2-inch loaf pan. Bake at 375 degrees for 25 to 30 minutes. Cool slightly. Remove from pans and cool on wire racks.

Yield: 2 loaves, or 34 slices

Preparation time: 30-35 minutes

Cooking time: 25-30 minutes

Rising time: 1 hour

Per 1/2-inch slice:
Calories...... 82
Protein (g)... 3
Fat (g)....... 1.4
Sat. Fat (g).. 0.1
Choles. (mg).. 0
Fiber (g)..... 1.8
Sodium (mg)... 100
%Cal-Fat...... 16%

PESTO-ONION BREAD

Per 1-inch slice:
Calories...... 73
Protein (g)... 2
Fat (g)....... 1.4
Sat. Fat (g).. 0.3
Choles. (mg).. 0
Fiber (g)..... 0.6
Sodium (mg)... 130
%Cal-Fat...... 17%

Dough for "Quick French Bread"
Pesto-Onion Filling:
1 cup fresh basil (loosely packed), chopped finely, or
   2 tablespoons dried
2 tablespoons egg substitutes
1 tablespoon olive oil
2 cloves garlic, crushed
1/4 teaspoon salt
1/2 cup onion, minced
3 tablespoons grated Parmesan cheese

Prepare dough for "Quick French Bread" (Recipe, page 347).

While dough is rising, prepare Pesto-Onion filling: Chop basil finely and combine with remaining ingredients.

After dough has risen for the first time, punch it down, and knead slightly. With a rolling pin press dough into a rectangle, about 11 x 14 inches.

Spread the basil-onion mixture over the dough, up to 1-inch from the edges. Starting with a long side, roll the dough into a cylinder. Place the cylinder in a crescent shape, seam side down, on a lightly greased cookie sheet. With a sharp knife, cut half way down through the dough at one-inch intervals. Allow the dough to rise for about 15 minutes.

Bake in preheated 400 degree oven 20–25 minutes or until bread is browned and sounds hollow when tapped on top.

Place bread on a rack to cool slightly. Serve warm for the best flavor.

Yield: 2 crescent-shaped loaves (24 slices).

Preparation time: 40–45 minutes.

Baking time: 20–25 minutes

Rising time: 1 hour, 15 minutes

DATE-NUT BREAD

1 8-ounce package chopped dates
2 teaspoons baking soda
2 cups boiling water
1 3/4 cups sugar
1/2 teaspoon salt
1/2 cup egg substitutes, slightly beaten
3 cups all-purpose flour
1 cup whole wheat flour
2 teaspoons baking powder
2 teaspoons vanilla
1/2 cup natural applesauce
1/2 cup walnuts, chopped

Per 1/2-inch slice:
Calories...... 131
Protein (g)... 2
Fat (g)....... 1.5
Sat. Fat (g).. 0.2
Choles. (mg).. 0
Fiber (g)..... 1.3
Sodium (mg)... 146
%Cal-Fat...... 10%

Preheat oven to 350 degrees.

Mix baking soda and dates in large mixing bowl. Add boiling water. Cool slightly.

After it cools, add sugar, salt and eggs. Mix well.

Combine all-purpose flour, wheat flour and baking powder. Add to date mixture. Add vanilla. Fold in applesauce and chopped walnuts.

Lightly spray two 8 1/2 x 4 1/2 x 2 1/2-inch non-stick loaf pans with a vegetable cooking spray. Pour batter into loaf pans. Bake at 350 degrees 55 to 60 minutes. Test for doneness by inserting toothpick into center of loaf. If toothpick comes out clean, it is done.

Yield: 2 loaves or 34 slices

Preparation time: 20-25 minutes

Cooking time: 55-60 minutes

LEMON TEA BREAD

1/2 cup whole wheat flour
1 1/2 cups all-purpose flour
3/4 cup sugar
2 1/2 teaspoons baking powder
1/4 teaspoon salt
3/4 cup skim milk
1/4 cup canola oil
2 egg substitutes (1/2 cup)
1 teaspoon grated lemon peel
1/2 cup chopped walnuts (optional)

Glaze:
2 teaspoons freshly squeezed lemon juice
1 tablespoon skim milk
Confectioners' sugar

Preheat oven to 350 degrees.

Combine the first five dry ingredients in large bowl. Stir until blended. Set aside.

Combine milk, canola oil and eggs in medium-size bowl. Add milk mixture to dry ingredients, mixing until well moistened. Stir in grated lemon peel, and walnuts, if desired.

Pour into non-stick loaf pan 8 1/2 x 4 1/2 x 2 1/2-inches. Bake in 350 degree oven 45 to 55 minutes or until done. Let cool for 10 minutes before removing from pan.

Meanwhile, make lemon glaze: Combine lemon juice and milk in a small bowl. Add enough powdered sugar to make a thick frosting. Spread the glaze over warm bread.

Bread may be served warm or cool. After it has reached room temperature, wrap and store in refrigerator.

Yield: l loaf, 17 1/2-inch slices

Preparation time: 25 minutes

Cooking time: 45-55 minutes

PUMPKIN BREAD

2 1/2 cups sugar
4 egg substitutes (1 cup)
3 1/2 cups all-purpose flour
1/2 teaspoon baking powder
2 teaspoons baking soda
1/2 teaspoon salt
1 1/2 teaspoons pumpkin pie spice
1/4 teaspoon cinnamon
1/3 cup canola oil
2/3 cup water
1 16-ounce can pumpkin

Per 1/3-inch slice:
Calories...... 82
Protein (g)... 1
Fat (g)....... 1.6
Sat. Fat (g).. 0.1
Choles. (mg).. 0
Fiber (g)..... 0.4
Sodium (mg)... 63
%Cal-Fat...... 17%

Preheat oven to 325 degrees.

In large mixing bowl, cream together sugar and eggs.

In another bowl, combine flour, baking powder, baking soda, salt and spices, mixing well.

Add dry ingredients, oil, water, and pumpkin to mixing bowl. Mix thoroughly with electric mixer.

Spray bottoms of two 9 x 5 x 3-inch loaf pans with a vegetable cooking spray. Pour batter evenly into both pans. Bake as 325 degrees for 65 to 75 minutes, or until toothpick inserted into center of loaf comes out clean. Cool. Remove from pans.

Yield: 2 loaves, or 54 slices

This is a delicious sweet bread that is low in fat, very moist and high in vitamin A. It tastes great toasted.

Preparation time: 20 minutes

Cooking time: 65-75 minutes

BANANA NUT BREAD

3/4 cup sugar
1 1/2 teaspoons baking soda
2 cups all-purpose flour
1/4 teaspoon salt
2 egg substitutes (1/2 cup)
1/4 cup canola oil
1/4 cup natural applesauce
1 teaspoon vanilla
3 tablespoons skim milk
3 ripe bananas, pureed
1/4 cup chopped walnuts

Preheat oven to 350 degrees.

Spray a 9 x 5 x 3-inch loaf pan with a vegetable cooking spray.

Combine sugar, baking soda, flour and salt in large mixing bowl. Mix well.

In a small mixing bowl, combine eggs (slightly beaten), canola oil, applesauce, vanilla and milk. Add egg mixture to dry ingredients. Add pureed bananas. Stir until combined, but do not over mix. Fold in walnuts.

Pour into loaf pan and bake at 350 degrees 40 to 50 minutes, or until toothpick inserted in center of loaf comes out clean.

Yield: 1 large loaf or 27 slices (1/3-inch thick).

Preparation time: 20 minutes

Cooking time: 40-50 minutes

ORANGE CORN BREAD

1 cup all-purpose flour
1 cup yellow cornmeal
1/2 teaspoon baking soda
1 tablespoon baking powder
1/3 cup sugar
1/4 cup orange juice
2 egg substitutes (1/2 cup)
1 cup skim milk
2 tablespoons canola or safflower oil

Per serving:
Calories...... 103
Protein (g)... 3
Fat (g)....... 2.2
Sat. Fat (g).. 0.2
Choles. (mg).. 0
Fiber (g)..... 0.8
Sodium (mg)... 106
%Cal-Fat...... 19%

Preheat oven to 425 degrees.

Combine dry ingredients in large mixing bowl. Set aside.

Combine remaining ingredients in medium-size mixing bowl. Add orange juice mixture to dry ingredients and stir until well moistened.

Pour into non-stick 9 x 9 x 2-inch pan. Bake at 425 degrees for 20 to 25 minutes. May be served warm or cold.

Yield: 16 2-inch square pieces.

Preparation time: 10-15 minutes

Cooking time: 20-25 minutes

GARLIC CRUSTINOS

1 French baguette (long, narrow French bread)
Vegetable cooking spray
Garlic salt

Per 2 slices:
Calories...... 30
Protein (g)... 1
Fat (g)....... 0.4
Sat. Fat (g).. 0
Choles. (mg).. 0
Fiber (g)..... 0.3
Sodium (mg)... 125
%Cal-Fat...... 12%

Preheat oven to 275 degrees.

Slice bread into 1/4-inch thick slices (as many slices as desired). Place slices on cookie sheet; spray them with vegetable cooking spray and sprinkle with garlic salt.

Bake at 275 degrees for 15 minutes, or until bread becomes

very crisp. Serve warm or at room temperature. After bread has cooled completely, store in air-tight container to keep crisp.

Yield: As desired

These crustinos are delicious served with soup, especially Bouillabaisse.

Preparation time: 5 minutes

Cooking time: 15 minutes

OAT BRAN-APPLE MUFFINS

1 1/4 cups oat bran cereal
1 cup oatmeal
1 1/4 cups all-purpose flour
1/2 cup brown sugar
1 teaspoon cinnamon
3 teaspoons baking powder
2 egg substitutes (1/2 cup)
1 cup skim milk
2 tablespoons canola oil
1 cup chunky applesauce

Preheat oven to 375 degrees.

In large bowl combine oat bran, oatmeal, flour, brown sugar, cinnamon, and baking powder.

In medium-size bowl, lightly beat egg substitutes. Stir in skim milk, canola oil, and applesauce until well blended.

Stir milk mixture into flour mixture until just moistened. Spoon batter into muffin tins lined with paper bake cups. Bake at 375 degrees for 15 to 20 minutes, or until lightly browned.

Yield: 16 to 18 muffins

Preparation time: 15-20 minutes

Cooking time: 15-20 minutes

Per serving:
Calories...... 122
Protein (g)... 4
Fat (g)....... 2.9
Sat. Fat (g).. 0.4
Choles. (mg).. 0
Fiber (g)..... 1.7
Sodium (mg)... 96
%Cal-Fat...... 21%

SOUTHERN-STYLE SPOON BREAD

2 cups skim milk
1/2 cup yellow cornmeal
1 tablespoon tub margarine
3/4 teaspoon salt
1 tablespoon sugar
1/2 teaspoon baking powder
2 egg whites

Preheat oven to 325 degrees.

Scald milk in top of double boiler. Gradually stir in corn meal with a wire whisk. Cook over medium heat until thickened, stirring frequently. Add margarine, salt, sugar and baking powder. Mix well.

Beat egg whites until stiff peaks form. Fold into cornmeal mixture. Spoon into nonstick 8 x 8-inch baking dish. Bake at 325 degrees for 30 minutes, or until mixture is set.

To serve, spoon onto plates.

Yield: 6 servings

Consistency is similar to a thick pudding.

Preparation time: 20-25 minutes

Cooking time: 30 minutes

Per serving:
Calories...... 101
Protein (g)... 5
Fat (g)....... 2.2
Sat. Fat (g).. 0.5
Choles. (mg).. 1
Fiber (g)..... 0.9
Sodium (mg)... 378
%Cal-Fat...... 20%

BLUEBERRY MUFFINS

Per serving:
Calories...... 143
Protein (g)... 3
Fat (g)....... 2.7
Sat. Fat (g).. 0.2
Choles. (mg).. 0
Fiber (g)..... 1
Sodium (mg)... 149
%Cal-Fat...... 17%

2 cups all-purpose flour
1/2 cup sugar
3 teaspoons baking powder
1/4 teaspoon salt
1 cup skim milk
1 egg substitute (1/4 cup)
2 tablespoons canola oil
1/4 cup natural applesauce
1 cup fresh or frozen blueberries, unthawed

Preheat oven to 400 degrees.

Combine flour, sugar, baking powder and salt in large mixing bowl. Mix well.

Combine milk, egg substitute, canola oil and applesauce. Add all at once to flour mixture. Mix just until moistened. Carefully fold in blueberries.

Spray non-stick muffin pans with cooking spray, or line with paper bake cups. Spoon batter into 12 muffin forms, filling 2/3 full. Bake at 400 degrees for 20 minutes or until golden brown. Remove from tin after 20 minutes.

Yield: 12 muffins

You may also use a 15-ounce can of blueberries in syrup, drained and rinsed. However, because they are softer, when you fold them into the batter, the blue color from the blueberry juice will marble throughout the batter.

Preparation time: 15 minutes

Cooking time: 20 minutes

CARROT BRAN MUFFINS

1 cup all-purpose flour
1 cup whole wheat flour
1/2 cup sugar
l tablespoon baking powder
1/2 teaspoon baking soda
1/4 teaspoon salt
2 egg whites
1 cup skim milk
1/4 cup natural applesauce
1 tablespoon canola oil
1 8-ounce can crushed pineapple, drained (no sugar
   added)
1 cup finely grated carrot
1/2 cup raisins

Per serving:
Calories...... 128
Protein (g)... 3
Fat (g)....... 1.2
Sat. Fat (g).. 0.1
Choles. (mg).. 0
Fiber (g)..... 2
Sodium (mg)... 140
%Cal-Fat...... 8%

Preheat oven to 400 degrees.

Grate carrots and set aside.

In large bowl combine flours, sugar, baking powder, baking soda and salt.

In medium-size bowl, lightly beat egg whites with a wire whisk or fork. Stir in milk, applesauce and canola oil until well blended.

Stir milk mixture into flour mixture just until moistened.

Fold in drained pineapple, grated carrots and raisins.

Spoon batter into non-stick muffin tins. Bake at 400 degrees for 15 to 20 minutes, or until golden brown and top springs back when touched.

Yield: 12 to 18 muffins, depending on size.

Ideal for a snack with either fruit juice or milk.

Preparation time: 20-25 minutes

Cooking time: 15-20 minutes

BRAN MUFFINS

Per serving:
Calories...... 120
Protein (g)... 3
Fat (g)....... 2
Sat. Fat (g).. 0.2
Choles. (mg).. 0
Fiber (g)..... 3.1
Sodium (mg)... 196
%Cal-Fat...... 15%

1 1/2 cups 100% wheat bran cereal
1 1/4 cups skim milk
1 1/4 cups all-purpose flour
1/2 cup sugar
1/4 teaspoon salt
1 tablespoon baking powder
1 teaspoon cinnamon
1/2 teaspoon ground cloves
1/2 teaspoon nutmeg
1 egg substitute (1/4 cup)
2 tablespoons canola oil
1/2 cup natural applesauce
1/2 to 3/4 cup raisins

Preheat oven to 375 degrees.

Combine cereal and milk in large mixing bowl. Let soak 5 to 10 minutes, or until cereal softens.

Meanwhile, stir together flour, sugar, salt, baking powder, cinnamon, cloves and nutmeg.

Add egg substitute, canola oil and applesauce to cereal mixture. Mix well. Add dry ingredients and mix just until moistened. Stir in raisins.

Prepare muffin tins by spraying with cooking spray or line with paper bake cups. Fill each muffin tin 2/3 full. Bake in preheated 375 degree oven for 15 to 20 minutes, or until golden brown.

Yield: 16 muffins.

For variety, raisins may be omitted, or other fruits may be substituted for the raisins, such as drained crushed pineapple or chopped dates.

Preparation time: 20 minutes

Cooking time: 15-20 minutes

CRUSTLESS SPINACH QUICHE

8 egg substitutes (2 cups)
1 12-ounce can evaporated skim milk
1/2 teaspoon salt
1/8 teaspoon cayenne pepper
1/2 teaspoon ground nutmeg
2 teaspoons olive oil
1/4 cup chopped onion
2 10-ounce packages frozen chopped spinach, thawed
   and drained (squeezed dry)
1 cup (4 ounces) shredded Swiss or Cheddar cheese
   (reduced-calorie)
2 tablespoons flour

Preheat oven to 350 degrees.

Combine egg substitutes, milk, salt, pepper and nutmeg in large mixing bowl. Beat slightly. Set aside.

Heat olive oil in medium-size saucepan. Add onion and saute until onion becomes translucent. Mix thawed and drained spinach with sauteed onion. Add to egg mixture.

Toss grated cheese with flour.

Sprinkle cheese evenly into two greased and floured 9-inch pie pans. Pour egg mixture over top.

Bake at 350 degrees for 40 to 45 minutes.

Yield: 16 servings (8 servings per pie).

Other ingredients may be added or substituted, such as lean ham, mushrooms, etc.

Preparation time: 20 minutes

Cooking time: 40-45 minutes

Per serving:
Calories...... 80
Protein (g)... 7
Fat (g)....... 3
Sat. Fat (g).. 1
Choles. (mg).. 1
Fiber (g)..... 1
Sodium (mg)... 215
%Cal Fat...... 33%

MAKE-AHEAD FRENCH TOAST

Per serving:
Calories...... 143
Protein (g)... 7
Fat (g)....... 2
Sat. Fat (g).. 0.4
Choles. (mg).. 1
Fiber (g)..... 0.6
Sodium (mg)... 199
%Cal-Fat...... 13%

4 egg substitutes (1 cup)
1/2 cup orange juice
1/4 cup skim milk
1/4 cup sugar
1/2 teaspoon vanilla
1/4 teaspoon ground nutmeg
8 slices French or Italian bread (3/4-inch thick)
Butter-flavored vegetable spray

Combine first six ingredients in medium-size bowl.

Arrange slices of bread in a single layer in a 9 x 13-inch pan or a jelly-roll pan. Pour egg mixture over the bread. Cover and refrigerator overnight.

The next morning, preheat oven to 400 degrees.

Spray a 9 x 13-inch pan or jelly-roll pan with a butter-flavored cooking spray. Transfer soaked bread slices to pan, arranging in a single layer.

Bake at 400 degrees for 20 minutes. Turn bread slices. Bake an additional 5 minutes.

Serve with lite syrup or warmed, cooked fruit over top.

Yield: 8 slices French toast

An ideal make-ahead breakfast for Sunday mornings or when entertaining out-of-town guests for the weekend.

Preparation time: 10-15 minutes

Cooking time: 25 minutes

CINNAMON FRENCH TOAST

4 egg substitutes (1 cup)
1/2 cup skim milk
1 teaspoon sugar
1/2 teaspoon cinnamon
8 slices whole wheat bread
Vegetable cooking spray

Spray skillet or griddle with cooking spray and place on stove at medium setting.

Combine egg substitutes, milk, sugar and cinnamon in shallow mixing bowl. Mix well.

Dip slices of bread in egg mixture and fry in preheated skillet or griddle until brown on both sides. Serve hot with syrup, and if desired, a small scraping of margarine.

Yield: 8 servings (1 slice each)

Preparation time: 10-15 minutes

Per serving:
Calories...... 104
Protein (g)... 7
Fat (g)....... 2.3
Sat. Fat (g).. 0.6
Choles. (mg).. 0
Fiber (g)..... 2.1
Sodium (mg)... 250
%Cal-Fat...... 19%

Desserts

CHOCOLATE BROWNIE PUDDING CAKE

2 1/2 cups all-purpose flour
1 1/2 cups sugar
1 teaspoon baking soda
1 teaspoon baking powder
1/2 teaspoon salt
3 tablespoons cocoa powder
2 egg whites, slightly beaten
1 1/4 cups skim milk
1 1/2 teaspoons lemon juice
3/4 teaspoon vanilla
1/2 cup chopped pecans
Amaretto Custard Sauce (Recipe, page 393)

Combine first six ingredients (dry ingredients) in a large mixing bowl. Stir to blend evenly. Add slightly beaten egg whites and skim milk, stirring until dry ingredients are moistened and batter is smooth. You may use an electric mixer. Stir in lemon juice, vanilla and pecans.

Spray a 1 1/2-quart pudding mold* with a vegetable cooking spray. Pour batter into mold and cover tightly with lid; or pour batter into a well-greased heatproof bowl and cover with a double layer of aluminum foil. Secure with string.

Position mold on a 1-inch rack in a large kettle placed over medium heat. Add boiling water, filling kettle one-third full. Cover and steam 2 1/4 hours. Water should boil gently during this time. Add more boiling water if necessary.

Lift mold from kettle. Remove lid to allow steam to escape. After 15 minutes, loosen sides with a knife and invert onto serving dish. Serve warm or cold with Amaretto Custard Sauce.

Yield: 8 to 10 servings.

A pudding mold is a metal dome-shaped mold with a lid that fastens down with clamps. It can be purchased at most kitchen accessory stores.

Preparation time: 20-25 minutes

Cooking time: 2 1/4 hours

CHOCOLATE CHIP BUNDT CAKE

2 1/2 cups all-purpose flour
2 cups sugar
1 cup cocoa powder
2 teaspoons baking soda
2 teaspoons baking powder
1/2 teaspoon salt
5 egg whites
1 1/3 cups skim milk
1 cup boiling water
2/3 cup applesauce
2 1/2 teaspoons vanilla
1/4 cup mini-chocolate chips (2 ounces)

Per serving with frosting:
Calories...... 182
Protein (g)... 3
Fat (g)....... 2.5
Sat. Fat (g).. 1
Choles. (mg).. 0
Fiber (g) 1.5
Sodium (mg)... 173
%Cal-Fat...... 10%

Preheat oven to 350 degrees.

Spray a 10-inch non-stick bundt pan with vegetable cooking spray.

Combine first six ingredients (dry ingredients) in a large mixing bowl. Mix well. Add remaining ingredients except chocolate chips. Beat at high speed for two minutes. Batter will be thin.

Pour into bundt pan. Sprinkle chocolate chips over top. Stir in slightly, letting some chips sink into batter. Bake at 350 degrees 40 to 50 minutes, or until toothpick inserted into center of cake comes out clean. Cool for 15 minutes before removing from pan. Cool completely before frosting with Chocolate-Coffee Frosting.

CHOCOLATE-COFFEE FROSTING
2 tablespoons light margarine, melted
1/2 teaspoon instant coffee grounds
2 cups powdered sugar
1/4 cup cocoa powder
Skim milk as needed (3 to 4 tablespoons)

In small bowl, melt margarine in microwave. Dissolve coffee grounds in melted margarine.

In mixing bowl, combine powdered sugar, margarine mixture, cocoa powder and 3 tablespoons skim milk. Beat until smooth. Add more milk as needed until desired consistency.

Yield: 24 servings.

Chocolate lovers will delight in this rich, moist chocolate cake.

Preparation time: 30 minutes

Cooking time: 45 minutes

CHOCOLATE ANGEL FOOD CAKE

Per serving:
Calories...... 123
Protein (g)... 3
Fat (g)....... 0.4
Sat. Fat (g).. 0.2
Choles. (mg).. 0
Fiber (g)..... 0.3
Sodium (mg)... 38
%Cal-Fat...... 3%

12 egg whites
1 1/2 teaspoons cream of tartar
2 teaspoons vanilla
1 cup sugar
1 cup sifted cake flour
1/3 cup unsweetened cocoa powder
3/4 cup sugar
1/4 teaspoon ground cinnamon
Amaretto Custard Sauce (Recipe, page 393)

Preheat oven to 375 degrees.

With an electric mixer, beat egg whites until foamy. Add cream of tartar. Beat until soft peaks form. Add vanilla, and gradually add 1 cup sugar. Beat until stiff peaks form.

Sift together flour, cocoa, 3/4 cup sugar and cinnamon. Fold into whites. Spoon batter into ungreased 10-inch tube pan.

Bake at 375 degrees for 35 to 40 minutes or until done.

Invert cake pan immediately and cool for 40 minutes. Loosen cake from sides and remove.

To serve, cut cake into slices. Top each slice with Amaretto Custard Sauce.

Yield: 16 servings

Preparation time: 20 minutes

Cooking time: 35-40 minutes

AMARETTO FUDGE CAKE

1 3/4 cups all-purpose flour
1 1/2 cups sugar
3/4 cup cocoa powder
1 1/2 teaspoons baking soda
1 1/2 teaspoons baking powder
1/2 teaspoon salt
4 egg whites
2/3 cup skim milk
1/3 cup Amaretto liqueur
1/2 cup applesauce
2 teaspoons vanilla
1 teaspoon almond extract
3/4 cup boiling water
1/4 cup mini-chocolate chips (2 ounces)
1/2 cup dark raisins (optional)

Per serving:
Calories...... 227
Protein (g)... 4
Fat (g)....... 1.8
Sat. Fat (g).. 0.8
Choles. (mg).. 0
Fiber (g)..... 1.8
Sodium (mg)... 297
%Cal-Fat...... 8%

Preheat oven to 325 degrees.

Spray a 9-inch springform pan with vegetable cooking spray. Combine the first six ingredients (dry ingredients) in a large mixing bowl. Mix well. Add remaining ingredients except chocolate chips and raisins. Beat at high speed for two minutes. Batter will be very thin.

Pour into springform pan. Sprinkle chocolate chips and raisins, if desired, evenly over top. (most of them will sink to the bottom.) Bake at 325 degrees 50 to 60 minutes, or until top of cake is firm to the touch.

Cool at least 30 minutes. Loosen edges of cake with knife before removing sides of springform pan. Cover to keep moist.

Yield: 12 servings

This cake resembles a chocolate cheesecake in its rich fudginess. The top may crack slightly, similar to a cheesecake.

Preparation time: 25-30 minutes

Cooking time: 50-60 minutes

NEW ORLEANS BREAD PUDDING

1 10-ounce loaf stale French bread (very hard)
1 12-ounce can evaporated skim milk
2 1/2 cups skim milk
4 egg substitutes (1 cup), slightly beaten
2 cups sugar
2 tablespoons vanilla extract
1 teaspoon cinnamon
3/4 cup golden raisins
1 apple, peeled and diced
1 tablespoon margarine, melted
Hard Sauce (optional)* (Recipe, page 392)

Preheat oven to 350 degrees.

In large mixing bowl, crumble bread into bite-size pieces. Pour evaporated milk and skim milk over bread. Soak until bread is completely softened.

Meanwhile, combine eggs, sugar, vanilla, cinnamon, raisins and diced apple. Add to bread mixture.

Spread melted margarine in bottom of 9 x 13-inch baking pan. Add bread pudding mixture, and bake until it is firm to the touch and the top is golden brown, approximately 40 to 45 minutes.

Cool slightly and cut into 3-inch squares. Serve either warm or cold. Place on individual dessert dishes. Drizzle Hard Sauce over top, if desired. Store in refrigerator.

Yield: 15 servings

The hard sauce converts a simple bread pudding into a rich, elegant dessert.

Preparation time: 25-35 minutes

Cooking time: 40-45 minutes

CARROT CAKE

1 1/2 cups sugar
1 1/2 cups all-purpose flour
1 cup whole wheat flour
1 1/2 teaspoons baking soda
1 1/2 teaspoons baking powder
1/2 teaspoon salt
2 teaspoons cinnamon
1 teaspoon allspice
4 egg whites
3/4 cup skim milk
1/2 cup natural applesauce
2 teaspoons vanilla
3/4 cup boiling water
2 cups finely shredded carrots (2 to 3 carrots)
Cream Cheese Frosting

Preheat oven to 375 degrees.

Grate carrots. Set aside.

Combine sugar, flours, baking soda, baking powder, salt, cinnamon and allspice in a large mixing bowl. Blend together well.

To same mixing bowl, add egg whites, milk, applesauce, vanilla and boiling water. Beat at high speed for 2 minutes. Fold in grated carrots.

Spray 10-inch bundt pan with vegetable cooking spray. Pour in batter. Bake at 375 degrees 35 to 40 minutes, or until toothpick inserted in center comes out clean. Remove from oven and cool slightly. Loosen edges of cake and invert onto serving plate. After cake is cooled completely, frost with Cream Cheese Frosting.

CREAM CHEESE FROSTING
3 ounces light cream cheese
1 tablespoon margarine
1 teaspoon vanilla
2 cups powdered sugar
3 tablespoons chopped walnuts

Mix together all ingredients except walnuts. Add small amount of skim milk if necessary for proper spreading consistency.

Per serving:
Calories...... 156
Protein (g)... 3
Fat (g)....... 1.8
Sat. Fat (g).. 0.7
Choles. (mg).. 4
Fiber (g)..... 1.3
Sodium (mg)... 148
%Cal-Fat...... 11%

Spread frosting on cake. Immediately sprinkle walnuts over top. (If you wait even a few minutes before sprinkling walnuts, frosting will be set, and the nuts will slip off.)

Yield: 24 servings

Preparation time: 35-40 minutes

Cooking time: 35-40 minutes

BANANAS FOSTER

4 bananas
2 tablespoons tub margarine
1/4 cup firmly packed brown sugar
Cinnamon
1/4 cup banana liqueur
1/4 cup light rum or brandy
4 large scoops vanilla frozen yogurt, or nonfat ice cream

Cut bananas in half crosswise; then slit down the middle. Set aside.

In saute pan, melt margarine with brown sugar. Heat until mixture begins to boil. Add bananas and saute until tender but still firm, about 1 1/2 to 2 minutes. Sprinkle with cinnamon.

Pour liqueur and rum or brandy over bananas. Heat until liqueur becomes very hot and ignite with a match.

As soon as flames disappear, serve immediately over frozen yogurt or nonfat ice cream.

Yield: 4 servings

Because of the spectacular flames from the ignited alcohol, this is an impressive dessert to serve. Since the flames shoot up fairly high, do not ignite near anything flammable.

Preparation time: 15-20 minutes

Per serving:
Calories...... 434
Protein (g)... 6
Fat (g)....... 6.5
Sat. Fat (g).. 1.5
Choles. (mg).. 0
Fiber (g)..... 2
Sodium (mg)... 155
%Cal-Fat...... 13%

STEAMED DATE-NUT PUDDING

2 cups all-purpose flour
1 cup sugar
1 teaspoon baking soda
1 teaspoon baking powder
2 egg whites, slightly beaten
1 cup skim milk
1 1/2 teaspoons lemon juice
3/4 cup chopped dates
1/2 cup chopped pecans
Brandy Sauce (Recipe, page 392)

Per serving:
Calories...... 277
Protein (g)... 5
Fat (g)....... 4.8
Sat. Fat (g).. 0.5
Choles. (mg).. 0
Fiber (g)..... 2.3
Sodium (mg)... 154
%Cal-Fat...... 15%

Combine flour, sugar, baking soda, and baking powder in a large mixing bowl. Add slightly beaten egg whites and skim milk, stirring until dry ingredients are moistened. Stir in lemon juice, dates and pecans. (If chopping your own dates, mix with 1 tablespoon flour, to avoid sticking together.)

Spray a 1 1/2-quart pudding mold* with a vegetable cooking spray. Pour batter into mold and cover tightly with lid; or pour batter into a well-greased heatproof bowl and cover with a double layer of aluminum foil. Secure with string.

Position mold on a 1-inch rack in a large kettle placed over medium heat. Add boiling water, filling kettle one-third full. Cover and steam 2 1/4 hours. Water should boil gently during this time. Add more boiling water if necessary.

Lift mold from kettle. Remove lid to allow steam to escape. After 15 minutes, loosen sides with knife and invert onto serving dish. Garnish with twisted lemon slices and serve warm or cold. To serve, place slice of pudding cake on dessert plate and top with Brandy Sauce.

Yield: 8 to 10 servings.

*A pudding mold is a metal dome-shaped mold with a lid that fastens down with clamps. It comes in various sizes and can be purchased at most kitchen accessory stores.

Preparation time: 20 minutes

Cooking time: 2 1/4 hours

MOCK CHERRY CHEESECAKE

Per serving:
Calories...... 260
Protein (g)... 8
Fat (g)....... 2.6
Sat. Fat (g).. 1
Choles. (mg).. 2
Fiber (g)..... 0.5
Sodium (mg)... 221
%Cal-Fat...... 9%

2 cups sugar
6 egg substitutes (1 1/2 cups)
2 teaspoons vanilla
3/4 cup self-rising flour
1 1/2 tablespoons yellow cornmeal
17 ounces evaporated skim milk
1/4 cup lemon juice
2 tablespoons light margarine, melted
1 21-ounce can cherry pie filling

Preheat oven to 350 degrees. Line outside of 9-inch springform pan with aluminum foil, shiny side out. (This is to slow down cooking process and minimize cracking of top.)

Combine all ingredients, except cherry pie filling, in large blender or food processor. Process on high until smooth and slightly foamy.

Pour into prepared springform pan. Bake at 350 degrees for 60 to 70 minutes, or until cheesecake is set (firm in center) and top is golden brown. Cool to room temperature.

Carefully remove sides from springform pan. Spoon cherry pie filling over cheesecake to within 1/2-inch of outside edge. Cover and refrigerate until ready to serve.

Yield: 12 to 14 servings

The batter is very thin so springform pan may leak slightly. This should not be a problem because the aluminum foil will catch any drips that may occur.

Preparation time: 10-15 minutes

Cooking time: 50-60 minutes

LEMON CUSTARD DELIGHT

1 cup sugar
3 tablespoons self-rising flour
1 cup skim milk
2 teaspoons canola oil
2 teaspoons egg substitute
2 drops yellow food coloring
1/4 teaspoon salt
Juice and grated zest of 1 lemon*
2 egg whites

Per serving:
Calories...... 179
Protein (g)... 3
Fat (g)....... 1.7
Sat. Fat (g).. 0.2
Choles. (mg).. 0
Fiber (g)..... 0.2
Sodium (mg)... 182
%Cal-Fat...... 8%

Preheat oven to 350 degrees.

In a medium-size bowl, combine sugar and flour. Mix well with a wire whisk. Add milk, canola oil, egg substitute, food coloring, salt, grated zest and lemon juice. Mix well with wire whisk.

In separate bowl, beat egg whites until stiff. Gently fold whites into lemon mixture until lumps have disappeared. Spoon mixture into 6 3-inch ramekins.

Set ramekins in a 9 x 13-inch pan and add hot water until it is halfway up the sides of the ramekins. Carefully place in oven and bake for 30 to 35 minutes or until a knife blade can be inserted into the center of ramekin and come out clean. Remove from oven. Cool 30 minutes. Invert ramekins onto a dessert plate. Serve immediately or make ahead and chill. Garnish with a twisted lemon slice and a sprig of fresh mint.

Yield: 6 servings

A zest of lemon is a small piece of the lemon peel. This dessert forms a light fluffy cake on the bottom and a rich "creamy" custard on top.

Preparation time: 25-30 minutes

Cooking time: 30-35 minutes

HAMILTON PIE

5 egg whites
1 teaspoon vanilla
1 cup sugar
1 package (36 crackers) nonfat soda crackers
1 teaspoon baking powder
1 can pressurized light whipping cream
3 cups fresh raspberries
4-6 tablespoons Chambord* or Amaretto liqueur

Preheat oven to 325 degrees. Spray 9-inch pie pan with vegetable cooking spray, covering surface well.

In large mixing bowl, beat egg whites until soft peaks form. Add vanilla. Gradually add sugar and continue beating until very stiff peaks form. Set aside.

Crush soda crackers with rolling pin. Transfer cracker crumbs to medium-size mixing bowl. Add baking powder to crumbs and mix well. Carefully fold crumb mixture into egg whites.

Pour into pie plate and bake at 325 degrees for 25 minutes, or until top is light golden brown. Cool completely.

Meanwhile wash raspberries. To serve, cut pie into eighths and place on individual plates. Top with whipping cream (about 1/4 cup per serving) and raspberries. Spoon approximately 2 teaspoons liqueur over each serving. Serve immediately.

Yield: 8 servings

A light, elegant dessert, which also tastes excellent with blackberries, blueberries or strawberries.

*Chambord is a raspberry-flavored liqueur.

Preparation time: 20 minutes

Cooking time: 25 minutes

STRAWBERRY SHORTCAKE

1 pint fresh strawberries, sliced
2 tablespoons sugar
1 1/4 cups all-purpose flour
2 tablespoons sugar
1 1/2 teaspoons baking powder
1/4 teaspoon salt
2 tablespoons light margarine
1 egg substitute (1/4 cup)
2 tablespoons skim milk
3 tablespoons natural applesauce
1 teaspoon finely shredded lemon peel (optional)
Vanilla frozen yogurt, nonfat or low-fat (optional)

Per serving:
Calories...... 221
Protein (g)... 6
Fat (g)....... 5.4
Sat. Fat (g).. 1.1
Choles. (mg).. 0
Fiber (g)..... 2.7
Sodium (mg)... 363
%Cal-Fat...... 22%

Preheat oven to 450 degrees.

Wash and slice strawberries. Sprinkle 2 tablespoons sugar over top and toss lightly. Sprinkle with 1 tablespoon water. Set aside.

Combine flour, 2 tablespoons sugar, baking powder and salt. Stir to blend. Cut in margarine with a pastry cutter until the consistency of course crumbs. Add egg substitute, milk, applesauce and lemon peel. Mix together, just until blended. Do not overmix. Divide dough into four equal portions. On a floured surface, roll each portion into a ball and flatten into a circle about 1/2-inch thick. Place on lightly greased cookie sheet and bake at 450 degrees for 8 to 10 minutes, or until golden. Remove from baking sheet and cool. Slit each biscuit.

Assemble 4 individual shortcakes. Place lower halves of biscuits on plates, followed by 1/2 of strawberries, then upper halves of biscuits, followed by remaining strawberries.

Top with vanilla frozen yogurt, if desired.

Yield: Serves 4

Preparation time: 20-30 minutes

Cooking time: 8-10 minutes

FROZEN YOGURT CHARLOTTE

Per serving:
Calories...... 254
Protein (g)... 6
Fat (g)....... 4.7
Sat. Fat (g).. NA
Choles. (mg).. 11
Fiber (g)..... 0.1
Sodium (mg)... 116
%Cal-Fat...... 17%

24 ladyfingers, split (2 packages)
1/4 cup Amaretto liqueur
1/2 cup chocolate wafer crumbs, divided
1 1/2 quarts black cherry frozen yogurt
1 1/2 quarts vanilla frozen yogurt
1 tablespoon rum
Fresh bing cherries for garnish, if desired

Let frozen yogurt thaw at room temperature approximately 20 minutes.

Meanwhile, split ladyfingers and lay flat, placing split side upward. Brush Amaretto over ladyfingers. Line bottom and sides of a 10-inch springform pan with ladyfingers, with cut side facing up or inward.

Sprinkle 6 tablespoons of wafer crumbs over the ladyfingers placed on bottom of pan.

Carefully spoon black cherry frozen yogurt over ladyfingers, spreading to the sides.

Combine vanilla frozen yogurt with 1 tablespoon rum. Spoon over black cherry frozen yogurt. Sprinkle with remaining 2 tablespoons wafer crumbs. Garnish with bing cherries, if desired.

Freeze until ready to serve. Remove sides from springform pan before serving.

Yield: 14 to 16 servings

Remove from freezer 10 to 15 minutes before serving, for greater ease in slicing.

Preparation time: 30-35 minutes

Additional time: 4 hours to freeze

ICE CREAM CAKE ROLL WITH BLUEBERRY SAUCE

2 egg substitutes (1/2 cup)
1 tablespoon canola oil
1/4 cup sugar
1 teaspoon vanilla
4 egg whites
1/2 cup sugar
3/4 cup all-purpose flour
1 teaspoon baking powder
1/4 teaspoon salt
1 quart vanilla ice milk or nonfat ice cream
Blueberry Sauce

Per serving:
Calories...... 297
Protein (g)... 6
Fat (g)....... 4.2
Sat. Fat (g).. 1.7
Choles. (mg).. 7
Fiber (g)..... 1
Sodium (mg)... 170
%Cal-Fat...... 13%

Preheat oven to 350 degrees.

Grease a 15 1/2 x 10 1/2 x 1-inch jelly roll pan. Line with waxed paper and grease again.

With an electric mixer, beat egg substitutes and oil until well mixed; gradually add 1/4 cup sugar and beat until mixture is frothy. Add vanilla and set aside.

Beat egg whites until soft peaks form. Gradually add 1/2 cup sugar and beat until stiff peaks form. Fold egg substitute mixture into whites.

Sift together flour, baking powder, and salt. Fold into egg mixture. Spread batter evenly in jelly roll pan.

Bake at 350 degrees for 10 to 12 minutes or until done.

Immediately invert cake onto a clean linen towel that has been liberally sprinkled with sifted confectioners' sugar. Remove waxed paper. Trim cake if edges are brown.

Starting at narrow end, roll cake and towel together. Cool completely on wire rack.

Meanwhile, soften ice milk by letting it stand at room temperature for 15 to 20 minutes.

Unroll cake in towel. Press carefully to flatten. Spread slightly softened ice milk up to 1/2-inch from outside edges of cake. Roll up. Spoon in ice milk at outside edges of roll where needed, to make ice milk flush with outside edge. Wrap with clear plastic wrap or aluminum foil and freeze until firm.

So serve, cut one-inch slices from roll, place on dessert plates, and top with warmed Blueberry Sauce.

Yield: Makes 10 1-inch slices.

Preparation time: 35-45 minutes

Cooking time: 10-12 minutes

Additional time: 4 hours to freeze

BLUEBERRY SAUCE

Per serving:
Calories...... 43
Protein (g)... 0
Fat (g)....... 0
Sat. Fat (g).. 0
Choles. (mg).. 0
Fiber (g)..... 0.3
Sodium (mg)... 1
%Cal-Fat...... 1%

1 cup sugar
2 1/2 tablespoons corn starch
1/4 teaspoon allspice
Dash salt
1 cup boiling water
1 pint fresh blueberries, washed
3 tablespoons lemon juice

In saucepan, combine sugar, cornstarch, allspice and salt. With a wire whisk, gradually stir in boiling water. Cook and stir until mixture thickens and boils. Cook 2 minutes more.

Add fresh blueberries and return to boiling. Remove from heat. Stir in lemon juice. Serve either warm or chilled.

Yield: Makes 3 cups sauce.

Instead of fresh blueberries, you may use one 10-ounce package frozen unsweetened blueberries, thawed and drained. Follow instructions as given above except increase cornstarch to 3 tablespoons.

Preparation time: 15 minutes

BLUEBERRY MERINGUE TORTES

Individual Meringue Shells:
3 egg whites
1 teaspoon vanilla
1/4 teaspoon cream of tartar
1 cup sugar
1/4 cup finely chopped almonds, toasted

6 cups low-fat or nonfat frozen yogurt (3/4 cup/serving)
Blueberry Sauce (Recipe, page 379)
Mint sprigs (optional)

Per serving:
Calories...... 435
Protein (g)... 8
Fat (g)....... 6.4
Sat. Fat (g).. 2.1
Choles. (mg).. 11
Fiber (g)..... 2
Sodium (mg)... 125
%Cal-Fat...... 13%

Preheat oven to 250 degrees.

Place egg whites in large mixing bowl. Add vanilla, cream of tartar, and dash salt. Beat until soft peaks form. Gradually add sugar, beating until very stiff peaks form. Stir in chopped almonds.

Cover baking sheet with waxed paper. Draw 8 circles, 3 1/2 inches in diameter, on waxed paper. Spread circles with approximately 1/3 cup meringue, using the back of a spoon to shape into individual shells.

Bake at 250 degrees for 45 to 60 minutes. Shells should be firm and dry, but still white. Turn off oven. Let shells dry in closed oven for 1 hour. Remove from paper while still warm.

Meanwhile make Blueberry Sauce. Cool slightly.

To serve, fill shells with frozen yogurt and spoon Blueberry Sauce over top. Garnish with mint sprigs, if desired.

Yield: 8 servings

Fresh strawberries and other fruits in season may be substituted for the Blueberry Sauce.

Preparation time: 35-40 minutes

Cooking time: 45-60 minutes

STRAWBERRY RUSSE

Per serving:
Calories...... 153
Protein (g)... 3
Fat (g)....... 3.8
Sat. Fat (g).. 2.3
Choles. (mg).. 14
Fiber (g)..... 1
Sodium (mg)... 57
%Cal-Fat...... 22%

20 ladyfingers, split
1/4 cup orange-flavored liqueur
2 envelopes unflavored gelatin
1/2 cup cold water
2 1/2 cups fresh strawberries, hulls removed, or 20 ounce
    pkg. frozen strawberries without syrup, thawed
3/4 cup sugar
4 tablespoons lemon juice
4 egg whites
1/2 cup whipping cream

Spray vegetable cooking spray on bottom only of 10-inch springform pan.

Split ladyfingers and lay flat. Sprinkle cut side with liqueur. Place ladyfingers, cut sides facing up and inward, around sides and in bottom of springform pan.

In small saucepan, soften gelatin in cold water. Stir over low heat until completely dissolved. Remove from heat.

Chop up strawberries in food processor, keeping mixture slightly lumpy. Transfer to a large bowl. Stir in sugar, lemon juice and gelatin mixture. Whisk until foamy. Refrigerate until mixture thickens slightly, about 10 to 20 minutes.

Meanwhile, in mixing bowl, beat egg whites until stiff peaks form. Fold into strawberry mixture.

In small bowl, beat whipping cream until stiff peaks form. Fold into strawberry mixture.

Pour into springform pan. Refrigerate at least 4 hours. Before serving, carefully remove sides of pan. Garnish with fresh strawberries, if available.

Yield: 12 servings

Preparation time: 35-40 minutes

Refrigeration time: 4 hours

BROWNIE BAKED ALASKA

1 quart vanilla ice milk or nonfat ice cream
1 cup sugar
1 1/4 cups all-purpose flour
1/2 cup cocoa powder
1 teaspoon baking soda
1/2 teaspoon baking powder
1/4 teaspoon salt
3 egg whites
2/3 cup skim milk
1/3 cup applesauce
1/2 cup boiling water
1 1/4 teaspoons vanilla
1/4 cup chopped walnuts

Meringue Topping:
5 egg whites
1 cup sugar

Per serving:
Calories...... 351
Protein (g)... 9
Fat (g)....... 6
Sat. Fat (g).. 2.8
Choles. (mg).. 12
Fiber (g)..... 1.8
Sodium (mg)... 291
%Cal-Fat...... 15%

Line an 8-inch cake pan with waxed paper, leaving an overhang around the edges. Pack slightly softened nonfat ice cream or ice milk into pan. Cover with foil. Freeze until firm (at least 3 to 4 hours).

Meanwhile make brownie. Preheat oven to 375 degrees.

Prepare 8-inch cakepan by spraying with vegetable cooking spray. Combine sugar, flour, cocoa powder, baking soda, baking powder and salt in large mixing bowl. Mix well. Add remaining ingredients except walnuts. Beat at high speed for two minutes. Batter will be thin. Fold in walnuts.

Pour into prepared cakepan. Bake at 375 degrees 30 to 35 minutes, or until toothpick inserted in center of cake comes out clean. Cool 20 minutes before removing from pan. Wrap in plastic wrap to maintain moisture. Refrigerate until ready to assemble.

To assemble:

Preheat oven to 500 degrees.

Prepare meringue topping: Beat egg whites until soft peaks form. Gradually beat in sugar. Continue beating until stiff peaks form. Set aside.

Place brownie cake on ovenproof serving dish. Invert frozen ice cream onto brownie layer, tugging at waxed paper to loosen from pan. Remove waxed paper. Spread meringue topping over top and sides, making sure the edges are sealed.

Bake at 500 degrees for 2 minutes or until meringue peaks are lightly browned. Serve immediately.

Yield: 10 to 12 servings

If you have difficulty removing frozen ice cream from container, dip container in lukewarm water for 30 to 60 seconds to loosen.

Preparation time: 50-60 minutes

Cooking time: 35-40 minutes

Additional time: 4 hours to freeze

FRESH PINEAPPLE WITH ORANGE LIQUEUR

1 ripe fresh pineapple, including shell
1/2 cup Triple Sec orange liqueur
1 orange
4 fresh strawberries

Cut leaves from pineapple. Next, cut lengthwise into four equal parts. Remove core from center of pineapple wedges; cut fruit away from rind into bite-size pieces, leaving it in the shell to serve. With a pastry brush, generously coat fruit pieces with orange liqueur.

Slice orange, crosswise, into four 1/4-inch slices. Cut a radius into the slice, twist, and place in center of pineapple wedge. Next, place 2 strawberry halves on either side of orange slice. Chill before serving.

Yield: 4 servings

A colorful, light dessert, ideal for lunch or brunch.

Preparation time: 10-15 minutes

Per serving:
Calories...... 135
Protein (g)... 1
Fat (g)....... 0.7
Sat. Fat (g).. 0
Choles. (mg).. 0
Fiber (g)..... 2.4
Sodium (mg)... 3
%Cal-Fat...... 5%

PEACH-RASPBERRY SUPREME

32-ounce can large peach halves, rinsed and drained
2 10-ounce packages frozen raspberries, defrosted and
drained
2 tablespoons Kirsch liqueur (cherry flavored)
Vanilla frozen yogurt or ice milk (optional)

Drain and rinse peach halves. Pat dry and set aside.

Defrost frozen raspberries. Drain liquid. Put drained raspberries in food processor. Add liqueur. Add one tablespoon sugar if no sugar is added to frozen raspberries. Process on and off until well chopped. Sauce will be thick.

Place each peach half on a small serving dish. (Stemmed glassware looks very elegant for this dessert.) Pour raspberry sauce over top, covering entire peach half. If desired, top with a small scoop of vanilla frozen yogurt or ice milk.

Yield: 8 servings.

For a variation, place a slice of pound cake or angel food cake as a foundation for this dessert. It is delicious.

Preparation time: 10-15 minutes

Per serving:
Calories...... 156
Protein (g)... 1
Fat (g)....... 0
Sat. Fat (g).. 0
Choles. (mg).. 0
Fiber (g)..... 4.4
Sodium (mg)... 8
%Cal-Fat...... 1%

PEACHES IN WINE

4 ripe peaches, peeled and sliced
1 1/2 cups Burgundy wine
1/2 cup sugar
1/2 teaspoon whole cloves
Lemon zest (narrow strips of lemon peel)

Peel peaches and slice into small slices. Place in medium-size bowl.

In small bowl, combine wine, sugar, cloves and lemon zest. Mix until sugar begins to dissolve. Pour over peaches. Cover.

Per serving:
Calories...... 215
Protein (g)... 0
Fat (g)....... 0
Sat. Fat (g).. 0
Choles. (mg).. 0
Fiber (g)..... 1
Sodium (mg)... 7
%Cal-Fat...... 0%

Marinate for at least 2 hours before serving. Stir occasionally. Refrigerate until ready to serve.

Yield: 4 to 6 servings

This tastes best if prepared the same day it is served. Marinating fruit between 3 and 6 hours is ideal. For best results, use fresh peaches at their peak of ripeness, neither too soft nor too hard.

Preparation time: 15-20 minutes

Marinating time: 3-6 hours

CUSTARD PIE

1 3/4 cups sugar
4 egg substitutes (1 cup)
1 teaspoon vanilla
1/2 cup self-rising flour
1 12-ounce can evaporated skim milk
1 1/2 tablespoons light margarine, melted

Preheat oven to 350 degrees.
Lightly spray 9-inch pie pan with vegetable cooking spray.
Combine all ingredients in blender or food processor. Process on high until smooth and slightly foamy.
Pour into pie pan. Bake at 350 degrees for 50 to 60 minutes, or until golden brown on top.

Yield: 1 9-inch pie, or 8 to 10 servings

Preparation time: 10-15 minutes

Cooking time: 50-60 minutes

Per serving:
Calories...... 239
Protein (g)... 7
Fat (g)....... 2.5
Sat. Fat (g).. 0.9
Choles. (mg).. 2
Fiber (g)..... 0.2
Sodium (mg)... 205
%Cal-Fat...... 9%

GRANOLA APPLE COBBLER

5 cups apples, peeled and sliced (4 to 6 apples)
1/2 cup chopped dates
3/4 cup sugar
2 tablespoons all-purpose flour
1/2 teaspoon ground cinnamon
1/4 teaspoon nutmeg

Topping:
1/2 cup rolled oats
1/2 cup whole wheat flour
1/4 cup firmly packed brown sugar
3 tablespoons light margarine
Low-fat vanilla frozen yogurt or ice milk

Per serving:
Calories...... 353
Protein (g)... 6
Fat (g)....... 5
Sat. Fat (g).. 1
Choles. (mg).. 0
Fiber (g)..... 3.5
Sodium (mg)... 58
%Cal-Fat...... 13%

Preheat oven to 350 degrees.

Peel apples and cut into thin slices. Place in 8-inch square baking dish. Add chopped dates.

In small mixing bowl, combine sugar, flour, cinnamon, and nutmeg. Pour over apples and mix well.

Prepare topping: Combine oats, flour, and brown sugar in mixing bowl. With a pastry cutter, cut in margarine until mixture is crumbly. Sprinkle over apples. Bake at 375 degrees for 45 minutes, or until apples are tender and topping is crisp. Serve warm or at room temperature.

To serve, spoon apple cobbler into individual bowls. Top with scoop of vanilla frozen yogurt or ice milk.

Yield: 8 servings

Preparation time: 20 minutes

Cooking time: 45 minutes

FROSTED APPLE COOKIES

Per 2 cookies with frosting:
Calories...... 125
Protein (g)... 2
Fat (g)....... 3.3
Sat. Fat (g).. 0.4
Choles. (mg).. 0
Fiber (g)..... 1.2
Sodium (mg)... 65
%Cal-Fat...... 23%

1 cup all-purpose flour
1 cup whole wheat flour
1 teaspoon baking soda
1/4 teaspoon salt
1 teaspoon ground cinnamon
1/2 teaspoon ground nutmeg
2/3 cup firmly packed brown sugar
1/2 cup skim milk
2 egg whites, slightly beaten
1/4 cup canola oil
1 cup raisins
1/4 cup chopped pecans
1 unpeeled apple, cored and finely chopped
Vanilla Frosting (recipe follows)

Preheat oven to 400 degrees.

Combine first seven ingredients in large mixing bowl. Set aside.

In small bowl, combine milk, egg whites, and canola oil. Add to ingredients in large bowl, mixing well. Fold in raisins, pecans and chopped apple.

Drop dough by rounded teaspoonfuls, 1 1/2 inches apart, onto greased cookie sheets.

Bake at 400 degrees for 12 to 15 minutes. Cool. Frost with Vanilla Frosting.

Yield: 4 1/2 dozen.

VANILLA FROSTING
1 1/2 cups powdered sugar
2 1/2 tablespoons skim milk
1 tablespoon soft tub margarine
1/2 teaspoon vanilla extract

Combine all ingredients in medium-size mixing bowl and beat until smooth. Makes enough frosting for 4 1/2 dozen cookies.

Preparation time: 35-45 minutes

Cooking time: 25-30 minutes

BAKED RICE PUDDING

4 egg substitutes (1 cup)
2 egg whites
3/4 cup sugar
1 3/4 cups skim milk
2 cups white or brown rice, cooked
1 teaspoon cinnamon
1/4 teaspoon nutmeg
1/3 cup raisins (optional)

Prepare rice according to package directions. Set aside.
Preheat oven to 400 degrees.
In large mixing bowl, combine egg substitutes and egg whites. Beat with wire whisk until slightly frothy. Beat in sugar. Add remaining ingredients including rice, and stir until well mixed.
Pour into a 2 1/2-quart casserole dish. Bake, uncovered, at 400 degrees 45 minutes or until custard is set. Serve warm or cold.

Yield: 6 to 8 servings

Preparation time: 15 minutes

Cooking time: 1 hour, 15 minutes

Per serving:
Calories...... 215
Protein (g)... 9
Fat (g)....... 1.5
Sat. Fat (g).. 0.4
Choles. (mg).. 1
Fiber (g)..... 0.3
Sodium (mg)... 112
%Cal-Fat...... 6%

RICE PUDDING (Stovetop)

1 1/2 cups brown or white rice (uncooked)
1 quart skim milk (4 cups)
1/2 to 3/4 cup sugar
3 tablespoons cornstarch
4 egg substitutes (1 cup)
2 teaspoons vanilla
1 teaspoon cinnamon
Raisins (optional)

Cook rice according to package directions.
Heat milk in large saucepan until warm.

Per serving:
Calories...... 256
Protein (g)... 10
Fat (g)....... 2
Sat. Fat (g).. 0.5
Choles. (mg).. 2
Fiber (g)..... 1.6
Sodium (mg)... 109
%Cal-Fat...... 7%

Meanwhile, with wire whisk, lightly beat together sugar, cornstarch and egg substitutes in bowl.

Add cooked rice and sugar mixture to warm milk. Add vanilla and cinnamon. Bring to a boil over medium heat, stirring frequently. Simmer until pudding thickens, about 2 minutes.

Serve warm or cold. Add raisins just before serving, if desired.

Yield: 8 to 10 servings

Preparation time: 15-20 minutes

Cooking time; 25 minutes

OATMEAL CRISPIES

For 2 cookies:
Calories...... 53
Protein (g)... 2
Fat (g)....... 1.4
Sat. Fat (g).. 0.1
Choles. (mg).. 0
Fiber (g)..... 0.6
Sodium (mg)... 43
%Cal-Fat...... 23%

3 egg whites
Dash of salt
1/2 teaspoon vanilla
1/2 cup granulated sugar
1 1/2 cups corn flakes
1 cup oatmeal
1/3 cup chopped nuts (walnuts or pecans)

Preheat oven to 350 degrees.

Combine egg whites, salt and vanilla in large mixing bowl. Beat until soft peaks form. Gradually add sugar; beat until stiff. Stir in corn flakes, oatmeal and nuts.

Drop batter from a teaspoon onto a cookie sheet sprayed with vegetable cooking spray.

Bake at 350 degrees for 18 to 20 minutes. Cool for 10 minutes and remove from cookie sheet.

Yield: 3 1/2 dozen cookies

These taste best if eaten soon after they are baked. They lose some of their crispness after a few hours.

Preparation time: 25 minutes

Cooking time: 35-40 minutes

LEMON-GLAZED SPICE BARS

1 cup all-purpose flour
1 teaspoon baking powder
1/2 teaspoon ground cinnamon
1/4 teaspoon ground cardamom
1 cup quick-cooking oats, uncooked
3/4 cup firmly packed brown sugar
1/3 cup canola oil
2 egg whites, slightly beaten
1 tablespoon lemon juice
1/2 teaspoon vanilla
1/4 cup chopped pecans
Lemon glaze (recipe follows)

Per serving:
Calories...... 52
Protein (g)... 1
Fat (g)....... 1.8
Sat. Fat (g).. 0.1
Choles. (mg).. 0
Fiber (g)..... 0.3
Sodium (mg)... 10
%Cal-Fat...... 31%

Preheat oven to 350 degrees.

Combine first 6 ingredients in large mixing bowl, mixing well. Add oil, egg whites, lemon juice, vanilla and pecans. Mix thoroughly.

Spoon batter into 9 x 13 x 2-inch non-stick baking pan.

Bake at 350 degrees for 25 minutes. Cool slightly.

Spread glaze over top while still warm. Cool. Cut into 2 x 2-inch bars.

Yield: 4 1/2 dozen.

LEMON GLAZE:
1 1/2 cups powdered sugar
1 tablespoon lemon juice
1/4 teaspoon ground cinnamon
3 tablespoons skim milk

Combine all ingredients in medium-size mixing bowl, mixing until smooth. Spread evenly over spice bars.

Preparation time: 25 minutes

Cooking time: 25 minutes

LOW-FAT LEMON BARS

Per 2x2-inch serving:
Calories...... 133
Protein (g)... 2
Fat (g)....... 4.4
Sat. Fat (g).. 0.4
Choles. (mg).. 0
Fiber (g)..... 0.4
Sodium (mg)... 35
%Cal-Fat...... 29%

1 3/4 cups all-purpose flour
1/2 cup oatmeal (uncooked)
1/2 cup powdered sugar
1/4 teaspoon salt
1/2 cup canola oil
4 egg substitutes (1 cup)
1 3/4 cups sugar
1/4 cup flour
5 tablespoons fresh-squeezed lemon juice
Powdered sugar

Preheat oven to 350 degrees.

Combine first four ingredients in medium-size bowl. Gradually pour in cooking oil, stirring until well blended. (Small lumps will be present. Large lumps can be broken up with fingers.) Press flour mixture into bottom of 9 x 13-inch non-stick pan. Bake for 15 minutes at 350 degrees.

Meanwhile, in a medium-size bowl, combine egg substitutes, sugar, flour and lemon juice. Beat with a wire whisk. Pour over hot pastry. Bake an additional 20 minutes at 350 degrees.

Remove from oven. Sprinkle with powdered sugar. Cut after cooled. Refrigerate until ready to serve.

Yield: 28 lemon bars, 2 inches x 2 inches, or 54 bars 1 x 2 inches.

These bars have less than half the fat of the classic lemon bar recipe, and the oil used is much less saturated than butter or margarine. These work out great when finger foods are preferable for dessert - picnics, buffet lunches, and cocktail parties.

Preparation time: 15-20 minutes

Cooking time: 35 minutes

BRANDY SAUCE

1/2 cup sugar
1 tablespoon cornstarch
1/4 teaspoon salt
2 cups skim milk
2 egg substitutes (1/2 cup)
1 teaspoon cooking oil
1/2 teaspoon vanilla
1/4 cup Brandy

Per 2 tablespoons:
Calories...... 43
Protein (g)... 2
Fat (g)....... 0.5
Sat. Fat (g).. 0.1
Choles. (mg).. 0
Fiber (g)..... 0
Sodium (mg)... 51
%Cal-Fat...... 11%

Combine sugar, cornstarch and salt in heavy saucepan. Stir in milk, egg substitute and cooking oil. Cook over medium heat, stirring frequently, until mixture begins to boil. Boil one minute longer, stirring constantly.

Remove from heat. Stir in vanilla and Brandy.

Serve warm or cold.

Yield: 2 1/2 cups sauce.

If time is limited, packaged vanilla pudding mix (3-ounce) may be used instead. Follow package directions, and after it is cooked, add Brandy.

Preparation time: 20 minutes

HARD SAUCE

1 tablespoon tub margarine
1 cup powdered sugar
2 tablespoons brandy
Water

Per 1 teaspoon:
Calories...... 35
Protein (g)... 0
Fat (g)....... 0.6
Sat. Fat (g).. 0.1
Choles. (mg).. 0
Fiber (g)..... 0
Sodium (mg)... 10
%Cal-Fat...... 15%

In a small mixing bowl, combine margarine, powdered sugar and brandy. Mix until smooth. Add a small amount of water, if necessary, to make a thin syrup, thin enough to spoon over desserts.

Yield: Approximately 1/2 cup sauce.

This is a very rich sauce, so only one to two teaspoons per serving is generally sufficient. If you prefer more, you will want to double the recipe.

Preparation time: 10 minutes

AMARETTO CUSTARD SAUCE

1/2 cup sugar
2 tablespoons cornstarch
2 cups skim milk
2 egg substitutes (1/2 cup)
1/4 teaspoon vanilla
1/4 cup Amaretto liqueur

Combine sugar and cornstarch in double boiler, placed over medium-high heat. Stir in milk and egg substitute, stirring frequently until mixture thickens to a pudding consistency.

Remove from heat and stir in vanilla and Amaretto. Serve either warm or chilled.

Yield: 2 1/2 cups sauce

This is a smooth and flavorful sauce, especially good spooned over slices of unfrosted cake. In preparing the sauce, a heavy saucepan (placed over medium heat) may be used instead of a double boiler, but the double boiler is much better for preventing scorching.

Preparation time: 20 minutes

YOGURT DESSERT TOPPING

2 cups nonfat or low-fat plain yogurt
1/4 cup firmly packed brown sugar
1/4 teaspoon cinnamon

Mix together yogurt, brown sugar and cinnamon. Serve over fruit desserts in place of whipped cream.

Yield: 2 cups dessert topping

Preparation time: 5 minutes

Per serving:
Calories...... 29
Protein (g)... 2
Fat (g)....... 0
Sat. Fat (g).. 0
Choles. (mg).. 0
Fiber (g)..... 0
Sodium (mg)... 23
%Cal-Fat...... 2%

Appendix A
Nutrient Analysis Of Fast Foods

	Cal	Pro	Fat	S.Fat	Chol	Na	%Fat
BURGER KING							
BK Broiler Chicken Sand.	267	22	8	2	45	728	27%
Bacon Dbl Cheeseburger	515	32	31	14	105	748	54%
Cheeseburger	318	17	15	7	50	661	42%
Chicken Sandwich (Fried)	685	26	40	8	82	1417	53%
Chicken Tenders (6 pc.)	236	16	13	3	46	541	50%
Croissan'wich, Egg, Ches	315	13	20	7	222	607	57%
Croissan'wich, Saus., Egg	534	21	40	13	268	985	67%
French Fries, medium	372	5	20	5	0	238	48%
French Toast Sticks	538	10	32	5	80	537	54%
Frozen Yogurt, Vanilla	120	2	3	2	10	40	23%
Hamburger	272	15	11	4	37	505	36%
Hamburger Deluxe	344	15	19	6	43	496	50%
Mini Muffins,Blueberry	292	4	14	3	72	244	43%
Ocean Fish Filet	495	20	25	4	57	879	45%
Salad, Chunky Chicken	142	20	4	1	49	443	25%
Salad, Side	25	1	0	0	0	27	0%
Shake, Vanilla	345	9	11	6	34	220	29%
Whopper	614	27	36	12	90	865	53%
Whopper w/Cheese	706	32	44	16	115	1177	56%
Whopper, Dbl w/Cheese	935	51	61	24	194	1245	59%
DOMINO'S PIZZA **(2 slcs, thin crust, 16")**							
Cheese Pizza	376	22	10	5	19	483	24%
Deluxe Pizza	498	27	20	9	40	954	37%
Dbl Cheese/Pepperoni	545	32	25	13	48	1042	42%
Pepperoni Pizza	460	24	17	8	28	825	34%
Sausage/Mushroom	430	24	16	8	28	552	33%
Veggie Pizza	498	31	18	10	36	1035	33%
HARDEE'S							
Bacon Cheeseburger	610	34	39	16	80	1030	58%
Big Deluxe Burger	500	27	30	12	70	760	54%
Big Twin	450	23	25	11	55	580	50%
Biscuit, Ham & Egg	370	15	19	4	160	1050	46%
Biscuit, Rise N' Shine	320	5	18	3	0	740	51%

Abbreviations used in this table are: Cal = calories; Pro = protein (g); Fat = total fat (g); S. Fat = saturated fat (g); Chol = cholesterol (mg); Na = sodium (mg); % Fat = % of calories from fat.

	Cal	Pro	Fat	S.Fat	Chol	Na	%Fat
Biscuit, Sausage	440	13	28	7	25	1100	57%
Cheeseburger	320	16	14	7	30	710	39%
Chicken Fillet	370	19	13	2	55	1060	32%
Chicken Stix, (6 pcs.)	210	19	9	2	35	680	39%
Cool Twist Cone, Vanilla	190	5	6	4	15	100	28%
Cool Twist Sunday, Fudge	320	7	12	6	25	270	34%
Crispy Curls (Fries)	300	4	16	3	0	840	48%
Fisherman's Fillet	500	23	24	6	70	1030	43%
French Fries, reg.	230	3	11	2	0	85	43%
Fried Chicken Breast	412	33	24	-	55	609	52%
Fried Chicken Leg	140	12	8	-	40	190	51%
Grilled Chicken Sand.	310	24	9	1	60	890	26%
Hamburger	270	13	10	4	20	490	33%
Hot Dog, All Beef	300	11	17	8	25	710	51%
Hot Ham N' Cheese	330	23	12	5	65	1420	33%
Muffin, Oat Bran Raisin	440	8	18	3	55	350	37%
Real Lean Deluxe	340	23	13	-	80	650	22%
Roast Beef Sandwich	350	26	11	-	58	732	28%
Roast Beef Sand., large	373	35	12	-	82	840	29%
Roast Beef, Big	360	24	15	6	65	1150	38%
Roast Beef, Regular	310	20	12	5	50	930	35%
Salad, Chef	240	22	15	9	115	930	56%
Salad, Garden	210	14	14	8	105	270	60%
Salad, Side	20	2	0	0	0	15	0%
Shake, Vanilla	400	13	9	6	50	320	20%
Turkey Club	390	29	16	4	70	1280	37%
Yogurt, Van., Frozen	160	6	4	3	10	75	23%

KENTUCKY FRIED CHICKEN

	Cal	Pro	Fat	S.Fat	Chol	Na	%Fat
Baked Beans	133	6	2	1	1	492	11%
Buttermilk Biscuit	235	4	12	3	1	655	45%
Chick Littles Sandwich	169	6	10	2	18	331	54%
Chocolate Pudding	156	2	7	6	2	127	43%
Cole Slaw	119	2	7	1	5	197	50%
Colonel's Chicken Sand.	482	21	27	6	47	1060	51%
Corn on the Cob	176	5	3	0	0	0	16%
Extra Crsp Center Breast	342	33	20	5	114	790	52%
Extra Crsp Drumstick	204	14	14	3	71	324	61%
Extra Crsp Side Breast	343	22	22	5	81	748	59%
Extra Crsp Thigh	406	20	30	8	129	688	66%
Extra Crsp Wing	254	12	19	4	67	422	66%
Kentucky Nuggets (6pc)	276	17	17	4	71	840	57%
Mshd Potatoes w/Gravy	71	2	2	0	0	339	20%
Orig Rec Center Breast	283	28	15	4	93	672	49%
Orig Rec Drumstick	146	13	8	2	67	275	52%
Orig Rec Side Breast	267	19	16	4	77	735	56%

	Cal	Pro	Fat	S.Fat	Chol	Na	%Fat
Orig Rec Thigh	294	18	20	5	123	619	60%
Orig Rec Wing	178	12	12	3	64	372	59%
Parfait, Strwbry Shtcake	230	2	9	5	20	162	34%
Potato Salad	117	2	12	2	14	497	59%

MCDONALD'S

	Cal	Pro	Fat	S.Fat	Chol	Na	%Fat
Apple Pie	260	2	15	4	6	240	52%
Big Mac	500	25	26	9	100	890	47%
Biscuit with Sausage	420	12	28	8	44	1040	60%
Biscuit w/Saus & Egg	500	19	33	10	270	1210	59%
Cheeseburger	305	15	13	5	50	710	38%
Chicken Brst Sand, Grld	252	24	4	1	50	740	14%
Chicken Fajitas	185	11	8	3	35	310	39%
Chicken McNuggets (6)	270	20	15	4	56	580	50%
Danish, Cinnamon Raisin	440	6	21	5	34	430	43%
Filet-O-Fish	370	14	18	4	50	930	44%
French Fries, med.	320	4	17	4	0	150	48%
Frozen Yogurt Cone	105	4	1	0	3	80	7%
Hamburger	255	12	9	3	37	490	32%
Hotcakes w/Marg & Syrup	410	8	9	1	8	640	20%
McLean Deluxe	320	22	10	4	60	670	28%
Milk Shake, Vanilla	290	11	1	1	10	170	4%
Muffin, Apple Bran, nofat	180	5	0	0	0	200	0%
Quarter Pdnr w/Cheese	510	28	28	11	115	1090	49%
Salad, Chef	170	17	9	4	111	400	48%
Salad, Chunky Chicken	150	25	4	1	78	230	24%

PIZZA HUT
(2 slices, medium pizza)

	Cal	Pro	Fat	S.Fat	Chol	Na	%Fat
Pan Pizza, Cheese	492	30	18	9	34	940	33%
Pan Pizza, Pepperoni	540	29	22	9	42	1127	37%
Pan Pizza, Supreme	589	32	30	14	48	1363	46%
Personal Pan Pepperoni	675	37	29	12	53	1335	39%
Personal Pan Supreme	647	33	28	11	49	1313	39%
Thin n'Crspy, Cheese	398	28	17	10	33	867	38%
Thin n'Crspy, Pepperoni	413	26	20	11	46	986	44%
Thin n'Crspy, Supreme	459	28	22	11	42	1328	43%

TACO BELL

	Cal	Pro	Fat	S.Fat	Chol	Na	%Fat
Burrito, Bean w/Red Sce	447	15	14	2	9	1148	28%
Burrito, Beef w/Red Sce	493	25	21	8	57	1311	38%
Burrito, Chicken	334	17	12	4	52	880	32%
Burrito, Fiesta	226	8	9	3	9	652	36%
Mexican Pizza	575	21	37	11	52	1031	58%
Meximelt, Chicken	257	14	15	7	48	779	53%
Nachos w/Cheese	346	7	18	6	9	399	47%
Salad, Chicken	125	8	8	4	32	252	58%

	Cal	Pro	Fat	S.Fat	Chol	Na	%Fat
Salad Dres, Ranch (2.5oz)	236	2	25	5	35	571	95%
Salsa, (1/3 oz.)	18	1	0	0	0	376	0%
Taco, Hard, Beef	183	10	11	5	32	276	54%
Taco, Hard, Chicken	171	12	9	3	52	337	47%
Taco Salad, w/Shell	905	34	61	19	80	910	61%
Taco Salad, no Shell	484	28	31	14	80	680	58%
Taco, Soft, Beef	225	12	12	5	32	554	48%
Taco, Soft, Chicken	213	14	10	4	52	615	42%
Taco Supreme	230	11	15	8	32	276	59%
Tostada, Fiesta	167	6	7	2	9	324	38%
Taco, Bean Burrito	630	25	25	7	41	1424	36%

WENDY'S

	Cal	Pro	Fat	S.Fat	Chol	Na	%Fat
Baked Potato, Brocli/Chs	400	8	16	3	-	455	36%
Baked Potato w/Cheese	420	8	15	4	10	310	32%
Baked Potato, Plain	270	6	0	0	0	20	0%
Big Classic	570	27	33	6	90	1085	52%
Big Classic w/Cheese	640	31	39	9	105	1345	55%
Big Classic, Dbl, w/Chs	820	50	51	14	170	1555	56%
Cheeseburger	410	28	21	9	80	760	46%
Cheeseburger, Double	590	47	33	14	145	970	50%
Chicken Club Sandwich	506	30	25	5	70	930	44%
Chicken Salad, (2 oz.)	120	7	8	1	0	215	60%
Chicken Nuggets (6 pc.)	280	14	20	4	50	600	64%
Chicken Sandwich, Fried	430	26	19	3	60	725	40%
Chicken Sand., Grilled	320	24	9	2	60	715	25%
Chocolate Chip Cookie	275	3	13	4	15	256	43%
Choc. Pudding, 1/4 cup	90	0	4	-	0	70	40%
Cottage Cheese, 1/2 cup	108	13	4	3	15	425	33%
Fish Filet Sandwich	460	18	25	5	55	780	49%
Flour Tortilla, 1	110	3	3	0	-	220	25%
French Fries, small	240	3	12	2	0	145	45%
Frosty Dessert, medium	520	10	18	6	65	286	32%
Hamburger, Double	520	43	27	11	130	710	47%
Hamburger, Plain	340	24	15	6	65	500	40%
Hamburger w/Everything	420	25	21	7	70	890	45%
Jr. Hamburger	260	15	9	3	34	570	31%
Jr. Swiss Deluxe	360	18	18	3	40	765	45%
Refried Beans (2 oz.)	70	4	3	1	0	215	39%
Salad, Chef	180	15	9	-	120	140	45%
Salad, Seafood (2 oz.)	110	4	7	0	0	455	57%
Salad, 3 Bean (1/4 c.)	60	1	0	0	-	15	0%

Note: A dash (-) means that data was not available.

Copyright 1991, CSPI. Reprinted from *The Completely Revised and Updated Fast-Food Guide*, which is available from CSPI, 1875 Conn. Ave., N.W. #300, Washington, DC 20009 for $7.95.

Bibliography

"A Barbecue Handbook," *USDA's Food News for Consumers*, U.S. Department of Agriculture, Summer, 1991.

"The Basic Four Food Guide," *Mayo Clinic Nutrition Letter*, Vol. 3, October 1990, pp. 4-5.

Blankenhorn, David H., "Beneficial Effects of Combined Colestipol-Niacin Therapy on Coronary Atherosclerosis and Coronary Venous Bypass Grafts," *The Journal of the American Medical Association*, Vol. 257, June 19, 1987, pp. 3233-3240.

"Breast Cancer," *Nutrition Action Healthletter*, Vol. 15, No. 2, March 1988, p. 1.

"But is Your Cholesterol Level What They Say it Is?," *Tufts University Diet and Nutrition Letter*, Vol. 6, February 1989, p. 7.

Castelli, W. P. "Epidemiology of Coronary Heart Disease: The Framingham Study," *The American Journal of Medicine*, February 27, 1984, pp. 4-12.

"Caffeine," *Mayo Clinic Nutrition Letter*, Vol. 3, October 1990, pp. 6-7.

"Chinese Restaurant Syndrome, Putting A Mysterious Ailment into Perspective," *Mayo Clinic Nutrition Letter*, Vol. 3, January 1990, pp. 4-5.

Cholesterol, Current Concepts for Clinicians, National Cholesterol Education Program, U.S. Department of Health and Human Services, National Institutes of Health, October 1, 1988.

Connor, Sonja L., et. al., "The Cholesterol-Saturated Fat Index for Coronary Prevention: Background, Use, and a Comprehensive Table of Foods," *Journal of the American Dietetic Association*, Vol. 89, No. 6, June 1989, pp. 807-816.

Connor, Sonja L. and William E. Connor, M.D., *The New American Diet* New York, Simon and Schuster Inc., 1986.

Cooper, Kenneth H., *Controlling Cholesterol*, New York, Bantam Books, 1988.

Diet Nutrition, and Cancer, by the Committee on Diet, Nutrition, and Cancer, National Research Council, Washington, D.C., National Academy Press, 1982.

"A Different Kind of Open-Heart Procedure," *Tufts University Diet and Nutrition Letter*, Vol. 8, No. 11, January 1991, p. 3.

"Eat to Swim . . . Bike . . . Run . . .," *Nutrition Action Healthletter*, Vol. 15, June/July 1988, pp. 1, 4-6.

"'Eat Your Vegetables' as Sound Today as Ever," Tufts University Diet and Nutrition Letter, Vol. 7, October 1989, pp. 1-2.

"Eating Out," *Mayo Clinic Nutrition Letter*, Vol. 2, February 1989, pp. 4-5.

Eating Smart, American Cancer Society, Inc., 1987.

"The Effects of Nonpharmacologic Interventions on Blood Pressure of Persons with High Normal Levels," The Trials of Hypertension Prevention Collaborative Research Group, Bethesda, Md., *The Journal of the American Medical Association*, Vol. 267, No. 9, March 4, 1992, pp. 1213-1220.

Enos, Major William F., et. al., "Coronary Disease Among United States Soldiers Killed in Action in Korea," *The Journal of the American Medical Association*, Vol. 152, July 18, 1953, pp. 1090-1093.

"Facts About . . . Exercise," The National Heart, Lung and Blood Institute, National Institutes of Health.

"Fast Food," *Mayo Clinic Nutrition Letter*, Vol. 2, July 1989, pp. 4-5.

"Five a Day," *Tufts University Diet and Nutrition Letter*, Vol. 6, February 1989, p. 2.

Gambino, Raymond, "NIH Consensus Development Conference on Triglycerides, High-Density Lipoprotein, and Coronary Heart Disease," *Lab Report*, Vol. 14, No. 3, March 1992, pp. 17-19.

"Genetic Factors Help Shape Your Shape," *Mayo Clinic Nutrition Letter*, Vol. 3, September 1990, p. 7.

Glueck, Charles J., "Pediatric Primary Prevention of Atherosclerosis," *The New England Journal of Medicine*, Vol. 314, January 16, 1986, pp. 175-177.

Gurkin, Kitty and Beth Kent, *The Dupac Nutrition Manual.*

Hamilton, Eva May Nunnelley, Eleanor Ross Whitney and Frances Sienkiewicz Sizer, *Nutrition: Concepts and Controversies*, St. Paul, West Publishing Co., 1985.

"High Blood Pressure," *Scientific American Medicine*, Vol. 1, October 1988, pp. 1-10.

"Hyperlipoproteinemia," *Scientific American Medicine*, Vol. 9, August 1986, pp. 1-4.

Ingersoll, Bruce, "U.S. Is Ready to Limit What Food Processors Can Claim on Labels," *The Wall Street Journal*, November 6, 1991, p. 1+.

"It's Never too Late to Start Exercising," *Tufts University Diet and Nutrition Letter*, Vol. 6, February 1989, p. 5.

"Label Language: Still Sounds a Lot Like Babel," *Tufts University Diet and Nutrition Letter*, Vol. 9, No. 8, October 1991, pp. 3-6.

Lefferts, Lisa Y., "Great Grilling," Nutrition Action Healthletter, Vol. 16, July/August 1989, pp. 5-7.

Liebman, Bonnie, "Roughing It: How Fiber Fights Cancer," *Nutrition Action Healthletter*, June 1984, pp. 5-9.

— "CSPI's Poultry Primer," *Nutrition Action Healthletter*, November 1986, pp. 8-9.

— and Anne Montgomery, "Dining Out in Beverly Hills, Seattle, Houston . . .," *Nutrition Action Healthletter*, Vol. 14, July/August 1987, p. 10.

— and Anne Montgomery, "Preventing Cancer," Nutrition Action Healthletter, Vol. 14, No. 6, July/August 1987, pp. 1, 4-6.

— and Robert Davis, "Eating for Your 80s," *Nutrition Action Healthletter*, Vol. 14, November 1987, pp. 1, 4-7.

— "Carrots Against Cancer?," *Nutrition Action Healthletter*, Vol. 15, No. 10, December 1988, pp. 1, 5-7.

— "Life in the Fat Lane," *Nutrition Action Healthletter*, Vol. 17, July/August 1990, pp. 8-9.

— "The HDL/Triglycerides Trap," *Nutrition Action Healthletter*, Vol. 17, No. 7, September 1990, pp. 1, 4-6.

— "Trans in Trouble," *Nutrition Action Healthletter*, Vol. 17, October 1990, p. 7.

"Lowering the Risk for High Blood Pressure," *Tufts University Diet and Nutrition Letter*, Vol. 5, No. 3, May 1987, pp. 3-6.

Naito, Herbert K., "Effect of Cholesterol Lowering on CHD Risk," *Consultant*, Vol. 28, June 1988, pp. 15-24.

Naito, Herbert K., "New Concerns on Detection and Treatment of Hypercholesterolemia," *Physicians Market Place*, Vol. 21, November 1987, p. 2.

Naito, Herbert K., "New Guidelines and Recommendations on the Detection, Evaluation, and Treatment of Patients with Undesirable Cholesterol Levels," *American Journal of Clinical Pathology*, Vol. 90, September 1988, pp. 358-361.

"New RDAs Call for More Calcium, Less Sodium," *Tufts University Diet and Nutrition Letter*, Vol. 7, January 1990, pp. 1-2.

Newman III, William P., et. al., "Relation of Serum Lipoprotein Levels and Systolic Blood Pressure to Early Atherosclerosis," *The New England Journal of Medicine*, Vol. 314, January 16, 1986, pp. 138-144.

Ornish, Dean, "Can Life Style Changes Reverse Coronary Heart Disease?," *The Lancet*, Vol. 336, July 21, 1990, pp. 129-133.

Piscatella, Joseph C., *Don't Eat Your Heart Out Cookbook*, New York, Workman Publishing Co. Inc., 1983.

"A Quick Consumer Guide to Safe Food Handling," U.S. Department of Agriculture, Food Safety and Inspection Service, September 1990.

"Recommendations for Treatment of Hyperlipidemia in Adults," (A Joint Statement of the Nutrition Committee and the Council on Arteriosclerosis), American Heart Association Special Report, Circulation 69, No. 5, 1984.

Recommended Dietary Allowances, Washington, D.C., National Academy of Sciences, 1980.

"Report of the Expert Panel on Detection, Evaluation and Treatment of High Blood Cholesterol in Adults," National Cholesterol Education Program, National Heart, Lung and Blood Institute, Archives of Internal Medicine, Vol. 145, 1988, pp. 36-69.

"Report of the Expert Panel on Detection, Evaluation and Treatment of High Blood Cholesterol in Adults," National Cholesterol Education Program, National Institutes of Health, U.S. Government Printing Office, 1989.

Rosenthal, Elizabeth, "Salt in Diet Might Be OK, Research Suggests," New York Times News Service, printed in *The News and Observer*, Raleigh, NC, December 31, 1991.

Ryan, Donna H., MD, and Barry M. Starr, "Vitamins in Prevention and Treatment of Cancer," *Contemporary Oncology*, January/February, 1992, pp. 45+.

"Smart Loser's Guide to Choosing a Weight Loss Program," *Tufts University Diet and Nutrition Letter*, Vol. 8, August 1990, pp. 3-6.

"Some Calories Count More Than Others," *Tufts University Diet and Nutrition Letter*, Vol. 6, November 1988, p. 2.

Strong, Jack P. M.D., "Coronary Atherosclerosis in Soldiers, A Clue to the Natural History of Atherosclerosis in the Young," *The Journal of the American Medical Association*, Vol. 256, November 28, 1986, pp. 2863-2866.

Strong, William B., "Cholesterol Screening for Children Is Warranted," *Clinical Chemistry News*, April 1989.

"Sugar Substitutes—Can They Help You Control Weight Safely?," *Mayo Clinic Nutrition Letter*, Vol. 3, August 1990, pp. 3-4.

"Tackling High Blood Pressure," *Nutrition Action Healthletter*, Vol. 16, May 1989, p. 1.

"Washing Away Sodium," *Nutrition Action Healthletter*, Vol. 16, June 1989, p. 13.

"What is Simplesse, The New Fat Substitute," *Mayo Clinic Nutrition Letter*, Vol. 3, April 1990, p. 8.

General Index

Alcohol:
  blood pressure and, 8, 10, 58, 107
  calories per gram, 28
  triglycerides and, 106-7
American Heart Association, 31-32,
    40, 122
  recommendations on cholesterol
    consumption, 32
  recommendations on fat consump-
    tion, 31
Angiotensin Converting Enzyme (ACE)
    inhibitors, 61
Anti-oxidant, 13
Artery spasm, 3
Artificial Sweeteners, *See* Sweeteners,
    artificial
Aspartic acid, 72
Aspertame, 72
Atherosclerosis, 3-8
  and cholesterol levels, 5-6
  development of, 3-4
  high blood pressure and, 8
  incidence of, 3
Athletes, diet tips for, 101
Au gratin, 123
Barley, 85
Beans:
  baked, vegetarian, 56
  benefits of, 85-86
  fiber in, 14, 54, 81, 85
  increasing intake of, 86
  as protein source, 54. 85, 91
  recommended daily servings of, 88
  as source of iron, 54
  as source of omega-3 fatty acids, 22
Bearnaise sauce, 123
Bechamel sauce, 123
Beta blockers, 61
Beta carotene, 12, 74-75
Blackened (meat or fish), 123, 125
Blankenhorn, David, 7

Blood Pressure, 8-10, 57-67, 110-13
  dietary influences on, 9, 57-60,
    112-13
  medical tests for, 102, 110, 112
  salt sensitivity and, 9-10, 57
Blood pressure, high, 8-9, 57-60, 110,
    112-13
  causes of, 8, 57-60
  in children, 112
  dietary factors and, 8-10, 57-60,
    107
  dietary treatment for, 112-13
  incidence of, in Japan, 9, 57
  incidence of, in U.S., 8
  medication for, 61, 113
  See also Blood pressure
Bordelaise sauce, 123
Bouillabaisse, 123
Braised, 123
Brown rice, 81, 84, 86, 139
Bulgur, 84
Buckwheat, 85
Burger King, 46, 395
Burkitt, Denis, 13
Caffeine, 137
Calcium:
  blood pressure and, 90, 60
  in chocolate milk, 136-37
  deficiency of, 60, 96
  supplements and blood pressure,
    60
Calcium entry blockers, 61
Calorie(s):
  average daily intake of, 41
  estimating personal daily intake of,
    41
  in fruits, 76
  needed to gain/lose one pound, 117-
    18
  low-, 26
  reduced-, 26,
  in selected foods, 44-46

in vegetables, 77
Cancer, 10-13
  beta carotene and, 12-13
  colon, 11-12
  fiber and, 11-12
  incidence of, 10
  dietary influences on, 10-13
Castelli, W. P., 5, 16, 106
Carbohydrates:
  calories in, 16, 27, 114
  as listed on food labels, 27
  See also Complex carbohydrates
Cheeses, 38-39
  CSI of, 36, 38
  ways to reduce fat from, 38-39
Children:
  desirable cholesterol level in, 108
  high blood pressures in, 112
  high cholesterol levels in, 107-9
  healthy snacks for, 133
Chinese Restaurant Syndrome, 63
Chinese Restaurants, 126
Cholesterol, blood, 17-18, 102-11
  children and, 107-9
  desirable levels, 7-8, 103
  diet and, 6-7, 31-32, 103, 105, 108-9
  estrogen and, 6-7
  HDL cholesterol, 17, 103-5
  heart attacks and, 5-8, 32
  increase in, with age, 109-10
  LDL cholesterol, 18, 104-5
  medical tests for, 102-3
  ratio, *See* Cholesterol ratio
Cholesterol, dietary, 17
  food labels and, 25
  recommendations on daily intake of, 29, 32
  sources in diet, 33-34
Cholesterol-lowering drugs, 110-11
  children and, 108
Cholesterol ratio, 106-7
Cholesterol-Saturated Fat Index (CSI), 34-40
  of cheeses, 36, 38-39
  of eggs, 36

of fats and oils, 36-37
of frozen desserts, 37
of meat, fish and poultry, 34-36
of milk products, 37
of salad dressings, 39-40
Cigarette smoking:
  HDL cholesterol and, 107
  as risk factor for heart disease, 8-9, 104
Complex carbohydrates, 74-86
  benefits of, 74-75
  cancer and, 12-13, 74-75
  fiber and, 80-83
  weight loss and, 75
  See also Fruits, Vegetables and Grains
Constipation, 13-14
Corn sweeteners, 71
Corn syrup, 71
Cornmeal, 85
Coronary heart disease, 3-8
  and cholesterol levels, 5-6
  development of, 4-5
  exercise and, 97-98
  incidence of, 3, 6-8
  reversal of, 7-8
  risk factors for, 104
Cottage cheese:
  on baked potato, 39, 56
  in cheese spread, 39, 56
Couscous, 84
Creamed, 123
Cruciferous vegetables, 12, 74, 78
Dairy products:
  cheeses, 38-39
  CSI of, 36
  fat in, 43, 45, 51
  protein in, 91
  recommended daily servings of, 88
Deficiencies, vitamins and mineral:
  calcium and effect on blood pressure, 60
  most common, 96
  definition of, 29, 96
Dextrose, 71
Diabetes mellitus, 16, 104

Diastolic blood pressure, high, 112-13
  treatment for, 113
Diet of 30% calories from fat, 31, 40
  calculating daily fat intake for, 42
  fat intake (based on total calories) for, 43
Diet of 20% calories from fat, 16, 31-32, 40, 88
  breakfast, lunch guidelines for, 51-52
  calculating daily fat intake for, 41-42
  dinner guidelines for, 53
  fat intake (based on total calories) for, 43
  National Institutes of Health (NIH) study regarding, 31-32
  sample daily menu, 50-51
  vs. 40% calories from fat, 16, 114-15
Diet Workshop diet plan, 120
Diuretics, 61
Diverticulosis, 13-14
Domino's Pizza, 46, 395
Eggs:
  cholesterol in, 33-34
  CSI of, 36
  cold storage of, 135
  in diet, 137
  protein in, 91
Electrocardiogram, EKG, 4
Enos, William, 4-5
Enriched, 25
Exercise, 96-101
  benefits of, 97
  blood pressure and, 58, 107
  calories burned in, 116
  children and, 108
  for conditioning heart and lungs, 98-100
  consult physician before, when to, 99-100
  heart rate Target Zone, 99-100
  and HDL cholesterol, 105, 107
  metabolism raised by, 115-16

triglycerides and, 106-7
types of, 98-99
and weight control, 115-17
Fast food(s):
  Appendix A, 395-98
  calorie content of, 46, 395-98
  fat content of, 46, 129-30, 395-98
  reducing fat from, 130
  restaurants, 46-47, 128-29
  salads, 46-47, 129
  sodium and, 63-64
Fat(s), dietary:
  breast cancer and, 11
  calculation of daily intake of, 42
  calories in, 16, 27, 114
  CSI of, 35-37
  computing percentage of, 27-28
  converting grams of fat to teaspoons of, 42
  daily minimum requirements of, 19, 31
  essential, 19, 31
  in fast foods, 46-47, 395-98
  fish oil, 20-22
  food labels and, 27-28
  in foods, 42-49
  heart disease and, 6, 8
  in poultry products, 34-35, 55
  recommended daily intake of, 31-32
  reducing intake of, 48-56
  sources of, in diet, 33
  in steak dinner, 47-48
  types of, 18-20
  weight control and, 114-15
  See also Monounsaturated fats, Polyunsaturated fats, Saturated fats, Diet of 30% calories from fat, and Diet of 20% calories from fat
Fiber, dietary, 14, 80-82
  benefits of, 14, 75
  in foods, 81
  in fruits, 76
  increasing intake of, 86
  insoluble, 14, 80
  insufficient, 13-14

Recipe Index

About the Author

A native of Burlington, Wis., Janet Chiavetta graduated from Marquette University with a degree in journalism. She worked as assistant director of public relations for the Mayo Clinic's St. Marys Hospital in Rochester, Minn.

Janet studied nutrition at Meredith College in Raleigh, N.C., where she now resides with her husband and two college age sons. Having been extensively involved in cultural and civic organizations, Janet has served as editor of several non-profit publications.

ORDER FORM

Eat, Drink and Be Healthy
Piedmont Publishers
P.O. Box 32296
Raleigh, NC 27622

Please send _____ copies of *Eat, Drink and Be Healthy* $ __24.95__ each

North Carolina residents add sales tax. $ __1.50__ each

Postage and handling $ 3.00 each

TOTAL ENCLOSED $ _____

Name_____

Address _____

City _____ State _____ Zip_____

Charge to: Acct. # _____ Exp. Date _____

☐ **Visa**   ☐ **Mastercard**

Signature _____ Phone (____)_____

Make checks payable to Piedmont Publishers.

— —

ORDER FORM

Eat, Drink and Be Healthy
Piedmont Publishers
P.O. Box 32296
Raleigh, NC 27622

Please send _____ copies of *Eat, Drink and Be Healthy* $ __24.95__ each

North Carolina residents add sales tax. $ __1.50__ each

Postage and handling $ 3.00 each

TOTAL ENCLOSED $ _____

Name_____

Address _____

City _____ State _____ Zip_____

Charge to: Acct. # _____ Exp. Date _____

☐ **Visa**   ☐ **Mastercard**

Signature _____ Phone (____)_____

Make checks payable to Piedmont Publishers.